Clinical Decision Making for Nurse Practitioners

A Case Study Approach

• • • • • • • • • • • • • • • •

Denise L. Robinson, RN, PhD, FNP

Associate Professor
Director, MSN Program
Northern Kentucky University
Highland Heights, Kentucky

Family Nurse Practitioner
Northern Kentucky Family Health Centers, Inc.
Covington, Kentucky

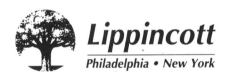

Lippincott
Philadelphia • New York

Acquisitions Editor: Lisa Stead
Assistant Editor: Claudia Vaughn
Project Editor: Gretchen Metzger
Production Manager: Helen Ewan
Production Coordinator: Patricia McCloskey
Assistant Art Director: Kathy Kelley-Luedtke
Indexer: Nancy Newman

9 8 7 6 5 4 3 2 1

Library of Congress Cataloging-in-Publications Data
Robinson, Denise.
     Clinical decision making for nurse practitioners : a case study
approach / Denise Robinson.
          p.   cm.
     Includes bibliographical references and index.
     ISBN 0–397–55459–1 (alk. paper)
     1. Nursing—Case studies.   2. Nursing—Decision making.
     3. Clinical competence.   4. Nursing—Problems, exercises, etc.
     I. Title.
     [DNLM: 1. Nursing Diagnosis—examination questions.   2. Diagnosis,
     Differential—nurses' instruction.   3. Clinical Medicine—case
     studies.   4. Patient Care Planning.   5. Decision Making.   6. Nurse
     Practitioners.   WY 18.2 R659c 1997]
     RT42.R63   1998
     610.73—dc21
     DNLM/DLC
     for Library of Congress   97–17251
                                                                        CIP

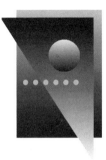

Contributors

Margaret Anderson, EdD, RN-C, CNAA
Assistant Professor and Director,
   BSN Program
Department of Nursing
Northern Kentucky University
Highland Heights, KY
   *Critical Thinking and Clinical
   Decision Making*

Alanna Andrus, MSN, PNP, FNP
Staff Nurse
Neonatal Intensive Care Unit
University of San Diego
San Diego, CA
   Case 18

Ellen Benton, MSN, RN, FNP
Asthma and Allergy Affiliates
Cincinnati, OH
   Case 35

Mavis Bechtle, MSN, WHP
Administrator
Skilled Nursing and Senior
   Services
St. Luke's Hospital
Fort Thomas, KY
FNP Graduate
Northern Kentucky University
Highland Heights, KY
   Case 40

Patricia Birchfield, DSN, ARNP
Associate Professor
College of Nursing
University of Kentucky
Lexington, KY
   Case 36

Rachel Broering, RN, MSN, FNP
Part-time Faculty
Northern Kentucky Family Health
   Centers, Inc.
Department of Nursing
Northern Kentucky University
Highland Heights, KY
   Case 8

Audricia I. Brooks, MSN, FNP
Ambulatory Care
Veterans Administration Medical Center
Cincinnati, OH
   Case 25

Sheila Carroll, MSN, FNP, CFNP
Summit Medical Group
Williamstown, KY
   Case 41

Christine Day, BSN, COGNP
Nurse Practitioner, Obstetrics and
   Gynecology
Group Health, Inc.
Group Health Association
Cincinnati, OH
   Case 26

Diane Enzweiler, MSN, RN-C, ARNP
Cardiology Associates, P.S.C.
Crestview Hills, KY
Case 11

Patsy L. Gephart, CNM, MSN
Nurse-Midwife
Michael R. Draznik, MD, Inc.
Cincinnati, OH
Case 3

Duff Halcomb, RN, MSN, FNP
School Health Coordinator
Laurel County School District
London, KY
Case 6

Jane Harley, RN, MSN, CFNP, CDE
Instructor
Family Nurse Practitioner Tract
University of Kentucky
Lexington, KY
Case 21

Barbara Heidt, MSN, RN, CS
Psychiatric Clinical Nurse
  Specialist
Nursing Administration
Children's Hospital Medical
  Center
Cincinnati, OH
Case 4

Judith Krogh Herrmann, MSN, RN, CS
Education Specialist
Education Service
Veterans Administration Medical
  Center
Cincinnati, OH
Case 37

Kim Hickok, MS, RN, FNP
Instructor
College of Nursing and Health
Wright State University
Denton, OH
Case 6

Laura Hearld Hoofring, MSN, CNS
Adolescent Medical/Psychiatric Services
Children's Hospital Medical Center
Cincinnati, OH
Case 4

Joyce Huffer, RN, MSN, FNP
Northern Kentucky Family Health
  Centers, Inc.
Newport, KY
Case 7

Sadie Hughes, MSN, RN, ANP
Nursing Home Care Unit
Veterans Administration Medical Center
Ft. Thomas, KY
Case 32

Delwin Jacoby, MSN, CFNP
Anderson Family Health Center
Lawrenceburg, KY
Adjunct Faculty
Family Nurse Practitioner Program
Spalding University
Louisville, KY
Case 15, Case 30

Deborah Johnsen, MSN, RN, ANP
Northern Kentucky Family Health
  Centers, Inc.
Covington, KY
Case 1

N. Elise Johnson, RN, MSN, FNP
Sardina Medical Center
Sardina, OH
Case 5

Pamela Kidd, RN, PhD, FNP, CEN
Family Nurse Practitioner, Associate Professor
College of Nursing
University of Kentucky
Lexington, KY
Director, MSN Program
Spaulding University
Louisville, KY
Case 6

Linda M. Kollar, RN, MSN, PNP
Director of Nursing
Division of Adolescent Medicine
Children's Hospital Medical Center
Cincinnati, OH
Case 13

Gary Loving, PhD, RN
Director, Acute Care Nursing Division
Associate Professor
College of Nursing
University of Oklahoma
Oklahoma City, OK
Critical Thinking and Clinical Decision Making

Lori McConlogue-O'Shaughnessy, MSN, RN, FNP
Northern Kentucky Family Health Centers, Inc.
Covington, KY
Case 7

Katherine McGee, MSN, RN, PNP
Baby Milk Fund—Treatment for Lead Exposed Children
Children's Hospital Medical Center
Cincinnati, OH
Case 2

Patricia McGowan, MSN, FNP
Ambulatory Care
Veterans Administration Medical Center
Cincinnati, OH
Case 37

Cheryl McKenzie, MN, RN, FNP
Associate Professor
Department of Nursing
Northern Kentucky University
Northern Kentucky Family Health Centers, Inc.
Highland Heights, KY
Case 24

Louise Niemer, PhD, RN
Assistant Professor
Department of Nursing
Northern Kentucky University
Highland Heights, KY
PNP Student
University of Cincinnati
Cincinnati, OH
Case 38

Cynthia A. Pastorino, MSN, RN
Department of Family and Community Medicine, Geriatrics Division
University of Louisville
Louisville, KY
Case 17

Betty Porter, EdD, CFNP
Chair
Department of Nursing and Allied Health Sciences
Morehead State University
Morehead, KY
Case 10

Veronica Weaver Renfrow, MSN, FNP
Domiciliary, Care for Homeless
  Veterans
Veterans Administration Medical Center
Cincinnati, OH
  Case 20

Angela K. Riley, MSN, RN, CCRN, ANP
Cardiology Associates P.S.C.
Crestview Hills, KY
  Case 27, Case 33

Denise L. Robinson, RN, PhD, FNP
Associate Professor
Director, MSN Program
Northern Kentucky University
Highland Heights, Kentucky
  Cases 12, 14, 16, 19, 22, 28, 29, 39

Karen Ruschman, MSN, RN, FNP
Ft. Thomas, KY
  Case 23, Case 34

Deborah Webb, RN, MSN, GNP
Clinical Coordinator, Nurse
  Practitioner
Bethesda Group Practice
Bethesda Hospital, Inc.
Milford, OH
  Case 9

Sandra Lee Woods, MSN, RN-C, WHP, FNP
Planned Parenthood
Cincinnati, OH
  Case 31

Nurse Practitioner Students Who Contributed to Case 5:

Kathryn E. Blednick, RN, MSN
University of Cincinnati
Cincinnati, OH

Janie Hague, RN, MSN
University of Cincinnati
Cincinnati, OH

Margaret Motz, RN, MSN
University of Cincinnati
Cincinnati, OH

Jim Mulloney, RN, MSN
Cardiac Surgery Recovery Room
University of Cincinnati
Cincinnati, OH

Barbara Neuman, RN, MSN
Clinical Research Nurse
Shriners Burns Institute
University of Cincinnati, College of
  Health and Nursing
Cincinnati, OH

June A. Stanley, RN, MSN
Clinical Specialist Clinical Care and
  Clinical Care Intern Program
  Director
The Christ Hospital
Cincinnati, OH

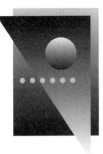

Preface

The purpose of this book is to help nurse practitioners (NPs) develop and refine the problem-solving skills needed to provide care for patients. In order to gain competence as NPs, students need to develop analytical skills. This book will help both the student NP and the newly practicing NP to develop skills in problem solving and making specific decisions about treatment for patients.

The text was conceived when I was an NP student. The faculty always tried to make sure each topic we talked about had clinical applicability. This was difficult, because no text gave enough detail or was based on clinical application. Frequently, the cases used as examples were not detailed enough, and students ended up regurgitating information from their textbooks. As a class assignment, four students gave a presentation on depression. Luckily, one of our fellow students had developed, with another colleague, a problem-focused self-directed modular learning method. We decided to use this technique for our presentation. As we developed the problem-focused case study on depression, it because apparent to me that this format was perfect to assist students in learning the diagnostic reasoning and clinical decision-making skills that are so vital for NPs. The problem-oriented method places responsibility for mastery of the content on the students, and allows them to proceed at an appropriate pace for their learning style and speed of learning.

The cases in the text were chosen based on actual practice, and on the research done by Pickwell (1993), which identified the types of patients family NPs commonly see in practice. It was difficult to choose the cases, because there are so many different types of problems that NPs frequently encounter. It was very tempting to include many more diagnoses and problems in the book; however, only the most common problems were chosen for the text. These case studies reflect what is seen in practice; in other words, they are based on real patients with multiple physical and social problems. It seems in practice that rarely, if ever, is a typical casebook example seen. The real-life perspective makes the cases more challenging, because it requires clinical judgment and critical thinking to sort through the large amount of data collected, and to develop an appropriate and pertinent plan.

This book uses the problem-oriented approach to therapy. This approach is used extensively by health care providers, and is a comprehensive and organized method for assessing and solving problems. The text utilizes the SOAP (S = subjective, O = objective, A = assessment, P = plan) format, which is commonly seen in practice. Each case presents a brief scenario about a patient. The development of critical thinking skills is enhanced by the thought processes used to identify tentative differential diagnoses at that point. Even with very little data, the NP begins to identify the possible pertinent diagnoses. The rest of the patient encounter revolves around obtaining, sorting, and organizing data to support or refute the potential differential diagnoses. Each case has questions to help identify questions needed at each level of data gathering, as well as more elaborate questions to help guide the NP in developing a thorough therapeutic plan of care.

The reader is encouraged to use a separate piece of paper to answer the questions for each patient. Writing the answers to each case will prove helpful in clinical decision making and in writing SOAP notes. Answer one section at a time, and then refer to the tutorial at the end of each chapter, which provides the answers to the questions.

Information in the text may become incorrect as new discoveries or drugs become available. Based on personal interpretation, each reader may not agree with the actions taken by the authors. Each author was chosen for expertise in his or her field. Health care providers frequently argue over the best way to do things. There are several correct answers to clinical problems, with the answers dependent on the expertise and background of the person providing the care. At times this is difficult for students to learn; it is much easier when there is just one way to do things. It is important to develop the most patient-specific plan by carefully utilizing all aspects of critical thinking and clinical judgment.

This text is appropriate for use by multiple audiences, including NP students, NPs preparing for certification examinations, and novice NPs. It may also serve as a review book for experienced nurse practitioners, who may need to update knowledge in a particular area as they move from one job to another with a different patient population.

The introduction to the text discusses the important issues of clinical decision making and critical thinking for NPs. Presented are suggestions regarding how the NP may learn to expand upon and improve his or her own clinical judgment skills with the use of this text. The remainder of the text consists of 41 case studies addressing patient issues and problems commonly seen by NPs in practice. Each case is presented using the SOAP format with appropriate questions. The tutorials present the answers to each of the questions. References are provided at the end of each chapter to assist the reader with information provided in the answers.

This text has been designed to present patient scenarios. It is not meant to be a comprehensive textbook on these topics. Instead, it presents reality-based learning with "need to know" content. Its goal is to facilitate the refinement of clinical decision making in nurse practitioners.

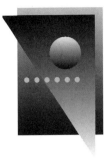

Acknowledgments

Development of this textbook has touched the lives of many people. I would like to give particular thanks to:

- the editors at Lippincott-Raven who facilitated the book's progress through the production phases
- my post–MSN FNP classmates at the University of Kentucky for working on the first case study
- Pamela Kidd who suggested the problem-focused method, and her colleague Kathleen Dorman Wagner, who used the problem-focused method extensively
- Lisa Stead for recognizing the potential of the case studies format and acting on it
- all the expert practitioners who contributed real-life case studies to the book
- my colleagues at Northern Kentucky University who helped in a variety of ways, knowing I was busy working on the book
- my family: John, Callie, Kristin, Mom, Robert, and Kim who patiently tolerated my absences during the crunch times and helped in any way they could.

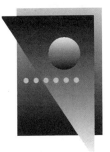

Contents

● *Critical Thinking and Clinical Decision Making*   *1*

● CASE **1**
  A 27-year-old woman with a chronic cough   *10*

● CASE **2**
  A 6-year-old boy with an itchy red eye   *27*

● CASE **3**
  A 38-year-old pregnant woman with vaginal bleeding   *36*

● CASE **4**
  An 8-year-old boy having difficulty in school   *48*

● CASE **5**
  A 55-year-old man with cough, fever, and SOB   *62*

● CASE **6**
  A 48-year-old woman with fatigue and headaches   *74*

● CASE **7**
  A 23-year-old woman with vaginal discharge   *91*

● CASE **8**
  A 36-year-old man with heartburn   *104*

● CASE **9**
A 65-year-old woman requesting a checkup 114

● CASE **10**
A 30-year-old woman with a headache 127

● CASE **11**
A 28-year-old woman with cough and fatigue 140

● CASE **12**
A 36-year-old woman with a breast lump 149

● CASE **13**
A 15-year-old boy requesting a well physical and sports examination 157

● CASE **14**
A 62-year-old man with a facial rash and a red eye 169

● CASE **15**
A 15-year-old boy with knee pain 179

● CASE **16**
A 17-year-old woman with abdominal pain 190

● CASE **17**
A 75-year-old woman with confusion and incontinence 199

● CASE **18**
A 3-week-old infant well-child check 215

● CASE **19**
A 4-year-old boy with a sore throat and earache 231

● CASE **20**
A 44-year-old man with chronic back pain   240

● CASE **21**
A 54-year-old man with blurred vision, polyuria, and fatigue   257

● CASE **22**
A 25-year-old woman with diarrhea and bloating   268

● CASE **23**
A 67-year-old man requesting a well physical   279

● CASE **24**
A 3-year-old girl with a rash   291

● CASE **25**
A 40-year-old woman with abdominal pain   299

● CASE **26**
A 25-year-old woman requesting birth control   310

● CASE **27**
A 20-year-old woman with burning during urination   324

● CASE **28**
A 5-year-old girl presents for a kindergarten physical   335

● CASE **29**
A 67-year-old man with a painful rash in the perineal area   345

● CASE **30**
A 26-year-old woman with eye pain and tearing   353

● CASE **31**

A 32-year-old woman with a lump under her arm   *364*

● CASE **32**

A 35-year-old man with LUQ abdominal pain with nausea and vomiting   *380*

● CASE **33**

A 25-year-old man with a 3-day history of rhinorrhea, frontal headache, and maxillary tooth pain   *391*

● CASE **34**

A 31-year-old woman with fatigue   *402*

● CASE **35**

A 68-year-old woman with severe dizziness   *414*

● CASE **36**

A 36-year-old woman with lower back pain   *429*

● CASE **37**

A 65-year-old man with elevated blood pressure   *441*

● CASE **38**

A 2-year-old boy presents for a well-child visit   *455*

● CASE **39**

A 55-year-old woman with a rash on her arm   *469*

● CASE **40**

A 29-year-old woman with a bump on her vagina with itching and discharge   *477*

● CASE **41**

A 29-year-old woman with an abnormal menstrual cycle and diarrhea   *487*

● *Index*   *499*

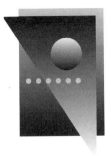

Critical Thinking and Clinical Decision Making

Educators, administrators, and experienced nurse practitioners often ask the question: How do I get professionals to actively think rather than to passively accept what is observed? Getting others to think is difficult but getting people to question the initial observations or conclusions often seems impossible.[1] The goal of this chapter is to offer some discussion surrounding critical thinking and clinical decision making and then offer some methods for encouraging it in one's self or in others.

Although some people may not differentiate between critical thinking and clinical decision making, there are some discernible differences.[1] The terms are frequently used synonymously and in that context are intended to mean the same thing. In the role of the nurse practitioner, not only is it important to differentiate the terms but it is also logical to assume that the development of critical thinking should improve or lead to more appropriate clinical decision making. Clinical decision making or critical clinical thinking is couched in the same assumptions used to support the teaching and enabling of critical thinking.

● CRITICAL THINKING

Some experts in the field of critical thinking make the point that without critical thinking, change (and therefore progress) in our society would not or could not have occurred.[4] Critical thinking by its very nature suggests questioning the *how* and *why* things are as they are and the development of improved methods for doing things differently. Brookfield[4] identifies nine critical thinking themes. The first five themes deal with the identification of critical thinkers. These characteristics include: 1) critical thinking as a productive and positive activity; 2) the context in which critical thinking occurs may change how critical thinking is seen; 3) critical thinking may be positive as well as negative; 4) emotions are often key to critical thinking; 5) and critical thinking is a process.[4]

Although some of these themes are fairly common, two are of particular interest here. One is that critical thinking is productive and positive and is an activity. This indicates that the critical thinker engages in a productive, positive activity. It is not passive; critical thinking involves doing something. Critical thinking produces something — a new way, a different way, a different stance or glance at a familiar methodology or assumption. Critical thinking is positive — it is not negating the organization or the facts but examining them in a different light or context. Critical thinking includes questioning the assumptions on which behavior, values, and action are based. The critical thinker asks the uncomfortable but necessary questions to understand how actions or decisions are made.[4]

The second theme of interest is the notion that critical thinking involves emotions. Critical thinking is often seen as dispassionate, distant, and coldly logical. Thus, emotional value or concern is eliminated by the process of thinking critically. Brookfield believes that "emotions are central to the critical thinking process" (p. 7).[4] The fear of consequences from the consideration of alternatives to the "usual way" or the consequences of questioning authority are powerful fears. The thrill of coming out of a critical thinking process intact or even healthier is also a powerful feeling. Critical thinkers consider the emotional fallout of change or progress rather than ignore it. Emotion is a part of the human experience and therefore based on values and assumptions. It is as important to examine the emotional aspect of the critical thinking process as it is to look at the logically based assumptions.[4]

Key to critical thinking is the thinker's ability to determine the assumptions underlying beliefs, values, and attitudes. When these assumptions are identified, the thinker has the opportunity and responsibility to examine them for appropriateness. Are the central assumptions culturally appropriate or logical? Are the assumptions based on current fact or fiction? Does the critical thinker see flaws in these assumptions? From this point, the critical thinker can make decisions and take action based on individual findings or beliefs about the assumptions. Again, this is a positive, productive activity because it examines long-held, culturally based beliefs that may no longer be appropriate. For example, one's assumption that a car will last 10 years may be rethought when the engine blows up and a new engine costs more than the car is worth. Rather than abiding by the original assumption, the owner may decide to purchase a different car because reexamination of the underlying assumptions reveals that they are no longer appropriate in the current context. This kind of critical thinking occurs in the lives of adults on a regular basis and is critical of logical thinking. Simply assuming the underlying assumptions still hold true is not rational or appropriate. Rather, to question or understand the underlying assumptions is the sign of mature, adult behavior. Figuring out what the underlying assumptions are is a step toward critical thinking. Examining these assumptions in the current context and then determining what action to take is the basic process of critical thinking. Although it is rather simplistic as stated, it is a difficult, involved, time-consuming process. There is a certain amount of fear involved in critical thinking. The examination of long-held beliefs, values, and attitudes implies a self-examination that is both exciting and frightening. What if one finds that one's long-held beliefs are not appropriate in the current culture? How does one go about replacing beliefs? How is a value system reordered? Of course, value systems are reordered frequently and often with little notice but once in a while an individual really feels the need to come to grips with some outmoded principles or values. As Brookfield points out, critical thinking can be stimulated by either positive or negative events in one's life or work.[1,4,5,7]

Once an individual has used the critical thinking process in one area of life or work, then it is more likely the individual will use the process in other domains. If an individual consistently practices critical thinking then critical thinking becomes a way of looking at the world and evaluating the context in which thoughts are generated. Getting people to think critically for the first time is a challenge. Once done, it is more likely to continue. Meyers suggests use of a nonthreatening, questioning approach.[7] Rather than accepting parroted answers or superficial discussion, a questioning, quiet, nonchallenging approach circumvents the naturally defensive attitude one takes when one perceives one's very existence is being challenged or negated. Subtlety permits the learner of critical thinking to feel safe and secure while examining the assumptions that maintain an orderly world. Examination of those assumptions in a protected environment produces a confident, secure individual unafraid of change or doubt yet sensitive to the fear or concern of others engaging (perhaps for the first time) in the critical thinking process.[7]

● CLINICAL DECISION MAKING

In the clinical arena, it is imperative for one to make the correct clinical decisions. The information presented in physical findings, history, and laboratory confirmation theoretically leads one to the correct decision. However, in some cases, differentiating one diagnosis from another is tedious and obscure. It is in this practice arena that accepting facts at face value may prolong the provision of proper treatment and care.[1]

The nursing process is a well-known and well-used tool to promote both critical thinking and critical clinical decision making. The steps of the nursing process are similar to the scientific method as well as a number of other problem-solving methodologies. The advantage of the nursing process for nurse practitioners is that most nursing practitioners are familiar with it and it encompasses the whole of nursing knowledge as a basis for treatment. By far the most important step of the process for the new practitioner is assessment. Either a focused assessment for the apparently well individual with a specific complaint, or an in-depth complete assessment for the first-time patient or the patient with vague complaints, is necessary. The nurse practitioner must make the decision regarding which assessment to begin and go from there. Of course, the nurse practitioner may need to switch from one type of assessment to another depending on what the data demonstrate.

As soon as a client offers some beginning complaint, the nurse practitioner is quick to begin entertaining some diagnoses and eliminating others.[1] As more information and physical findings become apparent, the nurse practitioner begins to narrow the possibilities of diagnoses. Eventually, one or more diagnoses are determined and the nurse practitioner begins to formulate a treatment plan. The decision to accept or reject diagnoses is the point at which critical clinical decision making becomes important.

● RELATIONSHIP OF CRITICAL THINKING AND CLINICAL DECISION MAKING

The relationship of critical thinking to clinical decision making is convoluted. If the premise that *critical thinking is a process* promotes skepticism, then it is appropriate to assume that skepticism and continual examination of data in the diagnosis and treatment of illness is also a process. And if the premise that *processes can be learned* is acceptable, then the assumption that *processes can be taught* is also appropriate. But how does one teach these processes? Is it necessary to teach one before the other or can they become concurrent learning experiences? Is it necessary to be a critical thinker in life in order to be a critical clinical decision maker or can one think critically clinically and transfer that experience to life? As simplistic as it may seem, the two processes are transferable and can be promoted from either direction. Critical thinking of some form is the goal of most educational and higher degree programs.[4] Therefore, critical thinking can be taught and can be transferred by the learner to other aspects of life.

● TEACHING CRITICAL THINKING AND CRITICAL CLINICAL DECISION MAKING

Again the question arises, how do educators, administrators, and experienced nurse practitioners encourage students to look beyond the obvious and question the common view of the data? It is not that the obvious may not be correct; it is that the less obvious may be more correct. Bates[2] outlines a succinct method for clinical thinking. She recommends **clustering symptoms and data** to **separate** the data of **concern from** the **normal or anticipated** data. It is at the time of clustering that the critical thinking process needs to intersect the clinical decision making process. This is the time at which the **obvious and less obvious** must be **examined** and **accepted or rejected**. Once the potential diagnoses have been critically examined, then data necessary to confirm, disconfirm, or differentiate can be obtained. To not examine the data critically is a disservice to the client. As stated earlier, it is important not to raise defenses and make defensiveness a barrier to learning.[7] Using a subtle approach and gently questioning how the nurse practitioner reached a conclusion or diagnosis will promote critical thinking. Helping the nurse practitioner develop a ~~healthy skepticism toward the obvious conclusion~~ will help the nurse practitioner regard skepticism as a ~~positive~~ feeling or characteristic rather than a negative one.[7] Seeing the relationship between one's ~~personal~~ value system and one's ~~professional~~ decisions requires gentle nudging and care. For example, the nurse practitioner who assumes that recurrent head lice in a child is the result of an uncaring or lazy mother is making an assumption about the mother not necessarily based on fact but rather on illogical premises about mothers. This nurse practitioner is not using all the nursing knowledge available to critically evaluate why the child has a recurrent condition. When using all that knowledge, the nurse practitioner may discover that the mother is unaware of how head lice are transmitted and the importance of thorough bed and house cleaning in addition to hair treatment. The nurse practitioner's personal value system may have provoked the attitude that lazy uncaring mothers do not treat head lice in the first place. In this example, getting the nurse practitioner to examine personal values will lead to reevaluation of the mother's knowledge base about head lice and its transfer.

Experienced critical thinkers ~~routinely examine their own thinking~~. One can view critical thinking as thinking about thinking in a way that improves one's thinking.[8] To examine one's thinking requires a set of ~~examination tools~~ and a questioning attitude. Two tools proposed by Paul[8] are ~~elements of reasoning~~ and ~~universal intellectual standards~~. Let's examine how the nurse practitioner can use these critical thinking tools in conjunction with the diagnostic reasoning process or clinical decision making.

Elements of Reasoning

The elements of reasoning provide a framework for the nurse nurse practitioner to break apart thinking. These elements ~~are purpose, question or issue, perspective or point of view, data, assumptions, concepts, inference, implication, and consequences.~~

When the nurse applies the diagnostic reasoning process, the nurse does so for a purpose. The overarching purpose for applying the process is to identify the basis for making diagnostic and treatment decisions about the patient. Specific purposes for specific decision-making activities, however, may vary. The purpose of the nurse's deliberations about diagnostic tests may be to rule out specific conditions from the differential diagnosis list. Or, the purpose for such deliberations about choice of test may be to maximize cost effectiveness for patient and/or provider. An economic perspective is a perspective from which the nurse practitioner must frequently reason. Consider Marie, the 20-year-old woman with burning during urination. When ~~prescribing antibiotics~~ for Marie, the nurse practitioner compares the ~~daily cost of three equally effective drugs~~. Relevant questions that the nurse practitioner might ask of self include: 1) What is my purpose for employing this diagnostic test? 2) Toward what end(s) am I considering this particular treatment option?

The questions or issues that arise during the diagnostic reasoning and treatment decision processes arise from data the nurse practitioner gathers during the patient encounter. One may gather data from many perspectives: a nursing perspective, a medical or pathophysiologic perspective, a psychological perspective, or a cultural perspective. It is important for the nurse practitioner to identify from what perspective or point of view the data is gathered. Sometimes it's more pertinent for the nurse practitioner to gather data from the patient's perspective or from the family's perspective. Consider John, the 15-year-old boy who presents for his sports participation physical. John has freely offered information to the nurse practitioner about experimentation with marijuana and alcohol. When deciding what to do with this information, the nurse practitioner must consider the confidence the patient has placed in the nurse practitioner. That is, the patient apparently views his drug use as benign. The nurse practitioner must also consider the possible implications or consequences of violating that confidence. The nurse practitioner's initial perspective might be to view the drug use with concern. Pertinent questions to self-examine thinking that the nurse practitioner might ask include: 1) Are there other data that indicate the drug use may be serious? 2) What is the basis for my concern? If there are not overt data to dispute the patient's perspective, the nurse practitioner should strongly consider the patient's perspective prior to divulging this confidential information.

One reason the nurse practitioner identifies multiple perspectives from which to interpret data is the fact that each of these perspectives operates on inherent assumptions. As discussed earlier, assumptions represent an element of reasoning not often explicitly identified in clinical reasoning. Assumptions can, however, have a profound effect on treatment decisions and thus on outcomes and consequences. The nurse practitioner may, for example, base the concern for John's drug experimentation on the assumption that any substance use is inherently pathologic and requires direct intervention. Acting on this assumption might lead the nurse practitioner to discuss John's marijuana use with his mother. If John's experimentation with marijuana was indeed merely experimentation, John would not be very likely to confide in any health practitioner in the near future. It's important to do some thinking about what assumptions one holds when making a diagnosis or a treatment decision. Personal value assumptions may not always be compatible with client behavior. John's personal values or culture may condone experimentation with certain drugs or it may be a part of normal teen growth and development.

Universal Intellectual Standards

Universal intellectual standards provide another useful tool with which the nurse practitioner can self-examine thinking. Intellectual standards include clarity and precision, depth, breadth, relevance, accuracy, and logic. Clarity is a relevant standard at many points in the diagnostic reasoning process.

Eliciting clear information from relevant data sources is crucial to the process. Clear communication of treatment decisions to the patient or other care givers may directly determine the success of the intervention(s). Key questions the nurse practitioner might ask of self during data collection include: 1) Are the data clear? 2) Do I need to clarify certain cues with the patient or other informants? 3) Am I clearly communicating treatment options or procedures with the client?

Precision, in addition to clarity, is often necessary. Precise communication of medication regimen, for example, may determine the patient's understanding of and subsequent compliance with the regimen. The nurse practitioner might instruct Marie, the 20-year-old with the urinary tract infection, to take TMP-SMZ twice daily. The nurse practitioner has been clear. Precisely when and on what schedule, however, should the patient take the antibiotics? With a 3-day course of antibiotics, it is important to maintain a serum level. To communicate precisely how such an outcome is achieved, the nurse practitioner would advise the patient to take the antibiotic at the same time every 12 hours and further advise the patient to take the drug at least 1 hour before or two hours after a meal. The nurse practitioner has then been precise.

Depth and breadth are sometimes important standards for assessing one's thinking in regard to particularly ambiguous data sets. Questions to self might help the nurse practitioner achieve depth and breadth when thinking through diagnostic or treatment decisions. Self-examination questions that promote depth and breadth respectively include: 1) Are there other important data elements that might support or refute my decision? 2) Are there other perspectives from which the data could be viewed? It is often tempting to accept superficial data as relevant diagnostic indicators. If one accepts superficial, first-pass data as the most relevant in situations where those data potentially represent a variety of diagnoses, that superficiality may cost the nurse practitioner diagnostic accuracy.

To determine that the diagnosis is indeed inaccurate may cost the nurse practitioner and the patient profoundly in time, money, or even pain and suffering. In situations where data are potentially ambiguous, nurse practitioners should ask themselves questions to assure that they base diagnoses on accurate and relevant data. Questions such as, "How could I check on the accuracy of these particular data?" might save valuable time in the long run.

The logic of a particular diagnoses is contained in the question, "Upon what cluster of data do I base this diagnosis?" Or, in the case of differential diagnoses, the logic of a particular diagnosis may be contained in the answer to, "From what conditions may I differentiate my patient's condition based on particular clusters of data?" The dysuria that Marie experienced could result from several possible diagnoses. There were not, however, any cues to cluster with the dysuria to support a diagnosis other than a lower urinary tract infection. If the nurse practitioner reflects upon the data underpinning particular diagnoses, and the data make sense with the diagnoses, then the diagnosis is probably accurate.

● CASE STUDIES AS A TEACHING AND LEARNING TOOL

Case study interpretation is a terrific method to use to teach and learn either critical thinking or clinical decision making. Case studies provide guidance in learning the next step in the nursing process; the diagnostic tests necessary to differentiate, confirm, or disconfirm diagnoses; the data findings and sorting of the data; as well as an opportunity to examine the underlying assumptions for both personal and professional values, beliefs, and attitudes. Case studies offer the opportunity for nonpersonal discussion because the threat of personalization is removed. Although the case study is based on and related to reality, it is not reality in the sense that the client is actually present in front of the nurse practitioner. Case studies offer a wonderful opportunity for discussion without the potential for defensiveness or the fear of error.

Case studies can be used to promote individual learning and data examination as well as group discussion and learning. Sometimes, individuals feel less threatened discussing values in groups because the individual does not have to defend personal values. The nurse practitioner can listen and then introspectively examine the context of personal values. Group discussion of diagnoses and differentiation is a rich environment for learning, free from the pressures of the clinical arena. It provides data for the nurse practitioner to consider in the privacy of the office and an opportunity to change without undue pressure or grief.

● CONCLUSIONS

Elements of reasoning and **universal intellectual standards** are but one way of viewing critical thinking and its relation to diagnostic reasoning and treatment decision making. Critical thinking embodies knowledge, experience, level of cognitive development, and a number of specific competencies and attitudes.[3,6,9] All of these critical thinking abilities require time and commitment from the nurse practitioner to develop. Maintaining a questioning, skeptical attitude will, however, assist the nurse practitioner to continue developing critical thinking abilities.

The use of case studies to promote individual and group examination of assumptions underlying assessment and diagnoses is a nonthreatening method to teach and learn critical thinking and decision making. The use of subtle, gentle questioning and prodding in combination with case studies offers the opportunity for growth without defensiveness and wariness on the part of the nurse practitioner. Learning to think critically is a difficult process that requires encouragement and support. Once the basic process is completed, then the transfer of the critical thinking process to either the personal or professional arena becomes easier and less fear-producing; over time, critical thinking becomes an automatic part of the diagnosis and treatment process.

REFERENCES

1. Bandman, E. L., & Bandman, B. (1995). *Critical thinking in nursing* (2nd edition). Norwalk, Connecticut: Appleton & Lange.
2. Bates, B. (1995). *A guide to clinical thinking.* Philadelphia: J. B. Lippincott Company.
3. Benner, P. (1984). *From novice to expert: Excellence and power in clinical practice.* Menlo Park, CA: Addison-Wesley.
4. Brookfield, S. D. (1987). *Developing critical thinkers.* San Francisco: Jossey-Bass Publishers.
5. Chaffee, J. (1994). Teaching for critical thinking. *National Vision:* 2(1), 24–25.
6. Kataoka-Yahiro, M., & Saylor, C. (1994). A critical thinking model for nursing judgment. *Journal of Nursing Education,* 33, 351–356.
7. Meyers, C. (1986). *Teaching students to think critically.* San Francisco: Jossey-Bass Publishers.
8. Paul, R. (1995). *Critical thinking: How to prepare students for a rapidly changing world.* Santa Rosa, CA: The Foundation for Critical Thinking.
9. Schon, D. (1983). *The reflective practitioner.* New York: Basic Books.

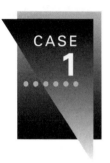

A 27-year-old woman with a chronic cough

SCENARIO

Shelly Pearl is a 27-year-old slender Caucasian female who presents today with c/o a chronic cough of more than 2 months and shortness of breath (SOB). Sometimes the cough produces a clear phlegm. Her episodes of SOB are occurring more often, up to several times a week, and it seems to take longer to recover. She has difficulty breathing at night and can sometimes hear a "wheezing sound." It occasionally feels like there is "a band around my chest and it is frightening." She also has been very tired lately, has a decreased appetite, and has been getting "my migraine headaches" more often. Shelly reports that she currently smokes 2 ppd, a habit she began at 15 years of age.

● TENTATIVE DIAGNOSES

Based on Shelly's presentation, what are your tentative differential diagnoses?

● HISTORY

What questions do you want to ask Shelly to assist you in developing a diagnosis?

● PHYSICAL ASSESSMENT

Based on the subjective data, what parts of the physical exam should be done, and why?

● DIFFERENTIAL DIAGNOSES

What are the significant positive and negative data that support or refute your diagnoses for Shelly?

● DIAGNOSTIC TESTS

Based on the history and physical, what, if any, diagnostic tests would you obtain for Shelly? Include your rationale for the tests.

● DIAGNOSIS

What subjective and objective data link with diagnostic test findings? What is your diagnosis?

● THERAPEUTIC PLAN

1. *What issues will you consider when deciding on treatment for Shelly?*
2. *What are the goals of therapy for Shelly?*
3. *What are the essential components of asthma management for Shelly?*
4. *What are the mainstays of pharmacological therapy for asthma?*
5. *What are environmental control measures to avoid allergens/irritants for Shelly?*
6. *What objective measures will help evaluate Shelly's lung function?*
7. *What education needs to be presented to Shelly and her family?*
8. *Based on the information given so far about Shelly, what impact do you think this situation has had on Shelly's family?*
9. *What would be appropriate interventions for Shelly's family?*
10. *Where can an NP obtain more information concerning asthma and/or additional resources for assisting asthmatic clients?*
11. *What other health care providers/professional disciplines could be included in a therapeutic plan of care for Shelly?*
12. *Shelly returns in 2 weeks. Her asthma symptoms have improved and she has gotten an air conditioning window unit, mattress covers for all beds, and has had a home visit from the visiting nurses to supervise her asthma management and environmental modifications. Shelly reports needing her albuterol MDI 3×/day, sometimes 4×/day. Her PEFR is usually around 80% of her personal best. She reports she had decreased her smoking to $1\frac{1}{2}$ ppd, and expresses a desire to quit. What modifications would you make for Shelly at today's visit?*
13. *How soon would you have Shelly return for follow up?*

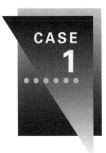

TUTORIAL

A 27-year-old woman with a chronic cough

SCENARIO

Shelly Pearl is a 27-year-old slender Caucasian female who presents today with c/o a chronic cough of more than 2 months and shortness of breath (SOB). Sometimes the cough produces a clear phlegm. Her episodes of SOB are occurring more often, up to several times a week, and it seems to take longer to recover. She has difficulty breathing at night and can sometimes hear a "wheezing sound." It occasionally feels like there is "a band around my chest and it is frightening." She also has been very tired lately, has a decreased appetite, and has been getting "my migraine headaches" more often. Shelly reports that she currently smokes 2 ppd, a habit she began at 15 years of age.

● TENTATIVE DIAGNOSES

Based on Shelly's presentation, what are your tentative differential diagnoses?

DIAGNOSIS	RATIONALE
Chronic bronchitis	Shelly is presenting with a chronic, productive cough, no fever, a history of allergies, and a 15-pack/year history of smoking. These are all contributing factors of chronic bronchitis.
Laryngeal dysfunction/ mechanical obstruction	Shelly is c/o wheezing, cough, and dyspnea, which are common symptoms of laryngeal dysfunction or mechanical obstruction.
Asthma	Shelly is c/o SOB, wheezing, cough, tightness in her chest, and a long history of smoking. Two additional risk factors are her lower socioeconomic bracket, and inner-city dwelling.

(continued)

DIAGNOSIS	*RATIONALE*
Pneumonia	Symptoms of productive cough, dyspnea, fatigue, anorexia, frequent URIs are suspicious of pneumonia. Absence of a fever does not rule this out.
CHF	Dyspnea, which is worse at night, fatigue, and decreased appetite are symptomatic of early CHF.
Drug-induced cough	A persistent bothersome cough is frequently symptomatic of the ACE inhibitors and selective beta-blockers.
GERD	A persistent cough, worse at night, and/or wheezing can result from aspiration of acid reflux. Patients frequently wake at night, coughing.

● HISTORY

What questions do you want to ask Shelly to assist you in developing a diagnosis?

REQUESTED DATA	*DATA ANSWER*
Allergies	NKDA History of allergies to dust mites, mold, ragweed
Medication	Metaprolol (Lopressor) 50 mg BID Ibuprofen 600 mg, q6h prn: prophylactic for headaches
Childhood diseases	Chicken pox
Immunizations	All childhood immunizations; last tetanus shot 2 years ago
Surgery/transfusions 　　Fractures/injuries/accidents	None
Hospitalizations	Vaginal childbirth ×2, 1990/1994 ED visits for URI/bronchitis, SOB
Adult illnesses	Frequent URI, bronchitis Headaches, migraine type
OBG History	LNMP: 7/4/96, normal flow, 5 days Pap/pelvic: 1 year ago, WNL BSE: no Mammogram: none GPA: 3/2/1
Last complete PE	Unsure

(continued)

REQUESTED DATA	DATA ANSWER
Weight changes	Lost about 5 lbs in past month
Appetite	Usually good; not very hungry lately
24-Hour diet recall	B: 4 cups coffee, black L: Canned soup, animal crackers, banana, soda (12 oz) D: Cheese pizza, applesauce, canned corn, 2 c coffee
Sleeping pattern	Bed around 10:30 PM, up at 6:45 am to get oldest ready for school. Occasional naps with 2-yr-old.
Family history	Fa: 52 y/o, HTN, smoker, obese Mo: 51 y/o, COPD, smoker, migraine headaches Bro: 30 y/o, smoker, obese, HTN Bro: 28 y/o smoker, asthma Two children: 6, female, good health; 2, female, good health
Social habits	Smokes 2 ppd, started at age 15. Tried to quit two times, unsuccessfully. No alcohol, 1 pot coffee/day, 2–3 sodas. Denies recreational drugs. Denies regular exercise, but lives on second floor of building in housing project in 2-bedroom apartment.
Social organizations	None
Relationship with husband	Separated from him for 18 mos, married for 8 yrs. Minimal contact when he picks up children every Saturday, returns children at noon on Sunday.
Relationship with children	Kids are important to her, but admits that it is hard being a single mom. Does not like to leave children with babysitter other than parents.
Relationship with parents/ siblings	Close to parents. Mother helps with girls. Dinner with parents every Sunday. Minimal contact with brothers: never very close.
Insurance/Income	Medicaid, food stamps, unemployed.
Education	Highest grade level: 11th grade. Has talked to social worker about obtaining GED. Wants to do this when youngest daughter goes to preschool.
Length of symptoms, effect on ADLs	Always had breathing problems, but worse in last 2 months. Difficulty climbing stairs, walking to grocery store, and getting oldest child to school.
What do you do for your cough, SOB?	Try to cut back on cigarettes, but can't. Tried OTC cough syrup, but with no relief.
Is there anything that makes your cough/SOB worse?	Smoking seems to cause increased wheezing. Symptoms seem to be worse since moving into apt. 2 months ago. Also, wheeze is more noticeable at night.

(continued)

REQUESTED DATA	DATA ANSWER
Is there anything that makes your SOB/cough better?	Nothing at present
How would you rate your overall health status?	Fair to good
How do you manage stress?	Watches TV, talks to her mother.

● PHYSICAL ASSESSMENT

Based on the subjective data, what parts of the physical exam should be done, and why?

SYSTEM	RATIONALE	FINDINGS
Skin color and character	With pulmonary symptoms, assess skin for color, diaphoresis, warmth.	Pale mucous membranes and pink nailbeds. Skin dry, no jaundice, bruises, scattered cherry angiomas on chest.
Vital signs	Baseline information, check temperature for indications of acute illness.	T 97.6, HR 94, R 20, B/P 104/64 Wt. 125 lbs Ht. 5'7"
Eye	Shelly had c/o migraine headaches so ophthalmic exam is indicated.	OD 20/30 OS 20/30 No glasses Visual fields and EOM intact Disc well marginated, no A/V nicking, no plaques.
Ears, nose , throat	Assess conjunctivae for anemia, oropharynx for laryngeal dysfunction/obstruction; nasal mucosa for allergic rhinitis vs rhinitis. Check for lymph nodes indicating immune response in infection. Assess accessory muscles used for breathing.	TMs: translucent, gray, light reflex and landmarks visible, no fluid. Nose: Mucosa pink, clear d/c, no polyps, septum midline. Mouth: Mucosa pink, no pharyngeal edema, exudate. No tonsillar edema, no lymphadenopathy. Thyroid: Nonpalpable, no carotid bruit.

(continued)

SYSTEM	*RATIONALE*	*FINDINGS*
Sinuses	Important to assess to r/o inflammation related to sinusitus.	No frontal/maxially sinus tenderness. Negative transillumination.
Lungs	Essential to assess in order to differentiate between possible diagnoses. Chief complaints, cough/SOB.	Resonant to percussion, lung expansion equal. No increase AP/lateral diameter. Diffuse expiratory, wheezes bilately. Fine crackles, Rt. base. No voice sounds or tactile fremitus.
Heart	Baseline information; with SOB may have increased HR.	$S_1 S_2$ WNL, no murmurs, gallops, or rubs.
Breasts	Not essential for this exam today; could omit; follow up at gynecological exam.	Symmetrical, no masses, tenderness or nipple d/c.
Abdomen	Helpful to r/o GERD; check for epigastric tenderness.	Nontender, no masses or guarding. No HSM. BS +.
Neurological assessment	Total neurological assessment not indicated here. Use only to determine if Shelly is not alert and oriented. May be detrimental if Shelly is in acute distress.	Gait normal, no tremors, strength 5/5. Negative Romberg. Tender paracervical muscles to palpation. DTRs 2+, Pain sensation intact. CN II-XII intact.
Extremities	Check for edema usually associated with CHF.	No edema, pulses 2+.
Pelvic	Not essential; will need to set up gyn. appointment.	Deferred.
Rectal	Not essential.	Deferred.

● DIFFERENTIAL DIAGNOSES

What are the significant positive and negative data which support or refute your diagnoses for Shelly?

DIAGNOSIS	POSITIVE DATA	NEGATIVE DATA
Chronic bronchitis	Chronic cough, cigarette smoker, progressive exertional dyspnea, wheezing, recurrent respiratory infections, fatigue, history of childhood allergies.	Weight loss, lack of libido, tachypnea, increased A/P chest wall diameter, decreased cardiac and breath sounds, hyperresonance on percussion, rhonchi, prolonged expiration, male, >50 years of age.
Laryngeal dysfunction/ mechanical obstruction	Wheezing, persistent productive cough, smoking, allergy.	Localized, fixed wheezing on auscultation, stridor. No history of FB.
Asthma	Cough, wheezing, chest tightness, dyspnea, recurrent URI, smoker, reversible and episodic fatigue, history of childhood asthma, tachycardia.	Seasonal/perennial pattern of symptoms, flexural eczema, use of accessory muscles, tachypnea, rhinitis, sinusitis, nasal polyps, allergic shiners.
Pneumonia	Productive cough, fatigue, dyspnea, anorexia, headache, crackles rt. base.	Abrupt onset of high fever, shaking, chills, pleuritic chest pain, myalgia, pharyngitis, localized diminished breath sounds, dullness to percussion, tactile fremitus, adventitious breath sounds.
CHF	Dyspnea worse at night, and on exertion, fatigue, decreased appetite, cough, pallor, mild tachycardia, exercise intolerance.	No JVD, S_3 gallop, peripheral edema, hemoptysis, orthopnea, inspiratory bibasilar crackles, weakness, nocturia, cyanosis.
Drug-induced cough	Nonselective beta blocker, persistent cough.	ACE inhibitor, dry cough.
GERD	Coughing worse at night with SOB.	Denies heartburn, no increase in heartburn when supine. No eating of meals late at night.

● DIAGNOSTIC TESTS

Based on the history and physical, what, if any, diagnostic testing would you obtain for Shelly and why?

DIAGNOSTIC TEST	RATIONALE	RESULTS
Spirometry	Good choice for obtaining objective measurement of lung function. This test can confirm the diagnosis of asthma, as well as establish a response to therapy. If Shelly is asthmatic, spirometry will show reduced expiratory flow rates and volumes, which can improve with bronchodilator therapy.	This is a test usually done in the outpatient department, not in the office.
PEFR	Good idea. This simple and reproducible measurement can be done in your center at the time of the visit. This will give you a quantitative value that correlates with the values obtained with a simple spirogram (FEV$_1$). The PEFR is portable and easy to do. You can teach and supervise Shelly at your office, ensuring understanding and correct technique. It is dependent on the amount of effort placed in the test.	Average 320 L/min with 3 attempts.
CXR	Not a bad idea if you suspect pneumonia, CHF, or infection as your primary diagnosis; however, it is time-consuming and costly. This adds little to the acute evaluation of asthma. Hyperinflation is the most common finding on CXR,	Not done.

(continued)

DIAGNOSTIC TEST	RATIONALE	RESULTS
	and it has no diagnostic or therapeutic value.	
Sinus radiograph	Interesting choice. This test will help you discriminate whether nasal polyps and sinusitis are complicating factors in your diagnosis. Shelly's history and PE to-day do not support rhinitis or recurring sinusitis, so choosing this test now is not indicated.	Not done.
Allergy tests	Good idea. Used to document specific allergens suggested by clinical history, confirm and reinforce the need for environmental control, and identify occupational aller-gens. This requires a refer-ral to an allergist, which is very costly. Testing may be indicated later for Shelly if first-line education about environmental controls as well as prescribed medica-tions do not improve her condition.	Not done.
CBC/TSH	Good thought. Shelly has not had any labs done for >1 year and is c/o fatigue and chronic URI. She may be anemic, hypothyroid, or have an acute infection at present. Also persons with chronic bronchitis typically have polycythemia as a compensatory mechanism for decreased PO_2. These tests would be a good choice.	CBC: WBC 9.6 RBC 4.2 Hgb 12.5 Hct 38 MCV 89.6 MCH 30.6 MCHC 34.2 RDW 13.3 Plat 250 TSH 3.1
Bronchoprovocation: Methacholine/ histamine	This test is costly and time consuming. Referral to a pulmonologist would be in-dicated if Shelly did not re-	Not done.

(continued)

DIAGNOSTIC TEST	RATIONALE	RESULTS
	spond to pharmacological therapy and environmental control. Bronchoprovocation is a 5-stage procedure with 5 different concentrations of methacholine/histamine administered. This diagnostic test is not indicated now (Gorroll et al., 1995).	
Occupational/ environmental allergen challenge	This test is a possibility because Shelly reports a worsening of her symptoms after moving to her new apartment. Patients with occupational asthma caused by toxic or irritant substances usually are able to report a direct relationship between exposure and onset of symptoms. They are symptom-free during days off from work. This is not indicated for Shelly.	Not done.
Pap smear/mammogram	Shelly is due for her yearly mammogram. A reminder today in your office is a good idea, and you can follow up at her next visit. The CBE today was WNL, and teaching BSE was done. No risk factors for breast cancer are present, so mammogram is not recommended until age 40.	Not done.

● DIAGNOSIS

After linking subjective and objective data with diagnostic test findings, what is your diagnosis?

Asthma, mild persistent

- episodic dyspnea
- chest tightness
- wheezing
- cough

Grading clinical severity of asthma by national education program guidelines, mild persistent

- Intermittent, brief (<1 hour) symptoms up to two times per week
- Infrequent nocturnal symptoms (<2 times per month)
- Asymptomatic between exacerbations
- Forced expiratory volume (FEV1) or peak expiratory flow rate (PEFR) > 80% baseline

● THERAPEUTIC PLAN

1. *What issues will you consider when deciding on treatment for Shelly?*

   Some issues to consider when deciding on treatment for Shelly:

   - Type of health insurance
   - Support systems in place
   - Socioeconomic status
   - Motivational factors to increase compliance
   - Stressors

2. *What are the goals of therapy for Shelly?*

   Goals of Therapy (Shapiro, 1996)

   - Maintain (near) "normal" pulmonary function rates
   - Maintain normal activity levels
   - Prevent chronic and troublesome symptoms
   - Prevent recurrent exacerbations of asthma
   - Avoid adverse effects from asthma medications

3. *What are the essential components of asthma management for Shelly?*

   - Objective measures of lung function
   - Pharmacological therapy
   - Environmental control measures to avoid allergens/irritants
   - Patient education

4. *What are the mainstays of pharmacological therapy for asthma?*

   A. Bronchodilators: Beta-2 agonists
      1. Albuterol
      2. Metaproterenol
      3. Pirbuterol
      4. Salmeterol (long-acting)
      5. Terbutaline
      6. Aminophylline (oral agent; not first line owing to systemic effects)

   Consider for Shelly what is covered on her insurance card, or if compliance will be a factor. Intially, albuterol MDI, 2 puffs QID, PRN. If bronchodilator is required more than 3–4 times/day then consider adding an anti-inflammatory agent.

B. Anti-inflammatory agents
   1. Nedocromil sodium (nonsteroidal anti-inflammatory)
   2. Cromolyn sodium (more effective for children)
   3. Inhaled corticosteroids
      a. Beclamethasone
      b. Funisolide
      c. Triamcinilone
      d. Other more potent MDIs have recently been released
   4. Oral corticosteroids, only for severe asthma exacerbation

Recent evidence indicates that anti-inflammatories may play an role earlier in the care of the asthmatic patient, thus preventing the long-term changes in the airways.

C. Acute exacerbations: albuterol (nebulizer 0.5 mgL/mL; 2.5 mg in 2 cc of saline 20–30 minutes ×3 (no comorbid cardiovascular disease), or epinephrine 0.3 mg subcutaneously ×3 over 60–90 minutes. In addition oral corticosteriods 60 mg immediately, then 60–120 mg per day in divided doses, tapered over several days.

5. *What are environmental control measures to avoid allergens/irritants for Shelly?*

A. Allergens
   1. Outdoor allergens:
      a. pollen
      b. mold

Consider getting room air conditioning, avoid going outside when mold and pollen count is up. Consider a social service referral for assistance in purchasing a room AC unit.

   2. Indoor allergens
      a. house dust mites

For Shelly and children, consider mattress covers for all the beds, wash bedding in 130 degree water, encase the pillows, remove carpets that are laid on concrete if possible.

      b. cockroach antigen

Studies demonstrate there is a rise in childhood asthma in the inner city areas where there is a high cockroach antigen concentration. Consider contacting the landlord for regular treatments/exterminations.

      c. animal dander

Shelly has no animals. Consider removing feather products, such as down pillows or comforters.

      d. mold/mildew

B. Irritants
   1. tobacco smoke (2nd-hand smoke exposure for children attributed to early age asthma onset/ frequent exacerbations)
   2. strong sprays/odors (perfume)
   3. air polllutants
   4. wood smoke

Consider approaching Shelly about a smoking cessation program. She has verbalized that "her children are her life" and has had several unsuccessful attempts at smoking cessation. This be a good time to start cutting back or identify a quit date. Be cautious as you may have too much information to discuss at the initial visit.

6. *What objective measures will help evaluate Shelly's lung function?*

   A. PEFR should be done daily in the AM and PM. The purpose of the PEFR is the early detection of airway obstruction, monitor response to therapy, investigate triggers, and facilitate provider/patient communication.
   B. Determine Shelly's personal best PEFR by having her do PEFR 2× day for 2–3 weeks. This will help you assess the progression of her asthma, her response to the therapy begun today, and the possible need for additional therapy.

   Zones are then established based on Shelly's personal best (PB):

   Green: 80–100% of PB: maintain current regimen or gradually reduce regimen over time.

   Yellow: 50–80% of PB: Acute exacerbation, may need to temporarily increase therapy.

   Red: below 50% of PB: Immediate bronchodilator treatment and ED if no improvement to yellow or green zone (Wiedemann & Kavuru, 1994).

7. *What education needs to be presented to Shelly and her family?*

   Shelly and her family members need to know/understand:

   - Asthma is a chronic, controllable disease
   - Asthma is an inflammatory disease
   - Asthma triggers symptoms
   - Action of asthma medications and adverse reactions
   - PEFR monitoring
   - Have access to additional community/educational resources

   Consider with Shelly the present stressors she has in her day-to-day situation. You may want to consider having her 6 y/o daughter come in with her for a visit, and her parents accompany her on another visit. It will be important to agree on goals for her therapy and management. Written instructions that are simple and uncomplicated may be helpful. Positive reinforcement and assistance in contacting community agencies may be necessary. Frequent return visits after the initial diagnosis are often needed to reinforce a patient's efforts. Observing Shelly's inhaler and PEFR techniques are an essential part of your education plan. Be careful to not overload Shelly with information. It would be helpful to determine what is "need to know" information that needs to be taught first, and what can wait until another visit.

8. *Based on the information given so far about Shelly, what impact do you think this situation has had on Shelly's family?*

Shelly is the primary care provider for her two young children, with minimal support from her estranged husband. This puts additional stressors on Shelly in the following ways:

- at risk for asthma excerbations requiring ED visits and inability to care for children
- chronicity of the disease/unpredictability of exacerbations
- familial nature of asthma
- financial strain owing to medication needs, environmental modifications
- possible insecure feelings/fears of her children over their mother's health
- complex treatment regimens

9. *What would be appropriate interventions for Shelly's family?*

Appropriate interventions for Shelly's family could include:

- educational program regarding asthma, including her 6 y/o child and parents
- smoking cessation program for Shelly and her parents. Education about the potential hazards of 2nd-hand smoke may be a motivational factor
- refer Shelly to an asthma support group, and/or receiving a monthly newsletter
- schedule regular free time for Shelly with parents as support
- utilize existing support systems/develop new ones
- assist Shelly with long-term goals for personal growth and financial independence

10. *Where can an NP obtain more information concerning asthma and/or additional resources for assisting asthmatic clients?*

Consider local organizations such as the American Lung Association with family asthma programs, local hospitals' outpatient support groups, books at the local library, checking the local newspaper for support groups, and asthma educational programs.

American Association for Respiratory Care
11030 Abales Ln.
Dallas, TX 75229-4524
214/243-2272

American Lung Association
1740 Broadway
New York, NY 10010
212/315-8700

Association for the Care of Asthma
Jefferson Medical College
1025 Walnut St. (ARD)
Philadelphia, PA 19107
215/928-8912

Asthma and Allergy Foundation of America
1717 Massachusetts Ave. NW
Suite 305
Washington, DC 20036
202/265-0265 or 1-800/727-8462

National Asthma Education Program
NHLBI Information Center
Box 30105
Bethesda, MD 20814-0105

National Center for Health Education
30 E. 29th St. (ARD)
New York, NY 10016-7901
212/769-1886

National Heart, Lung, and Blood Institute (NHLBI)
9000 Rockville Pike
Bethesda, MD 20892
301/951-3260

Parents of Children with Asthma
9450 Preston Trail East
Ponte Verde, FL 32082
904/285-1410

Allergy and Asthma Network/Mothers of Asthmatics, Inc.
1-800/878-4403

11. *What other health care providers/professional disciplines could be included in a therapeutic plan of care for Shelly?*

Consider referring Shelly to:

Home Health Agency: Several agencies now have specific asthma management programs included in their services to decrease the overall cost of health care and decrease the number of acute exacerbations. They provide nurses and/or respiratory therapists to help asthma management, assist in obtaining medications and equipment, and assess the environment.

Allergist/Pulmonologist: If Shelly's symptoms do not respond to optimal therapy

American Lung Association: Smoking cessation classes

Stress management/relaxation classes

Local single parent group for support/parenting skills

12. *Shelly returns in 2 weeks. Her asthma symptoms have improved and she has gotten an air conditioning window unit, mattress covers for all beds, and has had a home visit from the visiting nures to supervise her asthma management and environmental modifications. Shelly reports needing her albuterol MDI 3×/day, sometimes 4×/day. Her PEFR is usually around 80% of her personal best. She reports she had decreased her smoking to 1½ ppd, and expresses a desire to quit. What modifications would you make for Shelly at today's visit?*

Consider adding an inhaled anti-inflammatory agent based on her borderline PEFR and increase her albuterol to 3–4× day. (You may want to make sure the anti-inflammatory is covered on her insurance; it costs around $35–45/inhaler.) Once the anti-inflammatory is started (start with two puffs QID, and gradually decrease to TID, then BID), she may be able to decrease her use of the albuterol.

Observe Shelly's PEFR and inhaler technique. Consider inviting Shelly to attend your 7-week smoking cessation program at the health center.

Consider contacting her home care nurse for a telephone conference, after obtaining written consent (Bailey et al., 1994).

13. *How soon would you have Shelly return for follow up?*

Have Shelly return in 2 weeks again to determine her response to the added medications. You could have a phone conference with her if insurance or child care is an issue. Obtaining the PEFR data would provide good indication of how she was responding to the medication.

REFERENCES

Bailey W, Chung F, Lemanske R, Reed C. Asthma update: Better diagnosis, closer control. *Patient Care* 1994;(28):64–73.

Gorroll A, May L, Mulley A. *Primary Care Medicine*, 3rd ed. Philadelphia: Lippincott; 1995.

Reinke L, Hoffman, L. How to teach asthma co-management. *Am J Nurs* 1992;(19):40-48.

Shapiro G, Rachelefsky G, Williams P, Soler J. *Understanding and Managing Asthma; Update for the Managed Care Environment.* New York: Fisons Corp; 1996.

Uphold C, Graham M. *Clinical Guidelines in Family Practice*, 2nd ed. Gainesville, FL: Barmarrae Books; 1994.

Wiedemann H, Kavuru, M. *Diagnosis and Management of Asthma.* Cleveland, Ohio: Professional Communications, Inc; 1994.

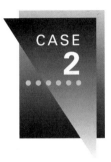

A 6-year-old boy with an itchy red eye

SCENARIO

Mary Jennings has brought her son Joe to your office. Joe is a 6-year-old Jordanian male. He presents with the complaint of an itchy red eye. Mary states that it was crusted with dry yellowish drainage several times this morning. Joe has complained to Mary frequently about pain in his eye.

● TENTATIVE DIAGNOSES

At this point, what tentative diagnoses can you identify based on Joe's presentation and Mary's brief history?

● HISTORY

What questions would you ask Mary and Joe that would facilitate in developing a diagnosis?

● PHYSICAL ASSESSMENT

Is a complete physical exam necessary?
   What parts of the exam would you include and why?
   How did your interpretation of the subjective data direct the physical examination?

● DIFFERENTIAL DIAGNOSES

List and prioritize the most probable differential diagnoses. List the positive and negative data that validate or refute each diagnosis.

● DIAGNOSTIC TESTS

What, if any, additional data should be obtained? Would any diagnostic tests be appropriate in this case? Include your rationale for the tests.

● DIAGNOSIS

What is your conclusive diagnosis?
What positive and negative data assisted you in arriving at your decision?

● THERAPEUTIC PLAN

1. *What therapeutic agent would you use in planning care for Joe?*
2. *What is your rationale for choosing this particular agent?*
3. *What are some alternatives to this treatment?*
4. *What education does Mary need to provide relief for Joe and decrease the risk of reinfection?*
5. *What follow-up care will Joe need?*

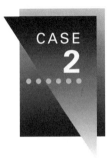

TUTORIAL

A 6-year-old boy with an itchy red eye

SCENARIO

Mary Jennings has brought her son Joe to your office. Joe is a 6-year-old Jordanian male. He presents with the complaint of an itchy red eye. Mary states that it was crusted with dry yellowish drainage several times this morning. Joe has complained to Mary frequently about pain in his eye.

● TENTATIVE DIAGNOSES

What are the potential diagnoses you have identified based on the preceding scenario?

DIFFERENTIAL DIAGNOSES   RATIONALE

DIFFERENTIAL DIAGNOSES	RATIONALE

Conjunctivitis
  Allergic
  Bacterial
  Chemical
  Viral
	Joe presents with itching, erythema, and pain in his OD. Mary has described a mucopurulent drainage from his OD. All of these symptoms are associated with conjunctivitis.

Corneal abrasion/eye trauma	Joe complains of erythema and pain in his OD. These symptoms and the unilateral involvement are associated with corneal abrasion and eye trauma.
Herpes simplex blepharitis	Joe's complaints of itching, erythema, and pain are associated with herpes simplex blepharitis. There is usually unilateral involvement with this diagnosis.
Iritis	Joe's complain of erythema, eye pain, and eye drainage are associated with iritis.
Glaucoma	Joe's complaints of pain and erythema of the eye are symptoms of glaucoma.

● HISTORY

What questions would you ask Mary and Joe that would facilitate in developing a diagnosis?

REQUESTED DATA	DATA ANSWER
Allergies	None known.
Medication	None.
Recent changes in health	No problems until present complaint. Last checkup 3 months ago.
Chief complaint: onset, location, quality, aggravating/alleviating factors	Joe describes burning, itching, and pain in OD. States that pain is not "too bad." Mary describes a thick yellow drainage. States it looks like pus. Joe's eyelids got stuck together by drainage. Joe denies a change in vision and blurred vision. Pain is bad when he looks at bright lights. Mary states warm wet washcloths have helped relieve burning.
Associated manifestations	No history of recent or concurrent respiratory infection.
Associated symptoms	Denies history of throat pain, ear pain, rhinorrhea.
History of exposure to conjunctivitis	None.
History of swimming in chlorinated or contaminated water	Has swam two times in the past week in nonchlorinated pool.
History of trauma to eye	None.
History of exposure to chemical	None.
Recent cold sores or exposure to herpes lesions	None.
Recent history of impetigo	None, but his younger brother was started on Keflex 3 days ago for impetigo on his face.
Family members with eye problems	Joe has two younger siblings who do not have any eye symptoms.
Past medical history	Normally healthy. No hospitalizations or surgeries.

● PHYSICAL ASSESSMENT

What parts of the physical exam would you perform? Is a complete physical exam necessary? What parts of the exam would you include and why?

SYSTEM	FINDINGS	RATIONALE
Skin	Skin is pink and supple, no lesion noted	Overall quick assessment of visible skin should be performed. Particular attention should be given to the face.
Heart sound	S_1 and S_2 normal, without murmur	Provides baseline information.
Breath sounds	Clear to auscultation	Allows the NP to determine if there has been respiratory involvement.
Vital signs	T (oral) 98, HR 84, RR 22, BP 88/56	Gives an indication of possible infection.
Ear, nose, throat	TMs pearl gray bilaterally. Nares patent and free of drainage. No pharyngeal erythema or edema. No oral lesions.	Gives an indication of possible infection.
Eyes	OS sclera white, without injection, erythema, or edema. OD edema of eyelids present. Crusted yellow drainage on lashes. Conjunctiva markedly inflamed. Cornea and eyelid margins without ulceration. PERL with positive red reflex bilaterally. Visual acuity reveals OD 20/20, OS 20/20.	Need to evaluate eyes thoroughly to identify possible diagnoses. Visual acuity should be completed for all patients with eye problems. It is vital for patients with decreased vision. This test may be painful if the child has photophobia.
Fundoscopic	Discs well marginated. No AV nicking.	Provides a quick indication of eye health. This test may be difficult owing to photophobia and constriction of pupils.
Lymphatics	No palpable lymph nodes in the head or neck.	Palpation of lymph nodes can provide an indication of infection.

● DIFFERENTIAL DIAGNOSES

List the positive and negative data that validate or refute each diagnosis.

DIAGNOSIS	POSITIVE DATA	NEGATIVE DATA
Allergic conjunctivitis	Conjunctiva inflamed. Itching and burning present. Cornea, pupil, and vision normal.	No watery discharge, profuse tearing, lymphadenopathy, bilateral involvement.
Bacterial conjunctivitis	Edema of eyelids; conjunctiva inflamed; itching, burning and pain present. Muco-purulent discharge; photophobia; cornea, pupil, vision normal. Unilateral involvement, history of recent impetigo in family.	No eyelid margin ulceration.
Chemical conjunctivitis	Burning, itching, and pain present. Photophobia and unilateral involvement.	Denies history of exposure to chemical. No excessive tearing or thin watery discharge.
Viral conjunctivitis	Edema of eyelids with burning and itching. Conjunctiva inflamed. Cornea, vision, and pupil normal.	Denies history of recent or concurrent URI or viral illness. No bilateral involvement. Profuse watery discharge not evident. No preauricular lymphadenopathy. No hypertrophy of lymphoid follicles of lower palpebral conjunctiva.
Corneal abrasion/eye trauma	Conjunctiva inflamed with itching, burning, and photophobia present. Unilateral involvement.	No history of trauma; cornea, vision, and pupil normal. No thin watery discharge.
Herpes simplex blepharitis	Conjunctiva inflamed with itching, burning, and photophobia. Unilateral involvement.	No history of herpes or herpes involvement. No thin watery discharge, corneal or lid ulcerations. No corneal or eyelid ulcerations, severe pain, or lymphadenopathy.

(continued)

DIAGNOSIS	POSITIVE DATA	NEGATIVE DATA
Iritis	Conjunctiva erythemic, with unilateral involvement. Complains of mild to moderate pain.	No decreased vision, severe pain, or decreased pupil sign with poor pupil reaction.
Glaucoma	Conjunctiva erythemic with mild to moderate pain.	No severe pain. Eye pressure normal. No cornea cloudiness, or marked decrease in vision. Pupil is not fixed or dilated.

● DIAGNOSTIC TESTS

Would any diagnostic tests be appropriate in this case? Include your rationale for the tests.

DIAGNOSTIC TEST	RATIONALE	RESULTS
Eye culture and gram stain	Would probably not be necessary for Joe at this point. If his infection is resistant or recurring this might be considered. Eye cultures should always be done on children less than 1 month of age. Cultures of the eye and nasopharynx should be done concurrently for gonococcal, chlamydial, and bacterial infections (Baker, 1996).	Test not done.

● DIAGNOSES

What diagnoses do you determine as being appropriate after a review of the subjective and objective data?

DIAGNOSES	RATIONALE
Conjunctivitis: bacterial	Positive history of exposure to causative bacteria. All of the symptoms Joe is experiencing can be effects of bacterial conjunctivitis. The negative finding of eyelid margin ulceration is not a consistent finding in patients with bacterial conjunctivitis, and does not eliminate this diagnosis.

● THERAPEUTIC PLAN

1. *What therapeutic agent would you use in planning care for Joe?*

   Sulfacetamide sodium ointment or solution.

2. *What is your rationale for choosing this particular agent?*

   It is both cost-effective and wide-spectrum. Use only in children more than 2 months of age. Discuss with Mary and Joe the choice of ointment or solution. Ointment is applied less frequently but can blur vision. Good for application at night because oily base stays in eye longer.

3. *What are some alternatives to this treatment?*

   Tobramycin ointment or solution or erythromycin ointment or solution would be alternative treatments for Joe. Gentamycin and neomycin are options for use but have a higher incidence of allergic reations (Merentstein, Kaplan, and Rosenberg, 1994).

4. *What education does Mary need to provide relief for Joe and decrease the risk of reinfection?*

   Medication Administration

   1. Clean the eye prior to medication administration. Wipe eye with a wet cotton ball from the inner to outer canthus. Throw cotton ball away.
   2. Sulfacetamide sodium ointment: Apply 4×/d and before bedtime, for 1 week. Sulfacetamide sodium solution 10%: instill two drops every 2–3 hours while awake, for 1 week. Drops may sting when first administered.

3. To apply or instill: Gently separate eyelids, pull down inner canthus or lower lid toward center of the eye. Place the drops or thin line of ointment in the pocket that is formed (Boynton, Dunn, and Stephens, 1994).
4. Infection should respond to treatment in 2–3 days.

Comfort Measures

1. Wet compresses, cool or warm per child's preference. Use cotton balls.
2. Joe may need distraction to keep him from rubbing or scratching his eye.

Infection Control

1. Good handwashing by entire family.
2. Have Joe keep his hands away from his face and eye.
3. Keep Joe's face cloths and towels separate from others. Use these linens one time only.
4. Monitor the siblings for symptoms.
5. What follow-up care will Joe need?

Joe should stay home from school until inflammation and discharge are gone.

Instruct Mary to call in 2–3 days if no improvement is seen. Instruct Mary to call if symptoms worsen or vision decreases. No follow-up visit is necessary if Joe responds to the medication. The infection should be resolved in 1 week.

REFERENCES

Baker RC. *Handbook of Pediatric Primary Care.* Boston: Little, Brown; 1996.

Boynton RW, Dunn ES, Stephens GR. *Manual of Ambulatory Pediatrics.* Philadelphia: JB Lippincott; 1994.

Merenstein GB, Kaplan DW, Rosenberg AA. *Handbook of Pediatrics.* Norwalk CT: Appleton and Lange; 1994.

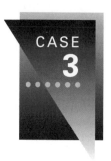

A 38-year-old pregnant woman with vaginal bleeding

SCENARIO

Kathryn Bradley is a 38-year-old Vietnamese female, G3P1A2, LMP 8/2/96. She has been attempting pregnancy for 6 months, with a positive home pregnancy test 2 weeks ago, 9/16/96. Kathryn is having the usual symptoms of pregnancy, including fatigue, breast tenderness, nausea and vomiting, and abdominal bloating. However, Kathryn woke up this morning with vaginal bleeding and she has continued to spot all day.

● TENTATIVE DIAGNOSES

Based on the information provided so far, what are potential diagnoses?

● HISTORY

1. *What are significant questions in the history for a pregnant woman with vaginal bleeding?*
2. *What are the key points to cover on the review of systems?*

● PHYSICAL ASSESSMENT

What are the significant portions of the physical examination that should be completed for Kathryn?

● DIFFERENTIAL DIAGNOSES

What are the significant positive and negative data that support or refute your diagnoses for Kathryn?

● DIAGNOSTIC TESTS

Based on the history and physical assessment, what, if any, diagnostic tests would you obtain? Include your rationale for the tests.

● DIAGNOSIS

What diagnoses are appropriate for Kathryn?

● THERAPEUTIC PLAN

1. *Calculate and identify where Kathryn is in the pregnancy.*
2. *What would your plan of care be for a woman in her first trimester with a threatened abortion?*
3. *What would you discuss with Kathryn in terms of nutrition during her pregnancy?*
4. *What influence would advanced maternal age have on your plan of care for Kathryn?*
5. *Kathryn is c/o abdominal bloating, nausea, vomiting, and fatigue. What suggestions and recommendations would you make for her?*
6. *What anticipatory guidance and instruction would you review with Kathryn regarding her pregnancy?*
7. *What are the warning signs you will review with Kathryn?*
8. *When should Kathryn return for prenatal care?*

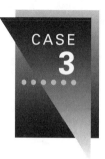

TUTORIAL

A 38-year-old pregnant woman with vaginal bleeding

SCENARIO

Kathryn Bradley is a 38-year-old Vietnamese female, G3P1A2, LMP 8/2/96. She has been attempting pregnancy for 6 months, with a positive home pregnancy test 2 weeks ago, 9/16/96. Kathryn is having the usual symptoms of pregnancy, including fatigue, breast tenderness, nausea and vomiting, and abdominal bloating. However, Kathryn woke up this morning with vaginal bleeding and she has continued to spot all day.

● TENTATIVE DIAGNOSES

Based on the information provided so far, what are the potential diagnoses?

DIAGNOSIS	RATIONALE
Spontaneous abortion	+ pregnancy test and presumptive signs of pregnancy with vaginal bleeding. + history of spontaneous abortion.
Ectopic pregnancy	+ pregnancy test. Consider ectopic pregnancy with any bleeding or abdominal pain within first 8 weeks of pregnancy.
Cervical cause such as polyps or erosion	Presence of vaginal bleeding.
Bleeding from other source such as genital trauma, rectal bleeding, UTI, etc.	Presence of vaginal bleeding.

● HISTORY

1. What are significant questions in the history for a pregnant woman with vaginal bleeding?

REQUESTED DATA	DATA ANSWER
Allergies	NKDA.
Current medications	None.
Surgery/transfusions	None/none.
Past medical history and hospitalizations/fractures/injuries/accidents	Chicken pox as a child. Hospitalized for a D&C 6 years ago; vaginal birth of child 5 years ago.
Adult illness	None.
OB/GYN history	Menarche: age 12. Cycle: q 28 days × 5 days, heavy flow first 2 days. LNMP: 8-2-96. Last pelvic: 10 months ago. Contraception: stopped OCs after last check up, used condoms. Has been attempting pregnancy × 6 months.
Appetite/weight changes	Good appetite, unsure of weight gain, but clothes seem tight since LMP, has had some nausea and vomiting, especially when she wakes in the morning. Sometimes also occurs in the evening too.
24-Hour diet recall	B: Juice, cereal with milk, toast with butter. L: Salad with dressing, tuna sandwich, milk. D: Spaghetti, salad with dressing, bread, water. S: Banana, milk.
Sleeping pattern	Goes to bed after daughter, falls asleep at 9:30 PM. Gets up at least once during night, sometimes difficulty in getting back to sleep. Up at 6:00 AM.
Social history	Tobacco: None, smoked socially in college, quit 10 yrs ago. Alcohol: Socially, likes glass of wine with dinner, stopped with + pregnancy test. Caffeine: Occasional coffee in AM, likes 1 soda/day. Drugs: None. Exercise: Tries to walk 2–3×/wk.
Family history	Father: 60, good health. Mother: 58, hysterectomy for heavy periods. Sister: 36, good health.

(continued)

REQUESTED DATA	DATA ANSWER
	Husband: 36, good health.
	Daughter: 5, good health.
Social organizations	Teachers' organization, women's church group.
Relationship with husband	Married × 10 years, good relationship.
Relationship with mother/ sibling	Good.
Income/insurance/home	Husband employed with a local firm. Kathryn teaches 2nd grade at a local school. Have medical and dental coverage through employer. Own their own home.
Length of symptoms/ confirmation of pregnancy	Attempting pregnancy × 6 months. + pregnancy test 6 days after missed period. Symptoms such as breast tenderness, fatigue started soon after + test.
Length of pregnancy	LMP 8-2-96: 7 weeks' gestation by dates.
Amount of bleeding	Awoke to find an 8 to 10-inch diameter spot of blood in bed. Now has spotting, wearing a light day pad, changed twice, not saturated. Has bleeding on tissue after urination.
Description	Initial episode was bright red, now seems to be more dark, like end of period. No clots, tissue, mucus, etc.
Associated symptoms	Occasionally feels some mild cramping but denies sharp or dull pain.
How has this affected ADLs?	No change until today. Resting today.

● PHYSICAL ASSESSMENT

What are the significant portions of the physical examination that should be completed for Kathryn?

SYSTEM	RATIONALE	FINDINGS
Vital signs	Provides baseline information.	B/P: 124/70
		HR: 80
		R: 16
		T: 97.8
		Ht. 5'6"

SYSTEM	RATIONALE	FINDINGS
		Wt. prepregnancy: 140 Today: 146
General appearance/skin	Gives overall guideline as to patient's condition.	Alert, NAD, appears anxious. Skin WNL.
Neck	Check for enlarged thyroid.	WNL.
Lungs	Provides baseline information.	CTA.
Heart	Baseline information.	Normal sinus rhythm, no MRG.
Abdomen	Baseline information.	BS+, soft, nontender, no masses.
CVA tenderness	Assessment for kidney tenderness.	Neg.
Pelvic	Important to assess for baseline information and to assess for source of bleeding.	Vulva/vagina: Normal appearance, no signs of trauma. Cervix: Cyanotic, closed, firm, small to moderate dark red blood from os. Uterus: Soft, enlarged about large egg-size, 7-week size Adnexae: WNL. Clinical pelvimetry: Deferred.
Rectal	Assess for rectal bleeding.	WNL.

● DIFFERENTIAL DIAGNOSES

What are the significant positive and negative data that support or refute your diagnoses for Kathryn?

DIAGNOSIS	POSITIVE DATA	NEGATIVE DATA
Pregnancy: threatened abortion	Child-bearing age, attempting pregnancy, missed period, + pregnancy test, + presumptive signs of pregnancy, vaginal bleeding.	No pain, minimal cramping.

(continued)

DIAGNOSIS	POSITIVE DATA	NEGATIVE DATA
Ectopic pregnancy	Child-bearing age, attempting pregnancy, missed period, + pregnancy test, + presumptive signs of pregnancy, vaginal bleeding, age 38.	No pain, adnexae WNL.
Cervical cause	None.	No obvious sign of polyp or cervical erosion. Cervix cyanotic, otherwise normal appearance.
Bleeding (other source)	Vaginal bleeding.	No obvious signs of trauma per history or exam. Rectal exam normal.

● DIAGNOSTIC TESTS

Based on the history and physical examination, what, if any, diagnostic tests would you obtain?

DIAGNOSTIC TEST	RATIONALE	RESULTS
Quantitative beta HCG	Provides a level of pregnancy hormone HCG. Repeat the test in 48 hours. Value should double in normal pregnancy. Abnormally low values of HCG may be indicative of ectopic pregnancy.	4221 mIU/L. 48 hours later 8710 mIU/L.
CBC	To detect anemia, presence of infections. Provides baseline information in routine prenatal care.	All within normal range.
RH typing/antibody titer	Determines need for RH immunoglobulins if Kathryn is RH negative. Also determines antibody level produced by RH-positive fetus.	Rh-positive. Antibody negative.

(continued)

DIAGNOSTIC TEST	RATIONALE	RESULTS
Blood type	Determines baseline data for pregnant woman to identify fetus at risk or ABO incompatibility.	Type A.
Rubella antibody titer	Determines immunity to rubella.	Immune.
Hepatitis virus screen	Identifies women with active disease or in carrier state.	Negative.
VDRL	Prenatal test required by state to identify pregnant women with untreated syphilis.	Nonreactive.
Pap smear	Screens for cervical intraepithelial neoplasia. Provides baseline data for pregnancy. Kathryn's last pap was 10 months ago.	WNL.
Genitourinary culture	Screens for asymptomatic infections: GC, chlamydia. Routine screening for pregnancy.	Negative.
U/A	Check for glucose and protein during pregnancy.	Glucose: Negative. Protein: Trace.
Urine for C&S	Identifies asymptomatic bacteriuria.	Negative.
Ultrasound	May be indicated if bleeding continues and serial quantitative HCGs are abnormal. May help to identify cause of bleeding. May identify intrauterine pregnancy to r/o ectopic. Ectopic pregnancy cannot be visualized with US (ACOG, 1990).	IUP 7.1 week. Fetal heart rate present, no evidence of bleeding.

● DIAGNOSES

What diagnoses are appropriate for Kathryn?

A. Probable intrauterine pregnancy: 7 weeks + pregnancy test, 7 week size uterus, cervical cyanosis, presumptive signs of pregnancy.

B. First trimester threatened abortion: Episode of bright vaginal bleeding followed by spotting. Slight cramping but not pain or continuous cramping. Cervix closed.

● THERAPEUTIC PLAN

1. *Calculate and identify where Kathryn is in the pregnancy.*

   A. Confirm pregnancy: Review labs and physical data with Kathryn.
   B. Calculate EDC and identify where Kathryn is in the pregnancy: Kathryn's LMP is 8-2-96. Using Naegele's rule, add 7 days to the LMP and subtract 3 months. For example:

$$
\begin{array}{l}
8 - 2 - 96 \\
\underline{+\ 7\ \text{days}} \\
8 - 9 - 96 \\
\underline{-\ 3\ \text{months}} \\
5 - 9 \\
\text{EDC} = 5\text{-}9\text{-}97
\end{array}
$$

Pregnancy is 40 weeks long from LMP and is divided into three trimesters. Kathryn is 7 weeks pregnant and in the first trimester.

2. *What would your plan of care be for a woman in her first trimester with a threatened abortion?*

   A. First trimester bleeding/threatened abortion: Obtain serial quantitative beta HCGs, 48 hours apart. Values should double in normal pregnancy. Watch for falling values, which may indicate pregnancy loss. Explain that vaginal bleeding can occur in 15–30% of all pregnancies (Pillitteri, 1995). Reassuring signs: The cervix is closed and not effaced and there is no pain or cramping. Rest for 48 hours. Observe for pain and/or increase in bleeding. Consider ultrasound if bleeding persists.

3. *What would you discuss with Kathryn in terms of nutrition during her pregnancy?*

   A. Nutrition during pregnancy: Good nutrition during pregnancy is essential for the growth of fetal and maternal tissues. Inform Kathryn of the need for good nutrition during pregnancy. Inform her that the average pregnant woman needs 1800–2200 calories per day or an increase of about 300 calories over her nonpregnant state (Kochenour, 1994; Varney, 1980).

Kathryn also needs to make sure she is getting adequate protein for fetal development. The RDA for protein is 60 gm, or an increase of 14 gm per day (Olds, London, and Ladewig, 1996).

Most of the recommended nutrients can be obtained by eating a well-balanced diet each day following the food guide pyramid. For example:

Dairy, 1 quart of milk or its equivalent every day; meat or meat alternatives, 3 servings daily; grain products, 6–11 servings daily; fruits and fruit juices, 2–4 servings daily; and vegetables and vegetable juices, 3–5 servings daily. Foodstuffs such as fat should be used in moderation; and sweets, sugars, and desserts are okay for occasional use (Olds, London, and Ladewig, 1996).

Other nutritional needs necessary for Kathryn during pregnancy include iron, folic acid, and calcium. The RDA for iron during pregnancy is 30 mg daily. 1 mg folic acid is recommended, as well as 1200 mg of calcium.

A prenatal supplement is ordered for Kathryn to take daily as a supplement to her diet. The vitamin should not be used in place of an adequate pregnancy diet. Kathryn may take vitamin with water or orange juice. If Kathryn has any nausea, encourage her to take the prenatal vitamin at bedtime.

Other dietary considerations include adequate fluid intake, which is necessary because of the increase in blood volume during pregnancy. Kathryn should drink 8–10 glasses of fluid daily. 4–6 glasses of the total should be water. Caffeinated beverages such as coffee, tea, and sodas should be used in moderation, as should Nutrasweet.

Ideal weight gain for pregnancy varies according to the prepregnant weight, but Kathryn should expect to gain 25–35 pounds during the pregnancy (Weiner, 1989).

4. *What influence would advanced maternal age have on your plan of care for Kathryn?*

  A. Advanced maternal age: Kathryn will be 38 years old by her EDC. Advise her of the risks of women delivering over age 35, such as increased chromosomal abnormalities. The risk for Kathryn would be about 4%, but inform her of the availability of testing, if desired.

Alpha fetoprotein screen is a blood test that can be drawn from Kathryn between 15–19 weeks of pregnancy. Levels of AFP are usually elevated in the presence of open neural tube defects, multiple gestations, and certain fetal abnormalities such as congenital nephrosis and cystic hygroma. Abnormally low values of APF have been associated with chromosomal disorders such as trisomy 21.

Amniocentesis is the aspiration of amniotic fluid from the amniotic sac. The fluid is collected with a needle through the abdomen and can be used to diagnose genetic disorders or abnormalities. The test is done during the second trimester.

Chorionic villus sampling (CVS) is another diagnostic technique that can be used to diagnose genetic disorders or abnormalities. The procedure involves obtaining a sample of chorionic villi from the developing placenta. CVS is done during the first trimester and the sample is obtained from a catheter inserted through the cervix or a needle inserted through the abdomen.

5. *Kathryn is c/o abdominal bloating, nausea, vomiting, and fatigue. What suggestions and recommendations would you make for her?*

A. Abdominal bloating: Explain to Kathryn that her abdominal bloating is a common discomfort in pregnancy owing to increased progesterone that causes reduced gastrointestinal motility. Kathryn should eat small frequent meals and chew foods slower and thoroughly. She should also establish regular bowel habits and avoid gas-producing foods and fatty foods. Once her bleeding has stopped, regular exercise such as walking will be helpful.

B. Nausea and vomiting of pregnancy: Explain to Kathryn that nausea and vomiting occur in 60–80% of women during pregnancy (Olds, London, and Ladewig, 1996). The causes of nausea and vomiting are unknown but may result from increased levels of HCG, alterations in carbohydrate metabolism, and decreased motility of the GI tract. Symptoms usually improve after 14 weeks.

Suggest that Kathryn eat small frequent meals without liquids. Drink liquids such as water, tea, sweet fruit juice (apple, grape, sport drinks, etc.) between meals.

Eat more bland foods such as dry toast, crackers, pretzels, and so on every 2–3 hours. Avoid fried, greasy, fatty foods. Also avoid odors and foods that seem to contribute to nausea.

Eat a protein snack at bedtime to help prevent nausea in the morning. Keep crackers and pretzels at the bedside if needed during the night or eat 2–3 in the morning before getting up.

If needed, Kathryn may try Vitamin B6 50 mg T po BID. Vitamin B6 was shown to be effective in early pregnancy (Kochenour, 1994). Phosphorated carbohydrate solution (Emetrol) may also be used. Take 1–2 tablespoons on arising and repeat every 3 hours PRN.

C. Fatigue: Explain to Kathryn that the cause of fatigue during pregnancy is probably due to metabolic changes. Fatigue is temporary during the first trimester and improves in the 2nd trimester. Take rest breaks during the day and go to bed early when possible.

6. *What anticipatory guidance and instruction would you review with Kathryn regarding her pregnancy?*

A. Anticipatory guidance and instruction: As Kathryn's prenatal care begins, make her aware of what will happen during prenatal visits and lab work that will be done in the future. Explain what additional physical changes and/or discomforts that Kathryn may experience between now and her next prenatal visit. Discuss comfort measures for the anticipated discomforts.

Instruct Kathryn to limit use of OTC medications.

Review fetal growth and development appropriate to her gestational age.

Provide community resources as needed.

7. *What are the warning signs you will review with Kathryn?*

Review warning signs:

1. Changes in vaginal bleeding
2. Facial and/or hand edema
3. Persistent vomiting for more than 24 hours
4. Fever, chills
5. Sudden, sharp, continuing abdominal pain
6. Sudden gush of fluid from vagina
7. Continuing severe headache
8. Cerebral or visual disturbance such as dizziness, spots, mental confusion
9. Changes in normal urination pattern
8. When should Kathryn return for prenatal care?

A. Follow-up: Appointments will be monthly until 28 weeks, then every 2 weeks until 36 weeks. During the last month, visits will be weekly.

REFERENCES

ACOG. American College of Obstetrics and Gynecologists, 409 12th St, Washington DC, 1989.

Kochenour NK. Normal pregnancy and prenatal care, in Scott JR, DiSaia PJ, Hammond CB, Spellacy WN (Eds). *Danforth's Obstetrics and Gynecology,* 7th ed. (pp. 67–104). Philadelphia: J.B. Lippincott; 1994.

Olds SB, London ML, Ladewig PW. *Maternal-Newborn Nursing: A Family-Centered Approach.* Menlo Park, CA: Addison-Wesley; 1996.

Pillitteri A. *Maternal and Child Health Nursing: Care of the Childbearing and Childrearing Family* (2nd ed.). Philadelphia: J.B. Lippincott; 1995.

Varney H. *Nurse-Midwifery.* Boston: Blackwell Scientific; 1980.

Weiner SM. *Clinical Manual of Maternity and Gynecologic Nursing.* St. Louis: C.V. Mosby; 1989.

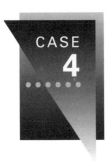

An 8-year-old boy having difficulty in school

SCENARIO

Jared Jones, an 8-year-old Caucasian male, was brought to the well child clinic for his regular checkup by his mother. Mother reports Jared has been in good health since his last checkup. He has always been a picky eater, preferring sweets and snacks over wholesome meals. During the visit Jared's mother reports that Jared is having a difficult time both in school and at home. He has had problems on the playground: He doesn't play games by the rules, often loses interest in games when he has to wait his turn, plays rough, and has frequent accidents. In the classroom he has difficulty following directions, and doesn't complete his work. He frequently gets into arguments with and interrupts his teacher and has received two detentions for this behavior this year.

At home Jared refuses to do anything his parents ask. Mother reports that he "just doesn't seem to listen." He bites his nails and is fretful. He blames his 10-year-old brother or 6-year-old sister for everything. Jared always wants to have his way and sulks when he has to compromise. His mother reports father and she both feel these behaviors have gone on long enough. They have tried to discipline Jared but always wind up feeling ineffective.

● TENTATIVE DIAGNOSES

Based on Jared's presentation, what are your tentative differential diagnoses?

● HISTORY

What additional information should be obtained from Jared and his mother to confirm or rule out the preceding diagnoses?

● PHYSICAL ASSESSMENT

What components of the physical exam should be done to assist in making the diagnosis?

● DIFFERENTIAL DIAGNOSES

What are the negative and positive data that assist in determining the appropriate diagnoses?

● DIAGNOSTIC TESTS

What diagnostic tests are appropriate to assist in your diagnoses?

● DIAGNOSIS

What is your conclusive diagnosis? What data support this decision?

● THERAPEUTIC PLAN

1. *What are issues to consider in the diagnosis of ADHD?*
2. *What medications are considered standard interventions for ADHD?*
3. *What evaluation data would indicate the medications are effective for Jared?*
4. *What counseling should be done for Jared and his family?*
5. *What interventions to increase Jared's success at school should be discussed?*
6. *What is the role of the NP in the care of children with ADHD?*
7. *What are resources that the family can use to adapt to ADHD?*
8. *Who should you refer to or consult with to provide Jared with expert care for ADHD?*

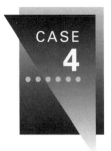

TUTORIAL

An 8-year-old boy having difficulty in school

SCENARIO

Jared Jones, an 8-year-old Caucasian male, was brought to the well child clinic for his regular checkup by his mother. Mother reports Jared has been in good health since his last checkup. He has always been a picky eater, preferring sweets and snacks over wholesome meals. During the visit Jared's mother reports that Jared is having a difficult time both in school and at home. He has had problems on the playground: He doesn't play games by the rules, often loses interest in games when he has to wait his turn, plays rough, and has frequent accidents. In the classroom he has difficulty following directions, and doesn't complete his work. He frequently gets into arguments with and interrupts his teacher and has received two detentions for this behavior this year.

At home Jared refuses to do anything his parents ask. Mother reports that he "just doesn't seem to listen." He bites his nails and is fretful. He blames his 10-year-old brother or 6-year-old sister for everything. Jared always wants to have his way and sulks when he has to compromise. His mother reports father and she both feel these behaviors have gone on long enough. They have tried to discipline Jared but always wind up feeling ineffective.

● TENTATIVE DIAGNOSES

Based on Jared's presentation, what are your tentative differential diagnoses?

DIAGNOSIS	RATIONALE
ADHD	Jared's mother reports problems at school and home: not completing his work, not following directions, not listening, interrupting teacher, not waiting his turn, losing interest in activities, and frequent accidents.

(continued)

DIAGNOSIS

RATIONALE

DIAGNOSIS	RATIONALE
Learning disability (LD)	Jared's mother reports a history of problems in school, especially not completing assignments.
Oppositional defiant disorder (ODD)	Jared's mother gives a history of refusal to do assignments, follow rules, and/or directions, or do anything his parents ask of him. Jared blames his siblings when he gets into trouble at home.
Organic/neurological problems	Jared's mother shares a history of frequent accidents. Frequent accidents may be the cause or result of a neurological disorder.
Generalized anxiety disorder	Habits such as nail biting and fretfulness could indicate an anxiety disorder.

● HISTORY

What additional information should be obtained from Jared and his mother to confirm or rule out the preceding diagnoses?

REQUESTED DATA

DATA ANSWER

REQUESTED DATA	DATA ANSWER
Allergies	None.
Medications	None.
Childhood illnesses/diseases	Chicken pox age 5. Otitis media: Several bouts from age 3 to 5, placement of PE tubes, age 4.
Immunizations	Up to date.
Hospitalizations	None.
Surgeries	Placement of PE tubes—outpatient.
Fractures/injuries/accidents	Age 2—fell, hitting head on coffee table, mild concussion, no fractures. Age 4—laceration to left temporal area, five stitches. Age 6—fell out of a tree, broken clavicle. Mother reports no history of seizures or seizure-like behaviors.
Prenatal history	39-week gestation. Normal vaginal delivery. No complications.

(continued)

REQUESTED DATA	*DATA ANSWER*
Developmental history	Met developmental milestones within normal range. Described as clumsy and demanding as far back as mother can remember.
Growth history	Has consistently been at the 25th percentile for height and weight.
Educational history	Attended preschool from age 3 to 5, had difficulty with social skills, not well accepted by peers. Performance in primary grades has been erratic, low achievement scores in 2nd-grade reading and language arts. Mother recently met with teacher for midterm report and was encouraged to pursue evaluation of Jared for learning and attention problems. A referral has not been made to the school psychologist.
Has Jared ever been in any type of special educational program? If so, for how long?	None.
Have any instructional modifications been made?	None.
Family history	Father: 11th grade education, failed 3rd grade and 6th grade, in good health, changes jobs frequently, short temper. Mother: 12th grade education, currently being treated for depression, on Fluoxetine (Prozac). H/O substance abuse in PGF and P uncle. Brother: age 10, healthy, doing well in school. Sister: age 6, healthy, doing well in school. Mother denies any family stressors at this time.
Marital relationship	Married 12 years. Many arguments about how to discipline the children. Dad loses his temper with Jared and is quick to spank. Mom is not comfortable with this and becomes angry with Dad. She prefers to remove Jared from the situation but has not found an effective way to do this.
Sibling relationships	Jared is competitive and often frustrated with his brother. He is close to his sister and they are able to play together with less conflict.
Social history and activities	Jared has one close friend at school. He does not get along with the kids his age in the neighborhood, often comes home crying. He enjoys shooting hoops, does better by himself, is most content at home playing video games by himself.

(continued)

REQUESTED DATA	DATA ANSWER
Sleeping patterns	Has difficulty settling down and going to sleep, but does sleep through the night once asleep.
Duration of symptoms	Has always had a lot of energy. Slept little as an infant. Active toddler.
Home setting	Jared lives with his biological parents in a three-bedroom home in a working class neighborhood. Jared shares a bedroom with his brother. There is a fenced yard and a basketball hoop in the driveway.
Family financial status	Dad works full-time as a carpenter's assistant. Mom works part-time at McDonalds while the children are in school. Mom denies financial problems at this time.
Insurance	Father carries health care insurance through his employer. It is a managed care plan that does provide for mental health services requiring precertification and a limited number of visits for outpatient therapy.
How do you feel about yourself?	"I don't have any friends, the kids at school make fun of me, I want to have friends but they don't want to play with me. I never get picked for the team when we play kickball or baseball."
How do you get along with your brother and sister?	"My brother always picks on me and when I get mad he yells for Dad and I get whipped. My sister lets me do things with her sometimes."
What is school like for you?	"I hate school. It's boring. My teacher never listens to me. I try real hard to do what I am told but I never seem to remember it all, or do it right. I never do anything right."
What do you really like about yourself?	"I'm real good at Nintendo."
What do you do that you are proud of?	"I shoot baskets good, but nobody wants to shoot with me; it's no fun to shoot by myself."
What makes you happy?	"I love Power Rangers."

● PHYSICAL ASSESSMENT

What components of the physical exam should be done to assist in making the diagnosis?

SYSTEM	RATIONALE	FINDINGS
General appearance	Provides overall view of Jared.	Alert, cooperative 8-year-old white male in no apparent distress. Ht: 28 3/4" (73 cm) Wt: 50 lbs. (23 K)
Vital signs	Baseline information.	B/P: 98/64 HR: 88 R: 20 T: 98.6
Skin	Well checkup—important to get overall screening exam.	No rash.
HEENT	Important to screen for neurological signs that may have an impact on his behavior.	NCAT PERRLA +RR DISC Margin well-defined and sharp, TM's thick (old scars) landmarks normal, + mobility. No nodes, neck supple, no masses.
Lungs	Baseline data for well physical.	Clear to auscultation.
Heart	Baseline data for well physical.	S1, S2 no murmur. Pulses 2+ symmetrical.
Abdomen	Well child exam.	Soft, + BS nontender/nondistended. No masses, no hepatosplenomegaly.
GU	Determine sexual growth and development.	Tanner I, circumcision WNL, testes both descended.
Neurological	Emphasis placed here to r/o a neurological/organic cause for behavior.	CN II-XII intact. Toes, no clonus, DTR 2+ symmetrical, gait symmetrical, negative Romberg, RAM's normal, equal strength, heel–toe walk, back straight.

● DIFFERENTIAL DIAGNOSES

What are the negative and positive data that assist in determining the appropriate diagnoses?

DIAGNOSIS	POSITIVE DATA	NEGATIVE DATA
ADHD	Has difficulty at home and at school, doesn't play games by the rules, has difficulty sustaining interest in games, demonstrates physical clumsiness and frequent accidents, has difficulty following directions, does not complete his work and doesn't listen, complains of being bored in school. Low self-esteem and poor social skills. School recommending further assessment for attentional difficulties and learning problems. Questionable positive family history.	Does **not** exhibit the behaviors associated with hyperactive type of ADHD, such as fidgets, often leaves seat in classroom, runs about or climbs excessively in situations in which it is inappropriate, "on the go" or behaving as if "driven by a motor," and often talks excessively. Jared does not blurt out answers before questions have been completed.
Learning disability	Family history suggestive of learning problems for father, documented problems in school with low achievement scores in reading and language arts.	Achievement in school to this point has been below expected. Jared has low scores on achievement tests but has demonstrated a skill level sufficient to be in his age-appropriate grade.
Oppositional defiant disorder	Argues with adults, actively defies or refuses to comply with adults' requests or rules, and often blames others for his mistakes or misbehavior.	Does not exhibit these behaviors associated with ODD: loses temper, deliberately annoys people, often touchy or easily annoyed by others, often angry and resentful, and often spiteful or vindictive.
Organic/neurological problem	History of repeated minor head traumas, learning difficulties, and behavioral difficulties.	Physical findings show no neurological deficits. No history of seizures.

(continued)

DIAGNOSIS	POSITIVE DATA	NEGATIVE DATA
Generalized anxiety disorder (GAD)	Difficulty falling asleep, and fretfulness and nail biting.	No evidence of excessive anxiety and worry, difficulty controlling worry; restless; easily fatigued; irritable; has difficulty concentrating; and muscle tension.

● DIAGNOSTIC TESTS

What diagnostic tests are appropriate to assist in your diagnoses?

DIAGNOSTIC TEST	RATIONALE	FINDINGS
Clinical interview to assess for DSM-IV-R criteria for ADHD, ODD, GAS, and LD.	Good choice. May be completed as part of the interview.	Meets DSM-IV criteria for ADHD, Inattention. Was noted to be very distractable during interview. Does not meet DSM-IV criteria for ODD, GAS, or LD.
Diagnostic tools: Conners Parent Questionnaire Conners Teacher Questionnaire ADHD Rating Scale	Good choices, depending on length of time you have to spend with the parent and child. These tools could be given to the parent and sent back to you for evaluation. It is helpful to have both parents complete parent questionnaires. Obtain written permission to communicate with the school personnel.	Conners Questionnaires distributed to mother and teacher.
Educational evaluation	Encourage mother to contact school and request that this be carried out there. Have permission in writing for school to send the reports to you.	Reports will be sent to provider.
MRI or CT scan of the head	Costly and time-consuming. No indication that there is a primary organic or neuro-	Not done at this time.

(continued)

DIAGNOSTIC TEST	RATIONALE	FINDINGS
	logical problem. May consider a neurological consult.	
Psychiatric evaluation	Good choice. Consultation with Child Psychiatric Clinical Nurse Specialist to assist in the evaluation of diagnostic information and development of behavior management program. Referral to child psychiatric clinical nurse specialist or child psychiatrist for evaluation of need for medication. Refer to neuropsychologist for additional evaluation based on findings reported by the school.	Consultation to assist with holistic treatment plan.

● DIAGNOSIS

What is your conclusive diagnosis? What data support this decision?

A. Findings strongly suggestive of ADHD, inattentive type.
B. Meets four of the six DSM-IV criteria for ADHD, inattentive type.
   1. Difficulty sustaining attention in tasks or play activities
   2. Often does not seem to listen when spoken to directly
   3. Often does not follow through on instructions and fails to finish schoolwork or chores
   4. Often avoids, dislikes, or is reluctant to engage in tasks that require sustained mental effort
   5. Often fails to give close details or makes careless mistakes in schoolwork or other activities
   6. Is often easily distracted by extraneous stimuli
C. Jared also demonstrates impulsive behaviors:
   1. Difficulty waiting his turn
   2. Interrupts or intrudes on others
D. Jared has associated features of children with ADHD, including:
   1. Family history
   2. Low self-esteem
   3. Poor social skills
   4. Clumsiness
   5. Demanding early temperament
   6. History of academic difficulty

It would be in the child's best interest to consult with a psychiatric clinical nurse specialist when you receive the screening forms back from the school. If the data obtained from the additional sources reinforce the diagnosis of ADHD, the child and family should be referred for appropriate treatment (Barkley, 1990; DSM-IV, 1994).

● THERAPEUTIC PLAN

1. *What are issues to consider in the diagnosis of ADHD?*

   A. Accuracy of diagnosis: Many children are quickly diagnosed with ADHD and placed on medication without a thorough evaluation. Some changes may be seen in the child's behavior, however, over a long period of time it will become evident that there are behaviors that are persistent. Many parents as well as health care providers are quite comfortable with the diagnosis of ADHD and will agree to medication as a quick fix. Many children diagnosed with ADHD actually fall within normal limits in terms of their behavior, based on their age and developmental level. Parents need education on developmental expectations and parenting skills.

   B. Coordination of diagnostic data: Look at the data from the various sources, talk with the people who have provided the data, and make sure that all data requested have been returned.

   Begin to build rapport with school personnel, as the care of this child will require participation of individuals from many disciplines.

   C. Comprehensive multidisciplinary approach will be needed to provide treatment.

   D. Parental participation will be necessary in various aspects of treatment.

   E. Clarify what services will be covered by the insurance company before making referrals.

   F. Be aware of your own limitations in evaluating the diagnostic data.

2. *What medications are considered standard interventions for ADHD?*

   The treatment for ADHD is multifaceted. The following treatment options are standard interventions. For additional information, a reliable source is Russell Barkley, *Attention-Deficit Hyperactivity Disorder: A Handbook for Diagnosis and Treatment.* The Guilford Press, New York, 1990.

   1. Methylphenidate (Ritalin) (77% positive response)
      a. dosage 5–20 mg (0.3 to 0.7 mg/kg)
      b. bid dose given early morning and midday
      c. tid dose give early morning, midday, after school
      d. example 8 AM–12 noon–4 PM
      e. maximum dose not to exceed 60 mg daily (National Inst., 1994)
   2. Ritalin SR one dose/day effect lasts 8 hrs.

3. Dextroamphetamine (Dexedrine) (74% positive response)
   a. dosage 2.5 to 10 mg bid/tid
   b. dosage intervals as for Ritalin
4. Dexedrine Spansules one dose/day
5. Adderall (efficacy unknown)
   a. dosage 5 mg qd/BID

All of the preceding drugs are schedule II drugs that require a written prescription.

6. Pemoline (Cylert) (73% positive effect)
   a. Dosage 18.75 mg to start; typical dose 0.5–3 mg/kg
   b. One dose/day

3. *What evaluation data would indicate the medications are effective for Jared?*

Jared should demonstrate an increase in his attention span and concentration as well as improved peer relations and an increase in compliance if the drug is working for him. Gradually increase dose weekly until desired effect is seen. Behavior changes and attentional changes should be noted within the first week of treatment, changes may be more obvious in the school situation. If no improvement is noted after 1 month of treatment, discontinue drug and try another. If no changes are noted even when dose is increased the child probably does not have ADHD.

4. *What counseling should be done for Jared and his family?*

Counseling is an integral part of the treatment for ADHD. These children are frustrating to those who interact with them, and the children themselves are frustrated by all the negative messages they receive regarding their behavior.

Suggested counseling would include:

Parent counseling and education about ADHD
Parent training in the area of behavior management
Parent counseling and training on environmental modifications or structuring
Parent education on medications and the role they play in treatment
Individual counseling with the child
Family therapy for the whole family
Couples/marital therapy for the parents

5. *What interventions to increase Jared's success at school should be discussed?*

Children with ADHD have difficulty in the area of academic performance and achievement. They demonstrate inattention, impulsive, and restless behavior in the classroom. They have difficulty staying seated, paying attention, working independently, and following directions and rules. The child with ADHD can be disruptive and interrupt class lessons as well as quiet work periods. They also lack organizational skills and have difficulty keeping track of their academic tools (books, pencils, and paper) and assignments.

The initial intervention with the school is to educate the teacher about the disorder. Once the teacher has working knowledge of the disorder, behavior management programs can be established. The behavior management program at school is an integral part of the overall behavior management program. Weekly or biweekly meetings between the parents, teachers, therapist are helpful in evaluating and monitoring the behavioral management program.

Needed areas of teacher education:

Teacher counseling and education about ADHD
Teacher training in classroom management
Teacher training in environmental modifications

6. *What is the role of the NP in the care of children with ADHD?*

The role of the NP will be to coordinate services and implement a comprehensive multidisciplinary treatment program. It is important to collaborate with the school and become knowledgeable of the services that can be provided in the school in the areas of special education and behavior management environmental modifications. NP caring for children will be able to provide a higher level of care if there are established relationships with professional peers to enhance the consultation process.

7. *What are resources that the family can use to adapt to ADHD?*

Attention Deficit Information Network (AD-IN)
475 Hillside Ave.
Needham, MA 02194

Provides up-to-date information on current research, and regional meetings. Offers aid in finding solutions to practical problems faced by adults and children with an attention disorder.

ADD Warehouse
300 NW 70th Ave.
Plantation, FL 33317
800 233-9273
Distributes books, tapes, and videos on ADHD

CHADD
National Headquarters
Suite 185
1859 North Pine Island Road
Plantation, FL 33322
305 384-6869
Parent Support Association

ADDA
4300 West Park Blvd.
Plano, TX 75093
Parent Support Association

Challenge
A Newsletter on ADHD
PO Box 2001
West Newbury, MA 01985
508 462-0495

8. *Who should you refer to or consult with to provide Jared with expert care for ADHD?*

It is advisable to consult with or refer to a child psychiatric clinical nurse specialist or a child psychiatrist.

REFERENCES

Barkley R. *Attention Deficit Hyperactivity Disorder: A Handbook for Diagnosis and Treatment.* New York: Guilford Press; 1990.

American Psychiatric Association. *Diagnostic and Statistical Manual of Mental Disorders,* 4th ed. Washington, DC: American Psychiatric Association; 1994.

National Institute of Mental Health. *Attention Deficit Hyperactivity Disorder: Care and Treatment.* National Institute of Mental Health; 1994.

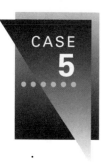

A 55-year-old man with cough, fever, and SOB

SCENARIO

John Kosich is a 55-year-old Caucasian male who presents with complaints of cough, fatigue, fever of 100°F, and increased shortness of breath with activity × 5 days. Cough is productive with large amount of thick tan sputum occurring day and night, worse at night when supine. Needs two pillows to sleep at night. Dyspnea with one flight of steps and intercourse. Has tried OTC Robitussin and Primatene Mist Inhaler with minimal relief. John states he has been smoking 1 ppd for 40 years.

● TENTATIVE DIAGNOSES

Based on John's presentation, what are your tentative differential diagnoses?

● HISTORY

1. *What questions do you want to ask John to assist you in developing a diagnosis?*
2. *What are the key points to cover on the review of systems?*

● PHYSICAL ASSESSMENT

What are the significant portions of the physical examination that should be completed for John?

● DIFFERENTIAL DIAGNOSES

What are the significant positive and negative data that support or refute your diagnoses for John?

● DIAGNOSTIC TESTS

Based on the history and physical assessment, what, if any, diagnostic tests would you do? Include your rationale for the tests.

● DIAGNOSIS

What diagnoses are appropriate for John?

● THERAPEUTIC PLAN

1. *What are the common bacterial etiologies causing an acute exacerbation of bronchitis?*
2. *What are the possible pharmacological treatments to choose from for John?*
3. *What alternative treatments might be appropriate during the acute exacerbation?*
4. *What long-term treatment might be appropriate for the underlying COPD?*
5. *What are issues of treatment that should be considered for John?*
6. *When should John return for follow up?*
7. *Based on information given about John, what impact do you think his illness might have on his family?*
8. *What would be appropriate interventions for John's family?*
9. *Where can a nurse practitioner obtain more information concerning bronchitis and COPD?*
10. *What other health care professionals might be involved in a therapeutic plan for John and his family?*
11. *John has improved from the acute exacerbation of bronchitis, but continues to smoke 1 pack per day and complains of fatigue and dyspnea on exertion. What adjustments would you make in the therapeutic plan based on this information?*

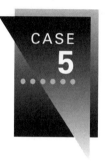

TUTORIAL

A 55-year-old man with cough, fever, and SOB

SCENARIO

John Kosich is a 55-year-old Caucasian male who presents with complaints of cough, fatigue, fever of 100°F, and increased shortness of breath with activity × 5 days. Cough is productive with large amount of thick tan sputum, worse at night when supine, occurring day and night. Needs two pillows to sleep at night. Dyspnea with one flight of steps and intercourse. Has tried OTC Robitussin and Primatene Mist Inhaler with minimal relief. John states he has been smoking 1 pack per day for 40 years.

● TENTATIVE DIAGNOSES

Based on John's presentation, what are your tentative differential diagnoses?

DIAGNOSIS	RATIONALE
Pneumonia	John is presenting with productive cough, colored sputum, DOE, SOB, fever, and fatigue. These are all symptoms of pneumonia.
Acute bronchitis	John c/o productive cough, colored sputum, fever, and fatigue.
COPD	John c/o cough, fatigue, and SOB. He has a 40-pack-year history of tobacco use.
Asthma	John c/o cough, worse when supine or on exertion. He has a + tobacco history.
Lung cancer	John c/o cough, SOB, and fatigue. He also has + smoking history.

(continued)

DIAGNOSIS	RATIONALE
TB	Complaints of cough, SOB, fatigue, and fever are all symptoms of TB.
Anemia	Fatigue, SOB.
CHF	John's symptoms of SOB, cough, orthopnea, fatigue, DOE, and history of tobacco use could put him at risk for CHF.

● HISTORY

What questions do you want to ask John to assist you in developing a diagnosis?

REQUESTED DATA	DATA ANSWER
Allergies	No known medical, food, or environmental allergies.
Current medications	Lisinopril (Zesteril) 10 mg QD Robitussin Primatene Mist × 5 d.
Surgery	Inguinal hernia repair (1985).
Past medical history and hospitalizations/fractures/injuries/accidents	Hx of HTN, tibia/fibula fx age 9.
Last complete PE	Not sure when it was.
Appetite	Normally good. Has gained weight in past year, but has not been hungry lately.
24-Hour diet recall	B: None. L: Soup/crackers for lunch. S: 2 Big Macs, large fries, milkshake for supper.
Sleeping	Difficulty sleeping lately owing to SOB/coughing.
Social history	Tobacco: 40-year-pack history. Alcohol: Denies.
Family history	Father: Died 69, HTN, lung CA, smoker. Mother: Living, age 76, CVA, NIDDM, obese. Daughter: 21 y/o, alive and well. Son: 25 y/o, alive and well.

(continued)

DIAGNOSIS	RATIONALE
Relationship with family	Family relationships: Married 30 years. Stable relationship with wife. Claims to have a good relationship with daughter who's in college; fair relationship with son who works at local factory. His mother lives locally. He visits her 2×/wk; considers this a burden on his time.
Income/insurance coverage	Earns $35,000/yr as an assembly line worker in a car factory. Has a good insurance coverage through union package.

What are the key points on the review of systems?

SYSTEM REVIEWED	DATA ANSWER
HEENT	Unremarkable.
Respiratory	c/o a morning cough productive of thick, whitish sputum × 18 months. Also admits to slowly worsening dyspnea and fatigue over past year. Denies night sweats or hemoptysis. Has 2-pillow orthopnea, and PND at night.
Cardiac	Unremarkable. Denies any edema.
GI	Denies constipation; diarrhea; black, tarry, or bloody stools.
GU	Denies dysuria, polyuria, retention.
Musculoskeletal	Occasional low back pain with heavy lifting.
Neurological	Denies syncope or weakness.

● PHYSICAL ASSESSMENT

What are the significant portions of the physical examination that should be completed for John?

SYSTEM	FINDINGS
Vital signs	B/P: 138/86 P: 90 R: 24 shallow

(continued)

SYSTEM	FINDINGS
	T: 99.8 Ht: 5'10" Wt: 250 lbs.
General appearance/skin color character	Skin warm, dry, intact without lesions. Ruddy facial complexion. Early fingernail clubbing. Capillary refill < 2 sec.
HEENT	TMs slightly opaque with light reflex and landmarks present. No nasal erythema or exudate, septum midline. Nontender frontal and maxillary sinuses. Pharynx mildly erythematous with no purulent exudate. Negative lymphadenopathy. Neck supple, thyroid symmetrical w/out enlargement, no carotid bruits, no JVD.
Lungs	AP: Lateral diameter > 1:2. Moderate use of accessory muscles. Bilat. tympany on percussion, decreased tactile fremitus. Diffuse coarse crackles and few scattered end expiratory wheezes throughout bilat. lung fields. Diminished breath sounds bilat. Negative lymphadenopathy.
Heart	S_1S_2 WNL, no murmur, gallop, or rubs.
Abdomen	Abdomen obese, BS +, negative bruits. No tenderness. No HSM or HJR.
Neurological	Alert and oriented.
Extremities	Increased pigmentation bilateral LE with mild varicosities and thickened toenails. PT pulses 1+, DP pulses 2+ bilaterally. No edema.

● DIFFERENTIAL DIAGNOSES

What are the significant positive and negative findings that support or refute your diagnoses for John?

DIAGNOSIS	POSITIVE DATA	NEGATIVE DATA
Pneumonia	Productive cough × 3 wks, SOB, fatigue, crackles, wheezes.	No bronchophony, egophony, whispered pectoriloquy, localized adventitious breath sounds, tactile fremitus, and percussion symmetrical bilat.

(continued)

DIAGNOSIS	POSITIVE DATA	NEGATIVE DATA
Acute bronchitis	Positive tobacco hx, increased productive cough, SOB, fever, fatigue, paroxysmal nocturnal dyspnea, two-pillow orthopnea; use of accessory muscles, diffuse coarse crackles and wheezes in bilateral lung fields.	18 month hx of fatigue, dyspnea & AM cough, increased AP: transverse diameter.
COPD	40-pack-year hx of tobacco use. Morning sputum production, ruddy complexion, clubbing of fingernails, moderate use of accessory muscles, increased AP: lateral diameter, wheezes, coarse crackles (Fromm & Varon, 1994).	Acute exacerbation of s/s, fever.
Asthma	Smoking hx, DOE, cough, fatigue; wheezing and use of accessory muscles.	Lack of childhood hx, Primatene Mist minimally effective; fever, amt/color of sputum production.
Lung cancer	Family hx, tobacco hx, 18 month hx of fatigue, SOB, cough; diffuse crackles and wheezes.	No weight loss, hemoptysis.
TB	SOB, cough, fatigue, tobacco; diffuse crackles, wheezes.	No weight loss, night sweats, hemoptysis.
Anemia	Fatigue, SOB.	No black or tarry stools, no paresthesia.
CHF	Paroxysmal nocturnal dyspnea.	No JVD, no hepatojugular reflux, no S_3; no fine crackles in bases, tan sputum, no peripheral edema.

● DIAGNOSTIC TESTS

Based on the history and physical examination, what, if any, diagnostic tests would you obtain?

DIAGNOSTIC TEST	RATIONALE	RESULTS
CXR	Good choice. This will help r/o pneumonia, TB, CA, CHF. It's also inexpensive, quick, and noninvasive.	No acute disease. CXR representative of chronic obstructive pulmonary disease.
Oxygen saturation	Good choice. Will help identify hypoxemia, and degree of compromise. Quick, inexpensive, and noninvasive.	92%.
PPD	Will r/o TB. Inexpensive and quick.	Negative.
Gram stain	Allows for more accurate treatment because it identifies causative organisms. It is often difficult to obtain adequate specimen and takes several days to get results.	NL flora.
EKG	Would do if suspicious of cardiac etiology or involvement. Relatively inexpensive, can be done in most offices.	NSR.
CBC with diff	Would not do on initial visit as fever is low grade, and patient is not in marked distress. However, might do on follow up if John has not improved. Would help differentiate viral, bacterial infection, as well as polycythemia.	Not done at this time.
ABGs	Will identify acidosis, chronic CO_2 retention, acid-base imbalance. Provides a more	Not done this visit.

(continued)

DIAGNOSTIC TEST	RATIONALE	RESULTS
	accurate assessment of oxygen level. Invasive, expensive, needs to be done in hospital lab.	
Pulmonary function tests	Good choice after acute exacerbation. Will differentiate restrictive versus obstructive disease, and identify severity of illness.	Not done at current time.
Electrolytes, LFT, renal, cholesterol	Provides baseline information about current status.	WNL.
H/H	Provides information about hemoglobin/hematocrit. Would help rule out anemia.	Hgb: 14.3.

● DIAGNOSES

What diagnoses do you determine as being appropriate after a review of the subjective and objective data (COPD with acute exacerbation)?

Data Supporting the Diagnosis of COPD with Acute Exacerbation

COPD consists of the following two entities:

1. *Emphysema:* A pathologic diagnosis based on a permanent abnormal dilation and destruction of the alveolar ducts and air spaces distal to the terminal bronchioles.

2. *Chronic bronchitis:* A clinical diagnosis based on the presence of a cough and sputum production occurring on most days for at least a 3-month period during two consecutive years. John probably has chronic bronchitis with an acute exacerbation. Very commonly, there are components of both emphysema and chronic bronchitis. In John's case the predominant symptoms seem to be of chronic bronchitis (Johannsen, 1994).

3. *Acute exacerbation:* Increased cough is the hallmark symptom. Client may also complain of fever, increased sputum production, increased SOB, and fatigue (Fromm & Varon, 1994).

● THERAPEUTIC PLAN

1. What are the common bacterial etiologies causing an acute exacerbation of bronchitis?

Most common etiologies of acute exacerbation of bronchitis:

- *Streptococcus pneumoniae*
- *Haemophilus influenza*
- *Moraxella catarrhalis*
- Viral (Fromm & Varon, 1994)

2. What are the possible pharmacological treatments to choose from for John?

Acute exacerbation of COPD:

A. Antibiotics:
1. Septra or doxycycline PO 100 mg BID
2. Amoxicillin—clavulanate (Augmentin) 250 mg PO TID × 10 days
3. Cefixime (Suprax) 400 mg PO QD × 10 days
4. Clarithromycin (Biaxin) 500 mg PO BID × 10 days
5. Azithromycin (Zithromax) 250 mg ii PO × 1 day, ii PO × 4 days
6. Ofloxacin (Floxin) 400 mg PO BID
B. Ipratropium (Atrovent) inhaler ii puffs QID
C. Albuterol (Proventil) inhaler ii puffs QID prn (provides immediate bronchodilation) (Fromm & Varon, 1994)

3. What alternative treatments might be appropriate during the acute exacerbation?

- Subcutaneous epinephrine 0.3 cc prn
- Prednisone with tapering dose if marked limitation of air movement; 40–80 mg daily in divided doses
- Mucokinetic agent for particularly thick secretions
- Expectorants
- Oxygen therapy with oxygen saturation <85% or PaO_2 <55

4. What long-term treatment might be appropriate for the underlying COPD?

- avoidance of irritants (discontinue smoking)
- pursed lip breathing/pulmonary rehab
- pneumonia vaccination
- annual influenza vaccination
- avoidance of respiratory infections
- nutrition: maintain adequate intake of calories and protein
- develop appropriate exercise program
- possible O_2 at home if O_2 saturation is < 85% (Jacobs, 1994; Uphold, 1994)

5. *What are issues of treatment that should be considered for John?*
   - Cost of medications: Septra and doxycycline are the two least expensive antibiotics.
   - Instruction in the proper use of inhaler.
   - Adherence: Return demonstration of proper use of inhaler important. Explain to patient that he will notice results from Ipratropium inhaler use in 2–4 weeks. This treatment modality will help improve and maintain adequate long -term oxygenation levels.

6. *When should John return for follow up?*

   Follow up within 24–48 hours by phone; follow-up visits weekly until acute exacerbation stabilized and then every 3–6 months.

7. *Based on information given about John, what impact do you think his illness might have on his family?*
   - Altered roles and responsibilities
   - Financial concerns
   - Emotional issues.

8. *What would be appropriate interventions for John's family?*

   Family counseling regarding the disease process, treatment modalities, and lifestyle alterations.

9. *Where can a nurse practitioner obtain more information concerning bronchitis and COPD?*

   American Lung Association, local smoking cessation classes, community hospital, pulmonary rehabilitation department.

10. *What other health care professionals might be involved in a therapeutic plan for John and his family?*

    Pulmonologist/physician for consultation and referral, oxygen supply company, counselor: individual or family as needed.

11. *John has improved from the acute exacerbation of bronchitis, but continues to smoke 1 ppd and complains of fatigue and dyspnea on exertion. What adjustments would you make in the therapeutic plan based on this information?*
    - Obtain ABGs
    - Continue to reinforce smoking cessation
    - Pulmonary function tests
    - Review pursed lip breathing
    - Increase Atrovent to iii puffs q4h
    - May consider steroid or theophylline inhaler (Jacobs, 1994)

REFERENCES

Fromm R, Varon J. Acute exacerbations of obstructive lung disease. *Postgrad Med 95* 1994;(8):101–106.

Jacobs M. Maintenance therapy for obstructive lung disease. *Postgrad Med 95* 1994;(8):87–96.

Johannsen JM. Chronic obstructive lung disease: Current comprehensive care for emphysema and bronchitis. *Nurse Pract 19* 1994;(1):59–67.

Uphold CR, Graham MV. *Clinical Guidelines in Family Practice.* Gainesville, FL: Barmarrae; 1994.

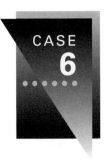

A 48-year-old woman with fatigue and headaches

SCENARIO

Florence McGee is a 48-year-old obese African-American female with complaints of fatigue, headaches, decreased libido, and irregular menses. She has also noticed increased skin dryness and sleep disturbances. Occasionally she notices that she shakes in the morning. Florence states that 3 months ago she lost her job as a paralegal. Her heachaches have worsened since she lost her job. She has been taking propranolol for the headaches, prescribed by a physician she saw 6 months ago. Florence says that her previous physical was over 2 years ago. She states she has gained about 15 pounds in the past 3 months.

● TENTATIVE DIAGNOSES

Based on Florence's presentation, what are your tentative differential diagnoses?

● HISTORY

What questions do you want to ask Florence to assist you in developing a diagnosis?

● PHYSICAL ASSESSMENT

Based on the subjective data you have obtained, what parts of the physical examination should be performed and why?

● DIFFERENTIAL DIAGNOSES

Examine all the data up to this point. Link the subjective and objective data to the appropriate differential diagnoses. What positive and negative data support or refute the diagnoses?

● DIAGNOSTIC TESTS

What additional data and/or diagnostic tests need to be performed to confirm the diagnosis?

● DIAGNOSIS

What is your conclusive diagnosis? What positives and negatives assisted you in your decision?

● THERAPEUTIC PLAN

1. *What are the issues to consider for Florence when deciding on treatment?*
2. *What are the possible treatments from which to choose?*
3. *What is the efficacy of each treatment?*
4. *What are alternative treatments that might be appropriate for Florence?*
5. *How often and when would you see Florence again?*
6. *Florence has shown little improvement after 6 weeks of treatment. What adjustments would you make in the therapeutic plan?*
7. *Based on the information given about Florence, what impact do you think this situation has had on Florence's family?*
8. *What would be appropriate interventions for Florence's family?*
9. *Where can a nurse practitioner obtain more information concerning depression and/or additional resources for assisting depressed clients?*
10. *What community resources can the nurse practitioner refer the depressed client and/or family to?*
11. *What other health care professionals should be involved in a plan of care for Florence? When should Florence be referred for more intensive therapy?*

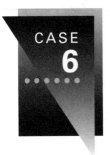

TUTORIAL

A 48-year-old woman with fatigue and headaches

SCENARIO

Florence McGee is a 48-year-old obese African-American female with complaints of fatigue, headaches, decreased libido, and irregular menses. She has also noticed increased skin dryness and sleep disturbances. Occasionally she notices that she shakes in the morning. Florence states that 3 months ago she lost her job as a paralegal. Her headaches have worsened since she lost her job. She has been taking propranolol for the heachaches, prescribed by a physician she saw 6 months ago. Florence says that her previous physical was over 2 years ago. She states she has gained about 15 pounds in the past 3 months.

● TENTATIVE DIAGNOSES

Based on Florence's presentation, what are your tentative differential diagnoses?

DIFFERENTIAL DIAGNOSES	RATIONALE
Brain tumor/primary neurological problem	Florence is presenting with headaches/decreased libido and irregular menses. These could be caused by a neurological problem.
Depression	Florence is presenting with fatigue, headaches, decreased libido, sleep disturbances, weight gain, and loss of job. These are all symptoms of depression.
Menopause	Florence is c/o irregular menses and decreased libido. Irregular menses may be the first symptom seen in perimenopause.

(continued)

DIFFERENTIAL DIAGNOSES   RATIONALE

DIFFERENTIAL DIAGNOSES	RATIONALE
Hypothyroidism	Florence is c/o fatigue and skin dryness, common symptoms for hypothyroidism.
Substance abuse	Florence is c/o shakiness in the morning, a sign seen when the body is lacking the abused substance, for example ETOH.
Anemia	Florence is c/o fatigue and skin dryness—possible indicators of anemia.
Decreased blood sugar	The symptoms of shakiness and fatigue could also lead one to suspect low blood sugar.

Note how many of the presenting symptoms overlap and could lead the NP to suspect many different problems.

● HISTORY

What questions do you want to ask Florence to assist you in developing a diagnosis?

REQUESTED DATA   DATA ANSWER

REQUESTED DATA	DATA ANSWER
Allergies	None.
Medications	Propranolol 20 mg po BID. Tylenol prn for H/A. Occasional laxative/antacid. No vitamins.
Childhood diseases	Asthma. Chickenpox.
Immunizations	Unsure about anything except tetanus/TB skin test: Done 5 years ago.
Surgery	Tubal ligation 12 years ago: 1983.
Transfusions	None.
Hospitalizations	Vaginal childbirth × 2: 1978, 1982.
Fractures/injuries, accidents	Fx radius at 7 y/o—no problems now. Fx ribs × 2—1986 slipped on ice.

(continued)

REQUESTED DATA	*DATA ANSWER*
Adult illness	Pneumonia, 1992. Costochondritis, 1990.
OBG history	LMP: 7-2-95, periods farther apart. Last pelvic: 2 years ago—WNL. Mammo: 2 years ago—WNL. SBE: Not regularly. G2P2A0.
Last complete PE	In 1982 when pregnant.
Weight changes	Has gained 10–15 pounds in the past month.
Appetite	Increased owing to "nerves," craves chocolate, eats what she wants, no special diet.
24-Hour diet recall	B: 2 glazed doughnuts, 2 cups coffee. L: Peanut butter crackers, apple, soda. D: Spaghetti, salad with no-fat ranch dressing, 2 pieces garlic bread, soda.
Sleeping pattern	Problems going to sleep and staying asleep—sleeps about 4 hours per night, naps occasionally during the day.
Family history	Father: Died 8 years ago at age of 59 of liver failure (admits father was alcoholic and sexually abusive to her). Mother: Living, age 76, mild HTN, nervous breakdown years ago. Two living brothers: 45, good health; 57 HTN. One living sister: 43, good health. Two children: 16, daughter, good health; 13, male, good health.
Social habits	Smokes $\frac{1}{2}$ pack/day × 25 years, occasional social drinker, drinks approx. 5 cups of coffee/day + 3 sodas/day. Denies recreational drugs, and does not exercise.
Social organizations	Church women's group, Jaycees; has not been to meeting in 3 months since losing her job.
Relationship with husband	Feels she and her husband do not talk much anymore. Thinks he is aggravated with her because she is not working. Having intercourse 1× every other week—little affection exchanged between them.
Relationship with children	Typical teenagers "who know it all," and "want to do it their way." Has a good relationship with them. They seem concerned about her.
Relationship with mother and siblings	Lives in different town than mother and sibs. Talks to mother 1× per week, sister 1× every 2 weeks, brothers 1× every 3–4 weeks. Mother and brothers live in Chicago. Sister lives in Durham, NC.

(continued)

REQUESTED DATA	DATA ANSWER
Income	Husband works as 1st shift supervisor at Lexington computer services. She is drawing unemployment. Things are tight now.
Insurance	Has medical and dental through husband's work.
Home	Own their own home—live about $3\frac{1}{2}$ miles from health center.
Length of symptoms	Last few months has been sad—really bad in last 6 weeks.
How has this affected your daily activities?	Seems hard to do anything, not as interested in things as I used to be, tired all the time, would rather just sleep. Sometimes I don't even get dressed. I'm also very shakey in the mornings until I really get started.
Losses in your life?	Job is probably a loss, wasn't really sad when Dad died, have lived away from my family for 15 years. Feel a loss in decrease in communication with husband; my children go their own way and do not need me as much as they used to.
How do you manage stress?	Watch TV, get off by myself, go to room, outside on deck or just driving, have tried praying.
Tell me about your heachaches.	I had them almost every day. I would get nauseated but did not vomit. They just pulled me down. The doctor put me on this medicine and it really seemed to decrease how many H/A I get now.
What do you do for your headaches?	Take propranolol every day. Tylenol or ibuprofen as needed. Sometimes have to lie down in quiet room; sometimes in the morning coffee or soda helps.
Do you ever think of hurting yourself?	No.
On a scale from 1 to 10, with 1 being terrible, and 10 being great, how do you feel?	3.
Have you ever felt this way before?	I've felt sad, but not for this long and this bad.
Are there situations and instances that make you feel worse?	I feel worse when I think about work or the loss of the closeness to my husband and my weight.
Do you feel bad all the time?	Pretty much. I have a few less sad times, but when I'm sad, I'm sad. I cry some, too.
Can you think of anything that would make you feel better?	Not really, not now. Maybe getting a job, getting back to normal, but I don't feel I have enough energy to work.

● PHYSICAL ASSESSMENT

Based on the subjective data you have obtained, what parts of the physical examination should be performed and why?

SYSTEM	RATIONALE	FINDINGS
Skin color and character	Provides overall indication of health. Also dry skin is an indicator of hypothyroidism. Pale skin is an indicator of anemia. Spider angiomas may indicate alcohol abuse, as do unexplained cuts and bruises.	Pale, but the mucous membranes and nailbeds are pink. No jaundice, bruises, spider angiomas. Skin dry.
Heart/peripheral pulses	Provides a baseline assessment of cardiovascular status.	S_1 and S_2 without murmur. No venous hum over neck. No carotid bruits. Pulses 2+, no edema.
Lungs	Provides a baseline assessment of respiratory status.	Clear to auscultation.
Vital signs	Provides a baseline assessment.	HR 72, R 20, B/P 116/86, Temp 99°F.
Cranial nerves	Needed to rule out neurological dysfunction.	II–XI intact.
Fundoscopic	Can indicate increased intercranial pressure and diabetic retinopathy.	No AV nicking. Disc with clear margins. No disc to cup ratio. No hemorrhages, cotton wool spots noted.
Mental status	Important system given her complaints of fatigue, and so on. Helps to rule out substance abuse, mental illness.	Mini Mental Status exam performed: Score of 30.
Motor function/muscle strength	Needed to rule out neurological dysfunction.	Gait normal, negative Romberg, extremities equal in strength, no tremors noted.
Sensation	Needed to rule out neurological dysfunction.	Pain discrimination intact in all extremities.

(continued)

SYSTEM	*RATIONALE*	*FINDINGS*
Reflexes	Needed to rule out neurological dysfunction, and identify baseline.	Biceps, triceps, brachioradialis, patellar, and ankle 2+ bilaterally.
Visual acuity	Only needed if complete physical exam is done, although may be gross screening for diabetic vision loss.	OD 20/30, OS 20/20 corrected with glasses.
Confrontation	Gross test for peripheral vision. May indicate neurological dysfunction.	Visual fields intact.
Abdominal	Provides information regarding abdominal function. If concerned about possible substance abuse, may indicate liver enlargement or tender abdomen owing to gastritis.	BS present all four quadrants. Abdomen obese and nontender. No HSM.
Breasts	Only would be done if time permits, and if you are concerned she may not return for annual breast/pelvic exam.	No masses or dimpling noted.
ENT	Looking for indications of substance abuse: nasal lesions; parotid gland enlargement; indications of anemia: pale mucous membranes.	Normocephalic, no sinus enderness, PERRLA, no pharyngeal erythema or oral lesions noted. Nasal septum midline. TMs gray with light reflex present.
Gynecologic	Would not usually be done— only consider if time permits, or you are concerned she may not return for annual exam.	Deferred.

● DIFFERENTIAL DIAGNOSES

Examine all the data up to this point. Link the subjective and objective data to the appropriate differential diagnoses. What positive and negative data support/refute the diagnoses?

DIAGNOSIS	POSITIVE DATA	NEGATIVE DATA
Hypothryoidism	Fatigue, weight gain, almost age 50.	No edema, bradycardia, decreased BS, decreased appetite, hyperflexia, hypotension, slurred speech, or hoarseness.
Diabetes	Shakes, fatigue.	No weight loss, visual changes, numbness, tingling of hands/feet; no history of fungal infections, nocturia, polyuria, or thirst.
Brain tumor	Change in personality/activities, headaches, and shakes.	No edema, papilledema, vomiting, change in gait, sensorium, reflexes, cranial nerves.
Substance abuse	Shakes, recent loss, decreased libido, dry skin, sleep abnormality, and fatigue.	No track marks, nasal lesions, GI complaints, vomiting, hepatomegaly, jaundice, palpitations.
Anemia	Shakes, fatigue, irregular menses, and pallor.	No family history, no bruising, hematuria, melena, splenomegaly, hepatomegaly, bone tenderness, murmur, pale mucous membranes.
Depression	Depressed mood, loss of interest or pleasure, weight gain, sleep disturbance, fatigue, feelings of worthlessness and sadness, irregular menses, decreased activity with organizations, and parenting of teenagers. Loss of job and mother's history of "mild" nervous breakdown.	No history of previous depression, suicide attempts, impaired concentration, psychomotor retardation.

● DIAGNOSTIC TESTS

What additional data and/or diagnostic tests need to be performed to confirm the diagnosis?

DIAGNOSTIC TEST	RATIONALE	RESULTS
Self-report depression scales: General Health Questionnaire, Zung Self-Rating Depression Scale, Beck Depression Inventory, Center for Epidemiological Studies Depression Scale	Good choice to help identify depression. Can complete in waiting area. Watch for false positive, where score indicates depression, but patient is not depressed. Do not include questionnaires in chart. Validity of test depends on people not having access to test prior to taking.	Florence scored 55 on the self-rating depression scale. This is equal to 69 on the Jung SDS.
Clinician completed depression scales: Hamilton Rating Scale for Depression.	Good choice. Depends on the amount of time you have to spend with this patient and your familiarity with the tools.	Not completed because self-report rating scale completed.
Clinical interview to assess for DSM IV-R criteria	Good choice. Can be completed as part of the interview or review of systems.	Interview revealed Florence to be depressed—meeting DSM criteria.
MRI or CT scan of the head	Very costly and time-consuming to get. Would only help if brain tumor was your primary diagnosis. Even in this case, a neurological consult may be warranted first, based on paucity of symptoms.	Not done.
Thyroid-stimulating hormone, T_4	Will help discriminate pituitary and thyroid disorders in combination with T_4. If TSH and T_4 both are low, an anterior pituitary disorder is suspected. If TSH is high or normal, and T_4 is low, a thyroid disorder is suspected. Requires a couple of days to get results.	TSH 2.2. T_4 8.

(continued)

DIAGNOSTIC TEST	*RATIONALE*	*RESULTS*
Sleep EEG	May help to r/o brain tumor or sleep disorder. Expensive and takes 1–2 hours to perform. Not warranted in this situation.	Not done.
Hemoglobin and hematocrit, CBC	It has been at least 2 years since Florence had this test. Because she is complaining of fatigue and irregular menses you could perform a fingerstick H&H. If abnormal send for outpatient CBC. Need to think in terms of what do you get from the CBC that you do not get from H&H.	HGB 14.8.
Blood glucose, electrolytes	Could do a fingerstick glucose because she is complaining of shakes in the morning and fatigue. Diabetes runs in her family. Weight gain and stress may precipitate diabetes. If BS high, arrange to have a glycosolated hemoglobin level drawn. Liver functions tests may provide data supporting substance abuse.	BS: 78. Na: 137. K: 3.8. Cl: 101. CO_2: 23. BUN: 11. Creat: 0.8. ALT: 20 U/L. AST: 10 U/L. Alk. Phos: 41. Bili: 1.0 mg/dL
Mammogram/pap smear	Florence is due for one. However, if you are busy today, you may have to arrange for these and a complete physical at another date. If Florence feels she lives too far away from the facility, you may wish to complete all health maintenance activities at this time. An issue of concern: Will Florence return for health maintenance activities since it has been > 2 years since her last full exam?	Not done. Appt. made for 2 weeks.

(continued)

DIAGNOSTIC TEST	RATIONALE	RESULTS
CAGE, SMASK	Screening questionnaires for alcohol dependence. Good choice. Can be integrated into interview.	Denies feeling angry because people criticize her drinking, has not ever felt guilty about drinking or has felt the need to cut down on drinking. Denies drinking first thing in morning as an eye opener to steady nerves.
U/A, drug screen	U/A may be appropriate if done as part of a routine yearly exam. If not, consider what data it will contribute to diagnosis. Drug screen probably not indicated because it was not supported by data in history.	Not done.

● DIAGNOSES

What is your conclusive diagnosis? What positives and negatives assisted you in your decision?

Depression, Nonsuicidal

Rationale: According to DSM IV criteria, five of following are present at same time:

One of the following two must be present:
- Depressed mood most of day or every day
- Markedly diminished interest or pleasure in almost all activities

Plus:
- Significant weight gain or loss
- Insomnia/hypersomnia
- Psychomotor agitation/retardation
- Fatigue
- Feelings of worthlessness
- Impaired concentration
- Recurrent thoughts of death or suicide

Six of preceding criteria are applicable for Florence, thus meeting DSM-IV criteria for depression (Depression Guideline Panel, vol. 1, 1993).

● THERAPEUTIC PLAN

1. *What are the issues to consider for Florence when deciding on treatment?*

   Some issues to consider when deciding
   on the treatment are:

   • Need to educate about illness, prognosis, and treatment plan
   • Ultimate selection of first treatment: collaborative process between patient and caregiver
   • Visits frequent enough to optimize adherence
   • Outcomes carefully assessed by interviews and self-rating scales

2. *What are the possible treatments from which to choose?*

   Effectiveness depends on cooperative effort to empower the patient, which helps increase compliance/adherence, and helps patient learn health maintenance strategies and gain coping skills. Choices for treatments include medications, psychotherapy, combined medications and psychotherapy, and electroconvulsive therapy (ECT).

3. *What is the efficacy of each treatment?*

   A. Medication
      1. Consider:
         a. side effect profiles
         b. history of prior response
         c. family history of response
         d. type of depression
         e. concurrent general medical or psychological illness
         f. other medications
         g. cost
         h. length of treatment: short versus long term
      2. Consider when:
         a. moderate to severe depression
         b. psychotic, melancholic or atypical
         c. patient requests
         d. psychotherapy not available
         e. prior positive response to medication
         f. maintenance is planned
      3. First and second line choices:
         a. Secondary amine tricyclics
            Nortriptyline (Pamelor); desipramine (Norpramin) 25–50 mg/day
         b. Bupropion (Wellbutrin) (heterocyclic)
         c. Fluoxetine (Prozac) (SSRIs) 20 mg/day
         d. Paroxetine (Paxil) (SSRI)
         e. Sertraline (Zoloft) (SSRI)
         f. Trazodone (Desyrel) (heterocyclic)

Side effects are most likely to occur at initiation or when meds increased; adaptation occurs over time.

Once-daily dosing at bedtime minimizes side effects and does not diminish efficacy, because one-half life is 24 hrs. The full therapeutic dosage is maintained until Florence has either responded or clearly failed to respond (evaluate at 6 and 12 wks).

B. Psychotherapy

Few clinical trials available demonstrating efficacy. Consider:

1. Useful for mild–moderate depression
2. When patient requests

C. Medication and psychotherapy

Consider when:

1. Either treatment alone only has partial response or poor interepisode recovery
2. Most patients do best when combined therapy is used

D. Electroconvulsive therapy (ECT)

Consider when:

1. More severe or psychotic forms
2. Other therapies have failed
3. Medication conditions precluding use of meds
4. Need for rapid response

Recommendations summarized from Depression Guideline Panel, 1993.

5. *How often and when would you see Florence again?*

Providing patient support and education optimizes adherence, facilitates dosage adjustment, minimizes side effects, and allows monitoring of clinical response. AHCPR recommends seeing more severely depressed patients weekly for first 6–8 wks. Less severe depressed patients may be seen every 10–14 days (Depression Guideline Panel, vol. 2, 1993).

6. *Florence has shown little improvement after 6 weeks of treatment. What adjustments would you make in the therapeutic plan?*

Failure to respond necessitates: reassessment of the adequacy of the diagnosis, and reassessment of the adequacy of treatment.

Ongoing, undisclosed substance abuse or underlying general medical condition are two common pitfalls.

Medication underdosing is common. Increasing doses of meds should be given in first few weeks for most antidepressants. Exception is fluozetine. Check blood level to determine therapeutic range, and indicate adherence level—if not within therapeutic dose, adjust appropriately.

Medication is recommended after acute episode for 4–9 months afterward. Reoccurances require longer treatment with medications. Those with greater than three recurrences may need to continue medications for life.

7. *Based on the information given about Florence, what impact do you think this situation has had on Florence's family?*

Although Florence has been depressed for an extended period of time, if the depression continues and/or becomes more severe, the impact will likely become more serious. Families with a member who is suffering depression frequently report feelings of:

- Grief over the loss of the person they once knew.
- Guilt that perhaps they are to blame for the illness.
- Anger at the behaviors/actions (or lack of), positive or negative directed at other family members as a release of frustrations.
- Powerlessness, a concern that the depression cannot be "cured" or that it may become a chronic condition.
- Fear of the unknown and future, and even of the depressed person.

Additionally, in Florence's and other similar cases, depression alters the emotional and functional equilibrium of the family by creating:

- Marital strain and stress.
- Altered communication/interaction patterns.
- Worry and concern by family members over Florence's lack of interest in personal hygiene, ADLs, usual activities and interests, altered social interactions, and feelings of hopelessness.
- Altered roles and responsibilities.
- Psychosocial impairment of spouse and increased risk of the children developing a psychiatric disorder.
- Fatigue and potential for burnout of caregivers.

8. *What would be appropriate interventions for Florence's family?*

Appropriate interventions for Florence's family could include:

- Education for the family concerning depression.
- Family/marital counseling (individual and/or group).
- Attending a community support group.
- Encourage continuation of normal activities/routines as much as possible.
- Family meetings to negotiate needed changes in shifting of responsibilities.
- "Time Out," providing breaks as needed to maintain balance.

- Utilize existing social support networks/develop new ones with help.
- Make sure "crisis hot line" phone numbers, and other needed phone numbers are near at hand for emergency use (Barker, 1994, Uphold, 1994).

9. *Where can a nurse practitioner obtain more information concerning depression and/or additional resources for assisting depressed clients?*

Look for numbers of local crisis/hot lines social support groups/hospitals with psychiatric units, or contact the following organizations.

National Alliance for the Mentally Ill (NAMI)
Arlington, VA
703 524-7600

National Depressive & Manic Association (NDMDA) Chicago, IL
312 642-0049

National Foundation for Depressive Illness
800 248-4344

National Mental Health Association Information
Center, 1021 Prince St. Alexandria, VA 22314
800 969-6642

Information Referral and Crisis Hotline
800 233-4357

American Psychological Association
202 336-6062

10. *What community resources can the nurse practitioner refer the depressed client and/or family to?*

As noted, the NP should have learned and identified the resources in his/her community that serve the needs of the depressed client and his or her family. This will be different in each community and will require research on the practitioner in advance of the need.

11. *What other health care professionals should be involved in a plan of care for Florence? When should Florence be referred for more intensive therapy?*

- Physician/Psychiatrist: for consultation and referral
- Psychologist: for referral for counseling/consultation
- Licensed clinical social worker, psychiatric nurse/specialist for consultation and referral

Florence should be referred to a specialist if her depression is severe, she exhibits suicidal ideation, if she requires multiple medications for control or improvement, or if you determine she has bipolar depression (Uphold, 1994).

REFERENCES

American Psychiatric Association. *Diagnosis and Statistical Manual of Mental Disorders.* Washington, DC: American Psychiatric Association; 1994.

Barker L, Burton J, Ziever P. *Principles of Ambulatory Medicine,* 4th ed. Baltimore: Williams & Wilkins; 1994.

Depression Guideline Panel. *Depression in Primary Care: Volume 1. Detection and Diagnosis. Clinical Practice Guideline, Number 5.* Rockville, MD: U.S. Department of Health and Human Services, Public Health Service, Agency for Health Care Policy and Research. AHCPR Publication No. 93-0550. April 1993.

Depression Guideline Panel. *Depression in Primary Care: Volume 2. Treatment. Clinical Practice Guideline, Number 5.* Rockville, MD: U.S. Department of Health and Human Services, Public Health Service, Agency for Health Care Policy and Research. AHCPR Publication No. 93-0550. April 1993.

Uphold C, Graham M. *Clinical Guidelines for Family Practice,* 2nd ed. Gainesville, FL: Barmarrae Books; 1994.

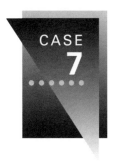

A 23-year-old woman with vaginal discharge

SCENARIO

Myra is a 23-year-old Caucasian female who presents with complaints of mild generalized aches and fatigue. She also c/o increased vaginal discharge with some itching. Her boyfriend has noticed an odor while having sex. She has a sensation of heaviness in the lower abdomen and admits to mild dysuria. Her last sexual contact was 3 days ago.

● TENTATIVE DIAGNOSES

Based on the information provided so far, what are potential differential diagnoses?

● HISTORY

1. *What are significant questions in the history for a woman with a vaginal discharge?*
2. *What are the key points to cover on the review of systems?*

● PHYSICAL ASSESSMENT

What are the significant portions of the physical examination that should be completed for Myra?

● DIFFERENTIAL DIAGNOSES

What are the significant positive and negative data that support or refute your diagnoses for Myra?

● DIAGNOSTIC TESTS

Based on the history and physical assessment, what, if any, diagnostic tests would you obtain? Include your rationale for the tests.

● DIAGNOSES

What diagnoses are appropriate for Myra?

● THERAPEUTIC PLAN

1. *What are your treatment choices for presumptive GC and chlamydia?*
2. *What obligation does the NP have concerning the CDC?*
3. *What symptoms should Myra be warned about related to her STD infection and immediate care?*
4. *What instructions should you discuss with Myra to help prevent the recurrence of a STD?*
5. *What follow up should Myra get related to the STD infection and when?*
6. *What psychological impact might the STD diagnosis have for Myra?*
7. *What recommendations can you make to Myra to help her deal with this situation?*
8. *What community resources are available for the NP related to STDs and patient information?*
9. *What long-term plan of care do you have for Myra?*

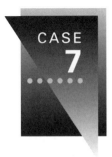

TUTORIAL

A 23-year-old woman with vaginal discharge

SCENARIO

Myra is a 23-year-old Caucasian female who presents with complaints of mild generalized aches and fatigue. She also c/o increased vaginal discharge with some itching. Her boyfriend has noticed an odor while having sex. She has a sensation of heaviness in the lower abdomen and admits to mild dysuria. Her last sexual contact was 3 days ago.

● TENTATIVE DIAGNOSES

What are the potential diagnoses you have identified based on the preceding scenario?

DIAGNOSIS	RATIONALE
STD (GC, chlamydia, trich)	Vaginal discharge with an odor.
Bacterial vaginitis	Vaginal discharge with odor.
UTI	Sensation of heaviness in lower abdomen with dysuria.
PID	Sensation of heaviness in abdomen, vaginal discharge.
Candida vaginitis	Vaginal discharge with itching.
Hypothyroid	Body aches and fatigue.
NIDDM	Candidiasis, fatigue, and urinary symptoms are consistent with DM.
Pregnancy	Heaviness in lower abdomen with dysuria (Johnson et al., 1996).

● HISTORY

1. What are significant questions in the history for a woman with vaginal discharge?

REQUESTED DATA	DATA ANSWER
Allergies	Sulfa: UTI as adolescent, treated with Bactrim: developed a rash and itching.
Current medications	OTC decongestant for nasal stuffiness.
Surgery/transfusions	None/None.
Past medical history and hospitalizations/fractures/injuries/accidents	Genital condyloma at age 16, treated with cryosurgery. No reoccurrences. No hospitalizations, fx, or injuries.
Childhood illness	None.
OB/GYN history	LNMP: One week ago. Spotting x 2 d followed by heavy flow that required new pad every 2–3 hours. Slight cramping. Previous menses 45 days ago (5 d duration, moderate flow). Cycle: 28d, 4–5 day duration. Menarche: 13 y/o. Age initial intercourse: 15. # Sexual partners: > 5 in lifetime, last year = 1. G0P0A0 Last pelvic/pap: 1 year ago. Had a problem—not sure what it was. Was supposed to repeat pap in 6 mos but did not. Contraceptive: OCs. Takes every morning when gets up. Denies missing pills. No barrier method of contraception. Denies rectal penetration or receiving oral fluids from partner. Believes partner is heterosexual. Unsure if he has ever been with prostitute in other parts of world.
Sleeping patterns	Right now gets 8–10 hours of sleep per night since she has gotten stuffy nose. Normally sleeps around 7–8 hrs. Denies night sweats.
24-Hour diet recall	B: 1 Pop-Tart, Mt. Dew. L: Hamburger, french fries, chocolate milk shake. D: Fried chicken, mashed potatoes, green beans, 8 oz Kool-Aid. S: Mt. Dew, Microwave popcorn.
Social history	Tobacco: None. Alcohol: Minimal (2–3 beers/mo).

(continued)

REQUESTED DATA DATA ANSWER

REQUESTED DATA	DATA ANSWER
	Caffeinated beverages: 2–3 12 oz cans Mt. Dew.
	Drugs: Marijuana every 2–3 mos. Experimented with crack and heroin 6+ years ago.
	Exercise: No regular exercise program.
Family history	Father: Unknown; not a part of family since Myra born.
	Mother: HTN since 35, now 43.
	MGM: IDDM.
	Siblings: 2 older step siblings: good health.
Education	HS graduate, enrolled in night school to learn computer programming.
Social organizations	Member of Southern Baptist Church since childhood. Attends church regularly and sings in choir. Many friends from church and high school.
Employment/finances/ insurance	Works full time in a clerical position at an insurance company. Hopes to be promoted when finishes computer course. Has marginal insurance through employer.
Housing	Myra lives with her grandmother in a small house in one of established communities of city. Her siblings live in area and she sees them frequently.
Relationships	Involved with a married man who is in the Air Force, stationed in adjacent city. Travel to other parts of country and world. He has told Myra he intends to divorce his wife. Myra sees him every 3 weeks when he is in the area for long weekends. Myra's mother and grandmother disapprove of this relationship and have encouraged Myra to stop seeing him. He denies having any discharge from penis or any problems.
Safety/prevention	Does not wear seatbelt. Smoke detector. No guns in house.

2. *What are the key points on the review of systems?*

SYSTEM REVIEWED DATA ANSWER

SYSTEM REVIEWED	DATA ANSWER
General	Feels as if she is getting a cold. Myra has been fatigued and achy all over.
HEENT	Has had scratchy throat, nasal congestion. Denies extreme thirst, or increased hunger.

(continued)

SYSTEM REVIEWED	DATA ANSWER
Gyn	Denies abdominal pain, pain on intercourse. Partner has no symptoms. He has been treated for an STD in past.
GU	Has dysuria, but no frequency or urgency or hematuria.
GI	No appetite changes, no weight changes.
Endocrine	Denies being told in past that she had "sugar." Denies feeling shaky if she hasn't eaten for a while. Had a sugar test and was told it was normal about 5 years ago.

● PHYSICAL ASSESSMENT

What are the significant portions of the physical examination that should be completed for Myra and why?

SYSTEM	RATIONALE	FINDINGS
Vital signs	Provide baseline data.	B/P: 136/82 P: 80 R: 16 T: 99.4°F Ht: 5'4" Wt: 170 lbs.
General appearance/skin	Gives overall view of patient/ assessment of skin is important when STD (such as syphilis) is a consideration.	White female, alert, cooperative in NAD. No skin lesions or rash noted.
HEENT	Important baseline information.	TMs gray, shiny, and mobile. Landmarks visible. Nasal passages with min. erythema and edema. Mild erythema of pharynx. No exudate. Sl. cervical adenopathy with mild tenderness. Thyroid nonpalpable.
Chest	Important baseline information.	Lungs CTA. Breasts symmetrical, no masses or nipple d/c. Axillary lymph nodes nonpalpable/nontender.

(continued)

SYSTEM	RATIONALE	FINDINGS
Heart	Important baseline information.	S$_1$S$_2$ WNL, no MRG. Peripheral pulses 2+.
Abdomen	System involved in chief complaint.	Rounded, nontender. BS+ No HSM. No guarding, no inguinal adenopathy.
Rectum	Important to obtain because provides for information related to uterus.	WNL sphincter tone, brown stool. No tenderness.
Pelvic	System involved in chief complaint (Dunnihoo, 1992).	Genitalia: Mildly excoriated, edematous. Vagina: pink, moist, mild erythema, thick, light yellow mucoid d/c. Cervix: Red, edematous, mucopurulent d/c from os, nontender. Uterus: Smooth, firm, nontender, negative CMT, normal size, negative Chadwick's or Hegar's signs. Adnexa: Nontender, no masses.

● DIFFERENTIAL DIAGNOSES

What are the significant positive and negative data that support or refute your diagnoses for Myra?

DIAGNOSIS	POSITIVE DATA	NEGATIVE DATA
STD	Vaginal d/c, mucopurulent d/c from os, no use of barrier methods, previous condyloma, edematous, erythemic cervix (Seller, 1996).	No labial pain, no fever, no abdominal pain, no pain when climbing steps.
UTI	Sensation of heaviness in lower abdomen with dysuria.	Denies urgency, frequency, or hematuria.
PID	Sensation of heaviness in abdomen, vaginal discharge, abnormal menses.	Negative CMT, no abdominal pain, no fever, no adnexal pain, no pain with intercourse.

(continued)

DIAGNOSIS	POSITIVE DATA	NEGATIVE DATA
Candida vaginitis	Vaginal discharge with itching.	Odor, white discharge, no recent antibiotic use.
Hypothyroid	Body aches and fatigue, irregular periods.	No dry skin, alopecia, weight gain.
NIDDM	Candidiasis, fatigue, and urinary symptoms. She also has a + FH of IDDM.	No weight loss, excessive thirst, or urination.
Pregnancy	Heaviness in lower abdomen with dysuria, fatigue, + sexually active, abnormal menses.	Uses OCs, uterus normal size, negative for Chadwick's/Hegar's signs.
URI	C/o of scratchy throat, nasal congestion, body aches, fatigue, low grade temperature, no exudate on tonsils, no cervical lymph node tenderness.	None.
Ectopic pregnancy	Heaviness in lower abdomen, irregular periods.	No abdominal pain, no adnexal pain or Chandalier's sign.
Bacterial vaginosis	Vaginal d/c with odor, itching.	No douching.
HIV	Fatigue, + sexual active, no barrier contraception, partner travels in different parts of world, previous hx of heroin use.	No opportunistic infections, denies night sweats, weight loss.

● DIAGNOSTIC TESTS

Based on the history and physical assessment, what, if any, diagnostic tests would you obtain?

DIAGNOSTIC TEST	RATIONALE	RESULTS
RPR	To check for presence of sphyilis in light of high-risk behaviors. Community has seen a dramatic increase in syphilis in past 4–5 years.	RPR, negative.

(continued)

DIAGNOSTIC TEST *RATIONALE* *RESULTS*

DIAGNOSTIC TEST	RATIONALE	RESULTS
Pap smear	For routine screening and HM related to increased incidence of cervical Ca with hx of HPV. Due to the inflammation, this test may need to be repeated at a later time once treatment for STDs has been completed.	Endocervical cells present, marked inflammation.
Wet mount/whiff test/pH	To check for presence of hyphae, pseudohyphae, clue cells, trichimonads. Whiff test is specific for BV and sometimes for trich. PH of BV is > 5.	+Clue cells. + Whiff. pH > 5. – Hyphae. – trichimonads.
Urine dip	Good choice, quick inexpensive test allowing a check for leukocytes, nitrites, blood, and glucose/ketones.	Negative dip.
Urine HCG	Quick, inexpensive way to check for pregnancy. Need to determine because Myra had a change in menstrual patterns and is sexually active.	Negative.
DNA probe	One test that indicates the presence of both gonorrhea and chlamydia. High sensitivity and less fragile than culture. Test results will not return for 2–3 days. May need to treat presumptively if concerned about compliance.	(+ GC when it returns 2–3 days later.)
TSH	Screening test for thyroid disorders.	TSH: 1.8.
H/H	Screening for anemia.	Hgb: 13.8.
HIV	HIV testing should be offered based on symptoms, at risk category, occupation of boyfriend, and his frequent travel.	Negative ELISA.

● DIAGNOSES

What diagnoses are appropriate for Myra?

Presumptive gonorrhea/chlamydia
Bacterial vaginosis
Mild URI
Emotional/family stress
Health maintenance needs

Data Supporting the Diagnosis

Presumptive GC and chlamydia: Mucopurulent d/c, edematous cervix, low grade fever, epidemiologically at risk because of age, sex, lifestyle behaviors, hx of STD, occupation of boyfriend and his travel.
Bacterial vaginosis: Vaginal d/c, itching, external appearance of vulva, clue cells, positive whiff test, pH > 5.
URI: Mild erythema, + cervical nodes, no exudate, lungs clear, nasal congestion.
Emotional/family stress: Lack of support by family for relationship with SO, marital status of SO, dissonance with strong religious beliefs.
Patient education needs: STDs, nutrition, exercise, CAD risk factors.

● THERAPEUTIC PLAN

1. What are your treatment choices for presumptive GC and chlamydia?

Azithromycin (Zithromax) 1 GM, po, now: One-time medication recommended by CDC for treatment of chlamydia because of increased compliance with a one-time dose. Other treatments include Doxycycline 100 mg PO BID × 7d.
Ceftriaxone (Rocephin) 125 mg/IM or Cefixime (Suprax) 400 mg PO: CDC guidelines for treatment of GC. Again, a one-time dose increases compliance.
Metronidazole (Flagyl) 2 GM ×1 or 500 BID × 7d. MetroGel or metronidazole and applicator qhs × 5.
Continue current OC product. Myra has used this method successfully without problems. Use back-up birth control × 1 month secondary to antibiotic therapy.

2. What obligation does the NP have concerning the CDC?

GC and chlamydia are reportable STDs. The information related to diagnosis, treatment, and partner notification are the responsibility of the NP or office manager to share with health department/CDC (Peter, 1994).

3. What symptoms should Myra be warned about related to her STD infection and immediate care?

The symptoms of PID should be reviewed with Myra carefully. If she would develop severe abdominal pain, fever, or pain on intercourse she should call the office ASAP (Seller, 1996).

4. *What instructions should you discuss with Myra to help prevent the recurrence of a STD?*
   - Use of condom at all times to decrease the risk of contracting STDs
   - Abstinence until test of cure and both partners are treated
   - No oral or rectal sex (Hawkins et al., 1995)

5. *What follow up should Myra get related to the STD infection and when?*

   Myra should return in 10 days. At this time:
   - Myra's symptoms should be diminished or gone.
   - You should discuss lab results with her.
   - You should also repeat the pelvic exam and cervical culture.
   - You should request that Myra give permission for her old records so documentation of her past pap smears, treatment of HPV, immunization records can provide a more complete data source on which to base Myra's care.

6. *What psychological impact might the STD diagnosis have for Myra?*
   - Will likely cause stress and strain on the relationship Myra has with current partner.
   - May cause grief over the loss of what Myra thought was a monogamous relationship.
   - May cause anger at self for trusting boyfriend, lack of confidence in her own judgment, particularly when family members did not approve.
   - May have fear of infertility after having STD.
   - Probable desire to keep this diagnosis from family members because they disapprove of the relationship.
   - May cause tension among Myra, her mother, and her grandmother (Jacobs & Gast, 1994).

7. *What recommendations can you make to Myra to help her deal with this situation?*

   Suggest that Myra consider going to a counselor to help her address some of the preceding issues. Most health departments have mental health professionals or contract out with a commercial agency. Reassure Myra that seeing a counselor or psychologist does not mean she is mentally ill. Explain about the effect of a loss and how the counselor can assist her to deal proactively with the situation.

8. *What community resources are available for the NP related to STDs and patient information?*

American Council for Healthful Living
439 Main St.
Orange, NJ 07050
201 674-7476

American Foundation for Prevention of Veneral Disease, Inc.
799 Broadway St., Suite 638
New York, NY 1003
212 759-2069

American Medical Association-
Order Department, OP-383
PO Box 821
Monroe, WI 53566
Ed. material on STDs

American VD Association
PO Box 22349
San Diego, CA 92122
619 453-3238
Asst in efforts to decrease STDs

Centers for Disease Control
Center for Infectious Disease
1600 Clifton Rd.
Atlanta, GA 30333
404 329-2401, 404 377-9563
Public info, research, policy formation

Citizens' Alliance for VD Awareness
222W Adams St.
Chicago, IL 60606
312 236-6339
Public info on STDs

VD National Hotline
260 Sheridan Ave.
Palo Alto, CA 94306
415 327-6465
Info and referral for service

World Health Organization Publications Centre, USA
c/o Lloyd Publications
49 Sheridan Ave.
Albany, NY 12210
518 436-9686
Educational materials on STDs

Consider contacting city, state, and county health departments; local STD treatment centers; and local Planned Parenthood (Clark, 1992).

9. *What long-term plan of care do you have for Myra?*

When Myra returns in 10 days, it will be important to discuss some health prevention/promotion issues with her. The following topics should be presented and discussed with Myra:

- Hepatitis B screen: Since sexually active and history of IVDA. Consider Hep B immunization series for Myra.
- Coronary Risk profile: +FH of heart disease, high-fat diet, increased weight-to-height ratio, FH of IDDM. Review symptoms of DM.
- Nutrition: Discuss areas of weight, high-fat diet, CAD risks, low calcium. Consider referral to health department for more extensive counseling/diet management.
- Exercise: Exercise will be very important to assist with weight management and reduce CAD risks.
- Lipid profile: Myra should return fasting if possible so a lipid screen can be done to help direct Myra in her diet and exercise efforts.
- BSE: Myra should be given a demonstration of BSE, and told when the best time is to examine her breasts.
- Safety: Encourage Myra to wear her seat belts and find out about the smoke detector in her home.
- Pap/pelvic: Discuss with Myra the importance of yearly follow up owing to her past history of HPV.
- Reinforce with written material on preceding topics if possible so Myra will have a reference (Carlson, 1996).

REFERENCE

Clark M. *Nursing in the Community.* Norwalk CT: Appleton Lange; 1992; 767–782.

Carlson K, Eisenstat S, Ziporyn T. *The Harvard Guide to Women's Health,* Cambridge: Harvard Press; 1996.

Centers for Disease Control and Prevention. *Sexually Transmitted Disease Treatment Guidelines,* 42; 1993.

DiPiro J. Sexually transmitted diseases, in DiPiro J, Talbert R, Hayes P, Yee G, Matzke G, Posey L (eds). *Pharmacotherapy: A Pathophysiological Approach,* 2nd ed. Norwalk, CT: Appleton Lange; 1993.

Dunnihoo D. *Fundamentals of Gynecology and Obstetrics,* Philadelphia: J.B. Lippincott; 1992; 164–167.

Glass R. *Office Gynecology,* Baltimore: Williams & Wilkins; 1993; 1–25.

Hatcher D. *Contraceptive Technology,* Salem, NH: Octal Publishing; 1994.

Hawkins J, Roberto-Nichols D, Stanley-Haney J. *Protocols for Nurse Practitioners in Gynecology Settings,* New York: Tiresias Press; 1995.

Jacobs A, Gast M. Sexually transmitted diseases. *Practical Gynecology.* Norwalk, CT: Appleton Lange; 1994.

Johnson C, Johnson B, Murray J, Apgar B. *Women's Health Care Handbook,* Philadelphia: CV Mosby; 1996.

Peter G. *Red Book: Report of the Committee on Infectious Disease.* Elk Grove Village, IL: American Academy of Pediatrics; 1994.

Seller R. *Differential Diagnosis of Common Complaints.* Philadelphia: W.B. Saunders; 1996.

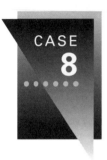

A 36-year-old man with heartburn

SCENARIO

Bill Star is a 36-year-old Caucasian male. He is employed as a stockbroker and works 60–70 hours a week. Frequently his job requires that he be out of town on short business trips. Bill presents with complaints of a midsternal burning sensation. His discomfort is often worse at night and he frequently wakes with a bad taste in his mouth. He has experienced no weight loss or change in appetite.

● TENTATIVE DIAGNOSES

Based on Bill's presentation, what are your differential diagnoses?

● HISTORY

What further information would you like to obtain from Bill to help with your subjective data collection?

● PHYSICAL ASSESSMENT

Based on the subjective data obtained, what should be included in the objective assessment of Bill and why?

● DIFFERENTIAL DIAGNOSIS

Having collected both subjective and objective data, now link the subjective and objective information to the appropriate differential diagnosis. Identify both positive and negative data that support or refute the diagnosis.

● DIAGNOSTIC TESTS

Are there diagnostic tests that will help to confirm the priority diagnosis or refute the differential diagnosis?

● DIAGNOSIS

Based on the subjective, objective, and diagnostic data you have gathered, what is your diagnosis of Bill? What data support this diagnosis?

● THERAPEUTIC PLAN

1. What lifestyle changes will be important for Bill to adopt?

2. What medications are appropriate for Bill to take?

3. How should Bill return for follow up?

4. At what point should Bill be referred to a physician?

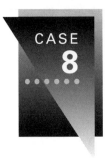

TUTORIAL

A 36-year-old man with heartburn

SCENARIO

Bill Star is a 36-year-old Caucasian male. He is employed as a stockbroker and works 60–70 hours a week. Frequently his job requires that he be out of town on short business trips. Bill presents with complaints of a midsternal burning sensation. His discomfort is often worse at night and he frequently wakes with a bad taste in his mouth. He has experienced no weight loss or change in appetite.

● TENTATIVE DIAGNOSES

Based on Bill's presentation, what are your differential diagnoses?

DIFFERENTIAL DIAGNOSIS   RATIONALE

Gastric or duodenal ulcer	Bill presents with a midsternal burning sensation, often associated with meals. He frequently takes 4–6 ASA qd. He smokes $1\frac{1}{2}$ packs of cigarettes a day. These factors can be significant for an ulcer.
GERD	Midsternal burning, associated with meals, waking during the night with a bad taste in his mouth, and his caffeine and cigarette use can all be associated with GERD.
Cardiac chest pain	Bill's midsternal pain and the fact that he smokes $1\frac{1}{2}$ packs of cigarettes a day could contribute to a cardiac etiology.

● HISTORY

What further information would you like to obtain from Bill to help with your subjective data collection?

REQUESTED DATA DATA ANSWER

History of present illness	Midsternal burning has been present for about 4–5 months. It occurs most often after a large meal and often in the middle of the night. There is no radiation of the discomfort, no shortness of breath, no diaphoresis. The discomfort is relieved somewhat by antacids. The discomfort can last for a couple of hours.
Allergies	None.
Medications	ASA as needed. Takes approx. 6/day for headache. Antacids, prn.
Surgery	Appendectomy, 1974.
Hospitalizations	Appendectomy, 1974. Kidney stones, 1989.
Transfusions	None.
Diet	Regular, no change in appetite, often eats fast food and conducts business over dinner.
24-Hour diet recall	B: 3 cups of coffee and danish at 6:30 AM. L: Hamburger, french fries, pop, sometimes a milk shake at 12:00 N. D: Steak, baked potato with butter and sour cream, salad with ranch dressing, coffee at 6–7:00 PM. S: Chips, soft drinks, candy bar in the midafternoon.
Sleep	No difficulty sleeping, goes to bed at 11–12:00 PM and wakes at 6:00 AM.
Social habits	Smokes $1\frac{1}{2}$ packs of cigarettes qd. ETOH 3–5 drinks every week. Caffeine, 4–5 cups of coffee, and four to five caffeinated sodas QD. No recreational drugs. No regular exercise.
Social history	Married to wife of 12 years, good relationship, 3 children. Works as a stock broker for 10 years, enjoys his job. Owns his own home. Income: $65,000 a year. Belongs to a country club, plays golf once a week in the summer and fall.

(continued)

REQUESTED DATA	DATA ANSWER
Family history	Father: Age 62, living, has HTN. Mother: Age 60, living, has had breast CA. Sister: Age 33, alive and well. Daughter: Age 10, alive and well. Son: Age 8, has epilepsy. Son: Age 5, has asthma and allergies.
Review of systems: General	Current health is good.
Cardiac	Denies chest pain, shortness of breath, orthopnea, history of HTN, edema.
GI	Denied weight gain or loss, vomiting, diarrhea, constipation, blood in stool, change in appetite, history of PUD.
GU	Denies change in pattern of urination, frequency, urgency, burning.
Neurological	C/o tension headaches for past 8 years, mainly during work week. Has associated neck tightness. No N/V, visual problems, or other associated symptoms.
Preventive health	Wears seat belt, has smoke detector in home. No guns in home. Has not had influenza vaccine. Has not had a checkup in past 5 years. Last dental exam 6 mos ago. Last vision exam 10 mo ago.

● PHYSICAL ASSESSMENT

Based on the subjective data obtained, what should be included in the objective assessment of Bill and why?

SYSTEM	RATIONALE	FINDINGS
Vital signs	Baseline information.	T: 98.4, P: 88, R: 18, B/P: 150/86
Height Weight	To establish general size and obesity status/weight loss or gain.	6' 245 lbs.
General appearance	Gives a general overview of Bill's status and urgency of complaint.	Slightly obese, well groomed, in no apparent distress.

(continued)

SYSTEM	RATIONALE	FINDINGS
HEENT	Not entirely necessary for Bill's problem. Will probably reveal no new information.	PERRAL, EOMs intact, TMs pearly with + light reflex, nares patent, neck supple, no adenopathy.
Cardiac	Prudent for routine exam, and needs to be ruled out as cause of chief complaint.	S_1, S_2 regular, no murmur, no S_4.
Respiratory	Prudent for routine exam.	Respirations even, unlabored. Breath sounds clear throughout.
Abdomen	Allows NP to r/o masses, fluid, ascites, organomegaly as well as confirm peristalsis with bowel sounds.	Bowel sounds present in four quadrants, abdomen soft, rounded, nontender, no hepato/splenomegaly, negative CVA tenderness.
Rectal	Prudent to evaluate for GI bleeding.	Prostate unremarkable; stool Hemoccult negative.

● DIFFERENTIAL DIAGNOSIS

Having collected both subjective and objective data, now link the subjective and objective information to the appropriate differential diagnosis. Identify both positive and negative data that support or refute the diagnosis.

DIAGNOSIS	POSITIVE DATA	NEGATIVE DATA
Peptic ulcer disease	Male, often awakened at night with discomfort, smoker, frequent use of ASA.	No family history of PUD, some relief with antacids, no change in weight.
GERD	Heartburn, specifically post-prandial. Some relief with use of antacids. Smokes, large caffeine intake, high-fat diet, overweight.	Usually does not eat late at night.
Cardiac chest pain	Substernal pain, smokes $1\frac{1}{2}$ packs of cigarettes every day. Blood pressure 160/92, No knowledge of cholesterol level.	Age (36), nondiabetic, no family history of coronary artery disease, pain is not brought on by exertion, no other associated symptoms.

● DIAGNOSTIC TESTS

Are there diagnostic tests that will help to confirm the priority diagnosis or refute the differential diagnosis?

DIAGNOSTIC TEST	RATIONALE	RESULTS
Endoscopy	Initially no diagnostic studies are necessary. UGI could help r/o PUD, however, endoscopy is the preferred test for PUD. The subjective and objective data will generally lead to the diagnosis of GERD. However, physician referral for endoscopy is recommended if any of the following "alarm" symptoms are present: odynophagia, dysphagia, nausea, vomiting, early satiety, weight loss, pulmonary symptoms, blood in stool, or chest pain (Horowitz & Fisher, 1995).	Endoscopy not done.
EKG	Because the patient is a heavy smoker and he is presently hypertensive, an EKG would be an acceptable test to help rule out a cardiac etiology (Uphold & Graham, 1994). (Bill's EKG was normal.)	EKG-NSR, no indications of ischemia or increased voltage.
Cholesterol	An increased cholesterol level will help to substantiate a differential diagnosis of a cardiac chest pain. A total cholesterol level is recommended every 5 years for persons without symptoms of coronary artery disease (American Academy of Family Physicians, 1992).	Bill's total cholesterol: Chol 158, LDL 100, HDL 38.

(continued)

DIAGNOSTIC TEST	RATIONALE	RESULTS
Helicobacter pylori	A test to detect the presence of *H. Pylori,* helpful in the diagnosis of PUD. Biopsy or breath test can be completed in office with appropriate equipment.	Not done.

● DIAGNOSIS

Based on the subjective, objective, and diagnostic data you have gathered, what is your diagnosis of Bill? What data support this diagnosis?

GERD

Rationale: Heartburn and nocturnal reflux of acid are hallmark symptoms of GERD (Horowitz & Fisher, 1995). Alcohol, obesity, smoking, high-fat diet, and caffeine all lead to decreased lower esophageal sphincter tone and reflux (Hixson, et al., 1992). Absence of the aforementioned "alarm" symptoms rules out other diagnoses. Additionally, Bill's EKG and total cholesterol were within normal limits. This, in addition to the lack of family history of CAD and no associated cardiac symptoms, help to rule out a cardiac etiology.

● THERAPEUTIC PLAN

1. *What lifestyle changes will be important for Bill to adopt?*

   Teaching lifestyle changes will play a large role for the nurse practitioner. Initially, GERD should be addressed nonpharmacologically in the following manner, known as phase I therapy:

   1. Normalize weight.
   2. Avoid large meals.
   3. Do not eat at least 2 hours prior to bedtime.
   4. Avoid alcohol, tobacco, caffeine, fatty foods, and chocolate.
   5. Elevate the head of the bed on blocks.
   6. Use antacids up to seven times a day.
   7. Avoid the following medications:
      Theophylline
      Calcium channel blockers
      Anticholinergics
      Beta-adrenergic agonists
      Alpha-adrenergic agonists

Narcotics
Nicotine
Estrogen
Progesterone

These medications decrease lower esophageal sphincter (LES) tone and should be avoided when possible (Hixson et al., 1992; Horowitz and Fisher, 1995; Uphold and Graham, 1994).

A two week trial of phase I therapy is recommended (Horowitz and Fischer, 1995).

2. *What medications are appropriate for Bill to take?*

Phase II therapy can be initiated after failure of phase I therapy. In phase II therapy pharmacologic agents are added to the already mentioned lifestyle changes. The first drug of choice in phase II therapy is an H_2-receptor antagonist (Horowitz & Fisher, 1995).

There are four equally effective H_2 antagonists (Robinson, 1995; Sontag, 1990; Uphold and Graham 1994):

Cimetidine (Tagamet) 400 mg BID
Ranitidine (Zantac) 150 mg BID
Famotidine (Pepcid) 20 mg BID
Nizatidine (Axid) 150 mg BID

H_2-receptor antagonists should be administered in BID doses, once in the AM and once after dinner (Sontag, 1990).

Antacids are considered second line treatment for GERD and are often initiated at the same time phase I therapy is started. They act to neutralize gastric acids and therefore increase the pH of refluxed gastric content. However, they offer only temporary symptomatic relief due to their short duration of action (Hixson et al., 1992). If utilized, dosing is recommended up to seven times a day, 1–3 hours after meals and at bedtime. Liquid antacids are recommended over chewable and they should not be administered within 2 hours of an H_2-receptor antagonist (Uphold & Graham, 1994).

Prokinetic drug therapy is another pharmacologic option for patients with GERD. In GERD there are several mechanisms that predispose the client to excessive esophageal acid exposure. These include: improper tone of the LES, impaired peristaltic contractions, gastric hypersecretion, and impaired gastric emptying, all of which can lead to reflux of stomach content. (Hixson et al., 1992; Robinson, 1995). Cisapride (Propulsid) is the recommended prokinetic agent. It may be used in conjunction with an H_2-receptor antagonist, particularly in patients proven to have motility abnormalities (Robinson, 1995).

Proton pump inhibitors are the option for refractory GERD. Omeprazole (Prilosec), and more recently lansoprazole (Prevacid), offer significant inhibition of acid secretion on a 24-hour basis. However, these drugs are expensive and once utilized it may not be possible to return to H_2-receptor antagonists (Robinson, 1995).

Whether H_2-receptor antagonists, antacids, or proton pump inhibitors are chosen, if improvement in symptoms is demonstrated, the chosen treatment should be continued for 6–8 weeks. The patient will need follow up after pharmacologic therapy is completed. It needs to be emphasized that the lifestyle changes initiated in phase I therapy need to become a way of life (Uphold and Graham, 1994).

3. When should Bill return for follow up?

Bill should return in 2 weeks to allow for evaluation of his symptoms. If the lifestyle changes have helped with reduction of symtoms, they should be continued. If there is no improvement in Bill's symptoms, phase II should be started.

4. At what point should Bill be referred to a physician?

If Bill were to experience any of the previously mentioned "alarm" symptoms: odynophagia, dysphagia, nausea, vomiting, early satiety, weight loss, pulmonary symptoms, blood in stool, or chest pain, immediate referral is indicated (Horowitz and Fisher, 1995). Referral is also indicated if two different medications have been tried without relief of symptoms. Additionally, any client who does not respond to therapy with H_2-receptor antagonists or proton pump inhibitors should be referred for further evaluation (Uphold and Graham, 1994).

REFERENCES

American Academy of Family Physicians, Commission on Public Health and Scientific Affairs. *Age Charts for Periodic Health Examinations.* Kansas City, MO: 1992.

Hixson LJ, Kelley CL, Jones WN, Tuohy CD. Current trends in the pharmacotherapy for gastroesophageal reflux disease. *Arch Int Med,* 1992; 152: 717–721.

Horowitz BJ, Fisher RS. Intervening in GERD: The phases of management. *Hosp Pract,* 1995; 15: 43–52.

Robinson M. Prokinetic therapy for gastroesophageal reflux disease. *Am Fam Phys,* 1995; 52(3): 957–961.

Sontag SJ. The medical management of reflux esophagitis. *Gastroent Clin N Am,* 1990; 19(3), 683–709.

Uphold CR, and Graham MV. *Clinical Guidelines in Family Practice.* Gainesville, FL: Barmarrae Books; 1994.

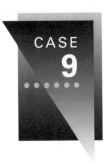

A 65-year-old woman requesting a checkup

SCENARIO

Ann Michaels is a 65-year-old widowed Asian female, first visit, requesting a physical exam for the Foster Grandparents Program. Ann has not seen a family physician since she went through natural menopause 17 years ago. She requested an appointment during the day because of difficulty driving at night, but is otherwise enjoying "good health."

● TENTATIVE DIAGNOSES

Based on Ann's presentation, what are your tentative differential diagnoses?

● HISTORY

What are significant questions you want to ask Ann in the history for an elderly physical exam that would assist in developing a maintenance and prevention plan as well as identifying any appropriate diagnosis?

● PHYSICAL ASSESSMENT

Based on the subjective data (history), what areas of the exam require closer scrutiny on the first visit and why?

● DIFFERENTIAL DIAGNOSES

Examine all data up to this point. Link the subjective and objective data to the appropriate differential diagnoses. Identify both positive and negative data that support or refute the diagnoses.

● DIAGNOSTIC TESTS

What screening and diagnostic tests would be appropriate for Ann?

● DIAGNOSES

What are your conclusive diagnoses? What is your rationale for concluding these diagnoses are correct?

● THERAPEUTIC PLAN

1. *What influence does Ann's + PPD have on her participation in the Foster Grandparents program?*
2. *What recommendations can you make for Ann in terms of immunizations?*
3. *What counseling would you do for Ann relative to her health promotion and prevention needs? Address the areas of:*

   Diet
   Injury prevention
   Dental health
   Hormone replacement therapy
   ASA therapy
   Regular health maintenance
4. *What therapy would you order for Ann for her osteoporosis?*
5. *What patient education is appropriate relative to the osteoporosis?*
6. *When would you have Ann return for follow up?*
7. *What referrals should be made for Ann?*

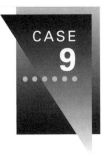

TUTORIAL

A 65-year-old woman requesting a checkup

SCENARIO

Ann Michaels is a 65-year-old widowed Asian female, first visit, requesting a physical exam for the Foster Grandparents Program. Ann has not seen a family physician since she went through natural menopause 17 years ago. She requested an appointment during the day because of difficulty driving at night, but is otherwise enjoying "good health."

● TENTATIVE DIAGNOSES

Based on Ann's presentation, what are your tentative differential diagnoses?

DIAGNOSIS	*RATIONALE*
Diagnosis not applicable at this time.	Well visit. When reviewing this case, keep in mind that the physical exam may be the only health maintenance visit for this elderly woman.

● HISTORY

What are significant questions you want to ask Ann in the history for an elderly physical exam that would assist in developing a maintenance and prevention plan as well as identifying any appropriate diagnoses?

REQUESTED DATA   DATA ANSWER

REQUESTED DATA	DATA ANSWER
Allergies	None.
Medications	Tylenol/Advil prn headache and arthritic pain; multivitamin with iron; infrequent Maalox.
Childhood diseases	Chicken pox, measles, mumps.
Immunizations	Unknown for childhood illness and tetanus. Has not received influenza, pneumococcal, or hepatitis B vaccines.
Surgery/transfusions	Appendectomy 25 years ago. None.
Hospitalizations	Vaginal delivery w/o complications × 2—1955, 1959.
Fractures, accidents, injuries	Mild cervical neck strain from MVA 1987 (seen at Urgent Care), no further problems.
Adult illness	Pneumonia, 1977; infrequent colds.
OB/GYN history	
LMP	1980.
Last pelvic/PAP	1979 or 1980.
Mammogram/SBE	Never/never.
Gravida/para	G2 P 2 A 0.
Last complete PE	Probably last pregnancy.
Last eye exam	4 years ago; began wearing bifocals at age 47; sees halos around lights at night.
Last dental exam	3 years ago; has all natural teeth.
Family history	Parents died 30 years ago in MVA; not aware of prior illness. Maternal grandmother: 98 y/o; "healthy" but has cataracts & arthritis. 1 living brother: 56 y/o; hypertension. 3 living sisters: 59 y/o, 61 y/o, 63 y/o; 1 w/ CAD & 1 w/ hypertension. 2 healthy children: 42 & 38 y/o men, good health.
Social habits	Nonsmoker, occasional social drink, drinks 1 cup of coffee & 1 cup of tea per day, no recreational drugs, walks several miles a day during nice weather and maintains her flower & vegetable gardens.
Social groups	Church choir; anticipating Foster Grandparents Program.

(continued)

REQUESTED DATA	DATA ANSWER
Relationship with family	Assists maternal grandmother w/shopping, lunch together weekly; siblings are supportive and interactive when possible but "very busy" with own families; sons very protective since death of their father, assist mother with house-hold chores, grandchildren visit at least weekly with sons.
Physical activity and functional status at home	Able to care for self: shops, cleans, performs all ADLs. Sons help with home repair and maintenance. Still able to drive own car, although does not like to drive at night anymore.
Insurance/income	Medical and dental insurance through AARP and Medicare; income through husband's pension and Social Security benefits.
Home	Owns her own home, ranch style w/basement, lives within five miles of both sons.
Appetite, 24-hour diet recall	B: Juice, toast, grapefruit or cereal with 2% milk, coffee. L: Soup and crackers or grilled cheese sandwich, fresh or canned fruit, 2% milk. D: Tea, baked potato with cheese, peas, cake. S: Yogurt.
Sleeping pattern	Sleeps 11/11:30 to 7/7:30. Usually up × 1 to void.
How do you handle stress? How would you rate your life on scale from 1 to 10 (10 best)?	Rating 3. Handles stress by increasing activities, and talking with friends and family.

● PHYSICAL ASSESSMENT

Based on the subjective data (history) what areas of the exam require closer scrutiny on the first visit and why?

SYSTEM	RATIONALE	FINDINGS
Vital signs	Provides baseline data for Ann. Gives quick view of cardiovascular/respiratory status. Recommended as yearly by	T = 97.6 (o), P = 80 and reg, R = 12 easy, B/P 160/92, RA sitting and standing, 158/90 LA sitting.

(continued)

SYSTEM	RATIONALE	FINDINGS
	United States Preventive Services Task Force (USPSTF).	Height: $64\frac{1}{2}$" Weight: 125 lbs
General appearance	Gives overall view of patient.	Well-nourished white female. Appears her stated age. Alert, oriented, affect appropriate.
Skin	Provides screening for malignancy, provides overall indication of health (Bates, 1983).	Warm and dry; no jaundice, bruises, ulcerations, rash. Negative for clubbing or cyanosis.
HEENT	Ann has not had an eye exam for 4 years and is experiencing visual changes. Restricts driving to daylight hours only because of "halos" around the lights and blurred vision. Patient is at increased risk for falls at home; particularly at night with artificial lighting. Alterations in vision and hearing are common changes with aging—they should be evaluated to determine if there are current or potential problems (Gorroll et al., 1995).	Normocephalic; normal hair distribution, PERRLA, sclera clear, conjunctiva pale, fundoscopic-bilateral lens opacification, red reflex present, unable to visualize retinal details, EOMs intact; Visual acuity 20/40 OS 20/60 OD with corrective lenses, TMs and canals clear, Weber lateralizes appropriately, Rinne AC > BC; nares patent, turbinates sl. pale and edematous; oropharynx clear, mucous membranes pink and moist, no ulcerations noted, tongue symetrical, uvula midline; negative sinus tenderness; neck supple, neg. adenopathy, tenderness, thyromegaly, bruits, JVD.
Cardiopulmonary	Ann has two siblings with hypertension and one with unspecified CAD. Her age and lack of post-menopausal estrogen replacement therapy also increases Mrs. Michaels' risk of CAD.	*Cardiac:* No chest wall abnormalities; neg. thrills, PMI at 6th intercostal space 1cm to left of MCL; reg rhythm w/ occas. extra systoles, S_1, S_2 (accentuated) w/ soft S_4. Grade II/VI systolic ejection murmur at left sternal border. *Lungs:* Diaphramatic excursion WNL, CTA, and percussion.

(continued)

SYSTEM	RATIONALE	FINDINGS
Abdomen	Increased incidence of GI problems with aging: dyspepsia, GERD, which may affect nutritional status. More serious diseases may also be evident.	Sl. rounded, striae present, BS × 4 quads, tympany throughout, soft, nontender, neg. mass or organomegaly, CVA tenderness.
Breasts	Clinical breast exam (CBE); review self-breast exam (SBE). There is controversy about the frequency of CBE and mammography. The USPSTF recommends mammography every 1–2 years from age 50 to 75. The American College of Physicians recommends CBE annually at age 40 and begin mammography every 1–2 years after age 50. To further cloud the issue, the American Cancer Society (and 11 other organizations) recommends CBE annually at age 40 and mammography every 1–2 years until age 50 and then annually.	Symmetrical, neg. dimpling, nontender, 1 cm mobile, firm nodule left breast in 6 o'clock position inferior to areola, neg. axillary or supraclavicular adenopathy or nipple discharge.
Genitourinary	It has been at least 17 years since Mrs. Michaels' last PAP and pelvic exam. Patient has not been educated in or performed SBE or had a CBE for the same period of time. Because of her age she is at increased risk for gynecological malignancy and breast pathology. This is a critical time to educate Ann on the importance of SBE and routine gynecological maintenance. Recommendations are fairly consistent for sexually active women or women over 18 years of age. Two to three years of consistently nor-	External genitalia w/o lesions, ulceration, or discharge. Vaginal vault neg. discharge, ulceration, min. erythema w/ sl.dry mucosa, cervix mild inflammation, PAP smear obtained with brush and spatula; neg. pain w/ cervical motion, adnexal mass or tenderness; uterus retroflexed approx. 8 weeks in size. Rectal: Good sphincter tone.

(continued)

SYSTEM	RATIONALE	FINDINGS
	mal annual PAP smears is sufficient to increase PAP smears to every 2–3 years until age 65. The American College of Physicians recommends continued PAP smears every 3 years in women 66–75 if they have not been screened in the last 10 years.	
Orthopedic	Increased incidence of osteoporosis with aging, and increasing risk of fractures and falls. It is important to evaluate her ROM.	ROM w/o pain or limitation of movement; neg erythema, edema, pain w/ palpation; click present right knee; peripheral pulses 2+ bilateral; cap. refill brisk.
Neurological	Assessment of sensory, cognitive, and functional status will provide a baseline for future. Safety issues for an elderly adult living alone can be based on neurological status.	CN II-XII intact, DTRs 2+ bilateral upper & lower extremities; no tremors noted; gait normal; Romberg neg; flexion & extension strength equal bilateral; discrimination of pain intact.

● DIFFERENTIAL DIAGNOSES

Examine all data up to this point. Link the subjective and objective data to the appropriate differential diagnoses. Identify both positive and negative data that support or refute the diagnoses.

DIAGNOSIS	POSITIVE DATA	NEGATIVE DATA
Hypertension	B/P 160/92 RA, + family history, elderly, abnormal cardiac exam.	First time visit, possible white coat HTN.
Decreased visual acuity: possible glaucoma	VA 20/40 OS, 20/60 OD with correction, sees halos around lights, wears bifocals, elderly.	Last exam 4 years ago.

(continued)

DIAGNOSIS	POSITIVE DATA	NEGATIVE DATA
Breast nodule	1 cm mobile, firm nodule in left breast at 6 o'clock position.	No previous personal or FH of breast cancer.
Osteoporosis	Female >65, poor dietary habits, Asian, some exercise, but not consistent, 17 years postmenopausal, no HRT.	No family history of fractures or osteoporosis.
Deficient gyn maintenance	No pap since menopause 17 years ago.	No FH of cervical cancer, no abnormal bleeding.
Deficient immunization	Has had chicken pox, measles, mumps.	Never had flu or pneumovax.

● DIAGNOSTIC TESTS

What screening and diagnostic tests would be appropriate for Ann?

DIAGNOSTIC TEST	RATIONALE	RESULTS
PPD skin test	Do PPD annually if household member with known tuberculosis or others at risk for close contact with the disease (health care professionals, nursing home staff, recent immigrants or refugees, etc.). Ann would qualify because of upcoming involvement as Foster Grandparent.	+ skin test, 10 cm induration.
U/A; CBC, electrolytes, renal panel, liver panel, uric acid, T4, TSH, non-fast. cholesterol & HDL	Baseline lab work. Other labs recommended by USPSTF yearly for those >65.	Cholesterol 247, HDL 32, otherwise WNL.
Mammogram	Baseline; characterize small nodule in left breast.	Benign calcification lt. breast. Recommend annual mammogram.
Fecal occult blood testing	The USPSTF does not recommend routine fecal occult testing. Fecal occult blood tests detect fewer than 50%	Negative hemoccult.

(continued)

DIAGNOSTIC TEST	*RATIONALE*	*RESULTS*
	of colon cancers. The American Cancer Society recommends annual rectal exam beginning at age 40, fecal occult testing annually at age 50, and sigmoido- scopy every 3–5 years after age 50.	
EKG	Electrocardiogram recom- mended for people with 2 or more cardiac risk factors. Abnormal cardiac exam & elev. B/P; if EKG shows LVH then proceed w/ echocardi- ogram.	EKG WNL.
Chest radiograph	Ann has elevated BP and a systolic murmur. The CXR will r/o cardiomegaly. If LVH present, obtain echocardio- gram.	CXR essentially normal with few scattered fibrotic changes.
Bone densitometry	Should be done to determine the extent of Ann's osteo- porosis and if she needs hormonal replacement. Be- cause she is 16 years post- menopause, >65, Asian, poor dietary habits?	Bone densitometry shows risk of fracture for age and osteo- penia.

● DIAGNOSES

What are your conclusive diagnoses? What is your rationale for concluding these diagnoses are correct?

Elevated Blood Pressure

Rationale: Ann's BP is elevated above the accepted normal. Because this is her first visit, she will need to return for serial B/P recheck before you can conclude she has HTN.

Visual Changes

Rationale: Ann's visual acuity reveals that she is not able to be corrected to 20/20. She is also experiencing halos around lights, and a decreased ability to see well at night. Again, she will require further testing before a firm diagnosis can be made. For safety issues, Ann should be cautioned not to drive at night. Keep areas of house well lighted.

Positive PPD Test

Rationale: Reading of PPD in 48 hours after placement revealed a 10-mm erythematous induration.

Osteoporosis

Rationale: Ann is 17 years postmenopausal. The rate of bone loss escalates without estrogen replacement and adequate calcium intake. Further evaluation may be appropriate to evaluate risk of fracture.

● THERAPEUTIC PLAN

1. *What influence does Ann's + PPD have on her participation in the Foster Grandparents program?*

   Mrs. Michaels' PPD skin test is positive. Her chest radiograph is negative for granulomas or calcifications. There is no family or personal history of TB. PPD reading 20 years ago was negative with no knowledge of recent exposure to TB. Initial data show Ann appears immunocompetent with no risk factors for HIV. Based on this information, Ann is not a candidate for prophylactic therapy, because the risk of INH hepatitis is comparable to developing active TB. However, if she becomes immunocompromised, receives long-term high-dose glucocorticoid treatment or develops renal failure, she should be treated with chemoprophylaxis. The Foster Grandparent program can be assured that Ann is not contagious.

2. *What recommendations can you make for Ann in terms of immunizations?*

   Recommend that Ann get:

   Td (tetanus-diptheria booster) now and every 10 years.
   Influenza vaccine—because she is over 65 years, repeated every year.
   Pneumococcal vaccine—because she is over 65 years she should receive one-time immunization.
   Hepatitis B—series recommended in health care occupations, high-risk behavior (IV drug abuse, homosexual men/women). Because Ann is not considered high risk she can determine if she wants the series. She should determine if her insurance will cover the cost of the immunizations.

3. *What counseling would you do for Ann relative to her health promotion and prevention needs? Address the areas of: diet, injury prevention, dental health, hormone replacement therapy, ASA therapy, regular health maintenance.*

Diet and exercise: Limit fats and cholesterol, grains, vegetables, fruits and adequate calcium intake for women (after menopause recommend 1500–2000 mg daily); exercise program (elevated heart rate 20 minutes three times per week).

Injury prevention: Falls, shoulder and lap belts, smoke detectors, smoking in bed, temperature of hot water heater, safety helmets, storage of firearms, CPR training.

Dental health: Biannual dental visits; flossing and brushing.

Hormone replacement therapy (HRT): Estrogen therapy for women at higher risk for osteoporosis is recommended. It would be appropriate to discuss the pros and cons of HRT with Ann, letting her make an informed decision. She could not start on HRT until the Pap results came back WNL.

ASA therapy: Because Ann is postmenopausal without HRT, ASA may decrease her risk for a cardiovascular event. One baby ASA (80 mg) QD is sufficient to obtain the desired results. Research data supporting the use of ASA in women are less conclusive than for men at this time.

Regular health maintenance: Discuss with Ann the importance to return yearly for CBE and gynecological maintenance. Demonstrate how to do an SBE and discuss the need to do monthly (Murphy, 1995).

4. *What therapy would you order for Ann for her osteoporosis? What patient education is appropriate relative to the osteoporosis?*

HRT achieves the most benefit if started within 1 year of menopause. However, HRT can be initiated at any time. The longer Ann takes HRT, the less likely she will get osteoporosis. Ann needs 1500 mg of calcium per day if she does not take HRT. Prior to menopause women need about 1000 mg of calcium per day. Bone loss can be determined with bone densitometry and apropriate treatment based on these findings and a serum calcium.

Ann needs to be educated on risk factors for osteoporosis:

Menopause < 48 y/o
Surgical oopherectomy
Decreased calcium in diet
Lack of exercise
Smoking
FH of osteoporosis
ETOH abuse
Small thin frame, fair skin
Hyperthyroidal
Steroid use

Review safety issues with Ann, such as to avoid loose rugs, wear flat rubber-soled shoes, use hand grips and mats in shower and tub, have a well-lit stairway, and use quadriceps for lifting while bending knees.

5. *When would you have Ann return for follow up?*

Ann would be asked to return for serial BP checks over 3–4 weeks. Weekly readings are preferred, then quarterly, then biannually.

6. *What referrals should be made for Ann?*

Ann should be referred for a complete eye exam. A complete eye exam including glaucoma screen and pupil dilation should be done because her last exam was 4 years ago and she is experiencing vision problems.

REFERENCES

Bates B. *A guide to physical assessment,* 3rd ed. Philadelphia: J.B. Lippincott; 1983.

Department of Health and Human Services. Healthy people 2000. *Report of the Department of Health and Human Services.* Washington, DC: Public Health Service.

Goroll AH, May LA, Mulley A Jr *Primary Care Medicine,* 3rd ed. Philadelphia: J.B. Lippincott; 1995.

Murphy P. Primary care for women: Screening tests and preventive services recommendations. *J Nurse-midwifery,* 1995; 40(2): 74–87.

U.S. Preventive Services Task Force. Guide to clinical preventive services. *Report of the U.S. Preventive Task Force.* Baltimore: Williams & Wilkins; 1996.

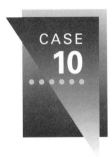

A 30-year-old woman with a headache

SCENARIO

Samantha Crosby, a 30-year-old African-American woman, presents in the clinic with a complaint of a headache that waxes and wanes. She reports that the headache has been present for about a year; however, she is uncertain of the exact onset. She describes the headache as occipital and bifrontal, usually steady but occasionally throbbing, and associated with dizziness and nausea when severe. The pain is generally not relieved by analgesics.

● TENTATIVE DIAGNOSES

Based on the preceding presentation, what are the tentative differential diagnoses?

● HISTORY

What additional history needs to be obtained from Samantha to assist in the development of a diagnosis?

● PHYSICAL ASSESSMENT

Based on the subjective data obtained, what components of the physical examination should be performed and why?

● DIFFERENTIAL DIAGNOSIS

Examine all of the data available to this point. Link the subjective and objective data to the appropriate differential diagnosis. Identify both positive and negative data that support or refute the diagnosis.

● DIAGNOSTIC TESTS

What additional data and/or diagnostic tests, if any, would you do? Include your rationale for the tests.

● DIAGNOSIS

Identify the definitive diagnosis with rationale for Samantha.

● THERAPEUTIC PLAN

1. *What is the usual treatment for chronic tension headaches?*
2. *What reassurance can you give Samantha regarding her headaches?*
3. *What lifestyle modifications might be appropriate for Samantha to help reduce her stress?*
4. *Discuss the concept of preventive versus abortive or symptomatic therapy.*
5. *What are issues to consider before prescribing pharmacologic therapy for Samantha?*
6. *What are pharmacologic choices for symptomatic and preventive therapy?*
7. *What are psychologic interventions that might be appropriate for Samantha?*
8. *What do you decide to prescribe for Samantha?*
9. *When should Samantha return for follow up?*
10. *What patient education should be discussed with Samantha?*
11. *Samantha returns in 2 weeks with little to no improvement in her headaches. She has tried the NSAID with little relief. Her headaches seem to be occurring less frequently since she began attending a yoga class now. What medication, if any, would you prescribe for Samantha?*

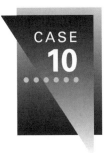

TUTORIAL

A 30-year-old woman with a headache

SCENARIO

Samantha Crosby, a 30-year-old African-American woman presents in the clinic with a complaint of a headache that waxes and wanes. She reports that the headache has been present for about a year; however, she is uncertain of the exact onset. She describes the headache as occipital and bifrontal, usually steady but occasionally throbbing, and associated with dizziness and nausea when severe. The pain is generally not relieved by analgesics.

● TENTATIVE DIAGNOSES

Based on the preceding presentation, what are the tentative differential diagnoses?

DIAGNOSES	RATIONALE
Analgesic rebound	Samantha c/o headache being present over a year. The continuous headache may be associated with withdrawal of pain medication being taken to relieve the headaches.
Cervical spondylosis	Samantha presents with chronic occipital head pain. This symptom may be associated with cervical spondylosis, which is a common cause of headache in middle or late life.
Hypertension	Samantha c/o occipital headache. Rare, however headaches may be associated with hypertension.
Anxiety	Samantha c/o occipital headache, which is frequently associated with cervical muscle contraction and anxiety.

(continued)

DIAGNOSES	*RATIONALE*
Cerebral tumor	Samantha presents with moderate to severe occipital and frontal headaches. Has dizziness, nausea, and vomiting when headaches are severe. Possible indicator of cerebral tumor.
Chronic tension-type headache	Samantha presents c/o a headache of over 1 year duration that is occipital and bifrontal, usually steady but occasionally throbbing and associated with dizziness, nausea, and vomiting when severe. These are all symptoms common to chronic tension-type headache.
Migraine headache	Samantha c/o occasional throbbing pain associated with dizziness, nausea, and vomiting when severe. These symptoms frequently are associated with migraine headaches.

● HISTORY

What additional history needs to be obtained from Samantha to assist in the development of a diagnosis?

REQUESTED DATA	*DATA ANSWER*
Allergies	None.
Previous diagnosis of headaches/ever been treated?	None previously diagnosed. However, reports having similar type of headaches at 16 years of age for about 2 years.
Tell me more about your headache—when and where does it start, how long does it last? Describe the pain.	Pain at onset starts in occipital and posterior region of the neck and progresses to the frontal area of the head. Headache is daily and continuous for over a year. Pain becomes bilateral. Pain is dull and pressing; however, when it becomes severe it is throbbing. Usually pain is better when lying down, gets worse later in day, and when she feels stressed.
Does the pain *prohibit* usual daily activities? Is the pain aggravated by mild physical activity?	Usually pain doesn't prevent activities. However, recently she has had to stop what she was doing with a few of the episodes. Coughing, sneezing, etc., do not increase the pain. Pain usually lasts about 4 days and has about six major episodes per month.

(continued)

REQUESTED DATA

DATA ANSWER

REQUESTED DATA	DATA ANSWER
Presence of associated features: nausea, vomiting, photophobia, phonophobia.	When severe, has nausea and vomiting. Sometimes has phonophobia and photophobia. Feelings of fatigue.
Presence of an aura; if yes, describe the aura.	No prodrome or aura.
Potential precipitating factors: dietary factors, relationship to menses, psychosocial stressors, other factors identified by the patient.	Headaches become more severe when there are conflicts and stress at home or at work.
Medication history: Drugs tried for *symptomatic relief* of headache (both over-the-counter and prescription medications). Prophylactic medications Current medications (include dose, length of time the drug has been taken, and effectiveness).	Excedrin Long-Acting. Presently taking no prophylactic medication or any other medications.
Nonpharmacologic therapies (e.g., biofeedback, hot or cold compresses, sleep). Note effectiveness.	Uses wet heat packs to neck and forehead, brings some relief.
Allergies	None.
Childhood illness/immunizations	Had all childhood illnesses and immunizations.
Past medical history/ surgeries/transfusions/ hospitalizations/fractures/ injuries/accidents	Usually healthy, only hospitalizations for childbirth.
OBG history	LNMP: 1/15/97. Last pelvic: 18 months ago. Last mammogram: None. G 2 P 2 A 0 Contraception used: tubal ligation.
Appetite/24-hour diet recall	B: Cereal with skim milk, sometimes coffee. L: Ham sandwich, pretzels, orange. D: Pizza, salad with ranch dressing, candy bar. S: Soda, popcorn.

(continued)

REQUESTED DATA	DATA ANSWER
Sleeping	Reports having difficulty sleeping, wakes up about 2 AM.
Social history	Tobacco: Used to smoke, quit about 5 years ago. Alcohol: Rare, social only. Drugs: Denies. Caffeinated beverages: 1–2 cups coffee, 1–2 sodas. Exercise: Sporadic. Social organizations: Goes to church, participates in church choir.
Family history	Father: 54, HTN. Mother: 52, has similar H/As. Sister: 32, has similar H/As. Spouse: 27, healthy. Children: Boy, 5, in good health; girl, 3, in good health.
Employment/finances/ insurance	Works as an accountant at a local medical center. She carries the health/dental insurance. She and her husband own their own home.
Relationship with husband, children, and family	Gets along well with family. She and her husband have been married for 9 years. The children were planned, and get along well with mother. At times feels stressed while trying to work and take care of home. Her family lives close, and they interact about 1×/week.
How do you handle stress?	Reports feeling anxious at times. Worried about what headaches may mean. Usually tries to get time by herself or lay down. Things stressful at work lately. She is worried about the medical center downsizing.

● PHYSICAL ASSESSMENT

Based on the subjective data obtained, what components of the physical examination should be performed and why?

SYSTEM	RATIONALE	FINDINGS
Height, weight, vital signs	Provides baseline data.	Ht. (without shoes): 5′ 4″ Weight (dressed): 136 lbs. T. 98.4 F., P. 80, regular, R. 18, BP: 124/82 rt. arm lying down,

(continued)

SYSTEM	RATIONALE	FINDINGS
		126/80 lt. arm lying down, 122/78 rt. arm immediately after getting up, 124/80 lt. arm immediately after getting up.
General/skin	Provides general overview of status of patient (Bates et al., 1995).	Appears fatigued but alert and cooperative, oriented and coherent. Somewhat anxious. Skin: warm to touch, no lesions, a 1-cm scar on rt. forearm.
HEENT	Brief screening. Important to evaluate anything that may have impact on H/As. Important to check for optic disc pressure or changes in visual field.	Normocephalic, no sinus pain. Vision corrected with glasses to 20/20 in each eye. Visual fields normal. Sclera clear. PERRLA, EOM intact. Disc margins sharp, red reflex present. No arterial narrowing or AV nicking. Rt. and lt. canals partially blocked with cerumen. TMs shiny gray with cone of light present. Trachea midline, thyroid nonpalpable, supple. No bruit. No LA.
Thorax and lungs	Provides baseline information.	CTA.
Cardiovascular	Provides baseline information.	Heart regular rhythm, no MRG.
Peripheral vascular	Brief screening information related to cardiovascular status.	No stasis pigmentation or ulcers of the lower extremities. Pulses 2+, no edema.
Abdomen	Checking for organomegaly.	Flat and symmetrical with good muscle tone. Bowel sounds +. No HSM; no CVA tenderness. No masses. No bruits.
Musculoskeletal	Important to determine tenseness of muscles in light of possible tension headaches.	Frontal, temporal, parietal, occipital, and pericranial muscles tight and tender on deep palpation. Normal gait and ROM.

(continued)

SYSTEM	RATIONALE	FINDINGS
Neurological	Important system to deter-mine if any pathological causes of headaches (Bates et al., 1995).	*Motor and sensory:* Gait nor-mal, muscle strength 5/5 throughout. Romberg nega-tive, pinprick, light touch, position, vibration, and stereognosis intact. Kernig's sign and Brudzin-ski's sign absent. *Cranial nerves I - XII:* Intact. *DTRs:* 2+.

● DIFFERENTIAL DIAGNOSIS

Examine all of the data available to this point. Link the subjective and objec-tive data to the appropriate differential diagnosis. Identify both positive and negative data that support or refute the diagnosis.

DIAGNOSIS	POSITIVE DATA	NEGATIVE DATA
Analgesic rebound	Headache over a year. Used analgesic medication for relief of H/As.	Associated with repetitive use of pain medication.
Cervical spondylosis	Chronic occipital head pain that worsens later in the day.	Occurs in middle or late life, no pain with neck movement. No crepitus.
HTN	H/As originating in the occi-pital area of the head, African-American.	B/P not elevated.
Cerebral tumor	Steadily worsening pain with N/V. H/A for over a year.	No neurological symptoms. H/A present on waking every day, decreasing after being up several hours.
Anxiety	Anxiety episodes. Difficulty handling stress at this time.	Alert, appropriate.
Migraine H/A	Unilateral throbbing pain assoc. with dizziness, N/V when severe. Increased with stress, light, and noise.	Aura.

(continued)

DIAGNOSIS	POSITIVE DATA	NEGATIVE DATA
	H/A when awakening from sleep +FH. Female.	
Chronic tension H/A	Frequent H/A, +FH. Bilateral dull aching, nonpulsating pain. Pain in occipital and cervical areas. + cervical muscle tightness, female, + FH.	N/V.

● DIAGNOSTIC TESTS

What additional data and/or diagnostic tests, if any, would you do? Include your rationale for the tests.

DIAGNOSTIC TEST	RATIONALE	RESULTS
Hemoglobin and hematocrit, CBC with differential blood chemistry	To rule out inflammatory and infectious conditions.	H/H: 14/38. All labs WNL.
Head CT or brain MRI.	No evidence of secondary type of headache. These tests are only indicated if a patient describes an atypical headache pattern, changes in headache pattern, or recent onset of persistent headaches.	Not done at this time.

● DIAGNOSIS

Identify the definitive diagnosis with rationale for Samantha.

Chronic tension-type headache mixed with migraine without aura (sometimes called mixed headache).

Diagnosis is based on the International Society for Headaches (ISH) diagnostic criteria for migraine without aura and tension-type headache (Couch, 1993; Dalessio, 1994; Diamond, 1992; Dubose et al., 1995; Olsen, 1988).

Supporting Data

Chronic tension-type headache:

- Increased tenderness of pericranial muscles demonstrated by manual palpation.
- Average headache frequency 15 d/mos (180 d/y) for 6 mos.
- Pressing quality of pain most of the time and does not inhibit activities.
- History and PE do not suggest a secondary cause of headache.

Migraine without aura headache:

- At least 5 attacks.
- Headache lasting 4–72 hours.
- Pulsating quality when severe.
- Occasionally has nausea and vomiting, photophobia, and phonophobia.

● THERAPEUTIC PLAN

1. What is the usual treatment for chronic tension?

Chronic tension-type headaches usually are treated with conservative modalities, pharmacologic agents, and in some cases psychologic intervention (Isselbacher et al., 1994).

2. What reassurance can you give Samantha regarding her headaches?

Samantha should be reassured that this is not a life-threatening disorder. She should be encouraged to actively participate in her own plan of care. It may take several trials to find the best therapy for her.

3. What lifestyle modifications might be appropriate for Samantha to help reduce her stress?

1. Topical heat or cold packs applied to affected muscles.
2. Respite (rest, sleep, vacation) from stressors.
3. Stress-reduction techniques (eg, regular exercise, sexual activity, relaxation therapy, physical therapy, electromyographic biofeedback, and/or hypnotherapy). Work and home stresses should be discussed and reduced if possible.
4. Dietary modifications: avoid chocolate, processed meats, and caffeine.

It is important to try lifestyle modifications first before considering medications. If H/As are disrupting Samantha's life or if the pain is severe, or if simple measures have failed then pharmacologic therapy should be considered (Diamond, 1992).

4. Discuss the concept of preventive versus abortive or symptomatic therapy.

Abortive or symptomatic therapy is used to treat symptoms once they occur or to prevent H/As after warning signs have appeared (aura). Preventive therapy is a prophylactic therapy to reduce the frequency of H/As. Preventive therapy should only be used after symptomatic therapy has failed. Samantha will need to understand the concept of preventive therapy and not take the medication to relieve acute pain.

5. *What are issues to consider before prescribing pharmacologic therapy for Samantha?*

The choice of pharmacologic therapy depends on the clinical situation. Consider:

- Side effects
- History of prior response
- Concurrent medical or psychological illness
- Other medications patient is taking
- Cost
- Length of treatment

Use the least potent and least addictive analgesic medication that relieves most of the patient's pain. Samantha has already tried Excedrin and it has not relieved her pain.

Headaches usually respond to medications such as ASA, NSAIDs. Sometimes combinations of ASA, caffeine, and a small of barbiturate can provide relief for moderate H/A when there is significant muscle contraction; however, daily use of this medication can cause a "rebound" H/A. Because of their addictive nature, narcotic medications should be avoided in treating H/As of a benign nature. Many patients report that narcotics do not themselves relieve the H/A, but allow them to go to sleep, and it is sleep that provides the best relief (Stevens, 1993; Weiss, 1993).

6. *What are pharmacologic choices for symptomatic and preventive therapy?*

Choices for Symptomatic Therapy for H/As

PAIN RELIEF OF MIGRAINE HEADACHES

Mild

ASA, NSAIDs, (with Reglan—enhances effectiveness of analgesic drugs) Isometheptene (Midrin)

Moderate–Severe

Ergotamine (Cafergot, Wigraine)
Dihydroergotamine (D.H.E. 45) recommended for severe pain
Sumatriptan succinate (Imitrex) 6 mg subq. or 25–100 mg oral

Choices for Preventive Therapy

PREVENTIVE OR PROPHYLACTIC THERAPY
....

Serotonin Inhibitors

Methysergide (Sansert)
Cyproheptadine (Periactin)

Beta-adrenergic Blockers

Propranolol (Inderal)
Nadolol (Corgard)
Atenolol (Tenormin)

Calcium-Channel Blockers

Verapamil (Calan)
Diltiazem (Cardizem)
Nifedipine (Procardia)

Antidepressants

Buspirone (Buspar)
Sertraline HCl (Zoloft)
Amitriptyline (Elavil)
Imipramine (Tofranil)
Trimipramine (Surmontil)
Doxepin (Sinequan)

Stevens, 1993; Weiss, 1993

---

7. *What are psychologic interventions that might be appropriate for Samantha?*

   Individual counseling or family counseling may be indicated when stressors at home are associated with the development of tension and migraine headaches.

8. *What do you decide to prescribe for Samantha?*

   After hearing the information presented, Samantha decides to try an OTC NSAID. She has used them for menstrual cramping and find they work well. She agrees to try some of the lifestyle measures to see if they help.

9. *When should Samantha return for follow up?*

   Samantha should make an appointment in 2 weeks to evaluate the effects of the medication and to determine if the recommendations for exercise, rest, relaxation techniques, and so on are helping. Explore further with Samantha any precipitant factors that may be associated with headaches.

10. What patient education should be discussed with Samantha?

Samantha should be told about headaches, dangers of drug overuse, need for stress reduction, and so on.

Encourage her to follow a healthy lifestyle, with good nutrition, regular exercise, and adequate sleep. Counsel Samantha to avoid situations and substances that are known precipitants. Recommend to Samantha that when pain occurs, she use physical measures (as well as medications) such as relaxation techniques, application of cold or heat at site of pain, and decrease environmental stimuli.

11. Samantha returns in 2 weeks with little to no improvement in her headaches. She has tried the NSAID with little relief. Her headaches seem to be occurring less frequently since she began attending a yoga class. What medication, if any, would you prescribe for Samantha?

Since Samantha's H/As are usually mild to moderate, Midrin will be tried as a symptomatic pain reliever. If this relieves her pain, but she continues to have H/As, the next step would be to discuss preventive medications. For severe H/As with N/V, the option of Imitrex self-injections might be an option.

REFERENCES

Bates B, Bickley LS, Hoekelman RA. *A Guide to Physical Examination and History Taking,* 6th ed. Philadelphia: J.B. Lippincott; 1995.

Couch JR. Headache to worry about. *Med Clin N Am,* 1993; 77(1): 141–167.

Dalessio DJ. Diagnosing the severe headache. *Neurology* 1994; (suppl 3): 21–30.

Diamond S. Acute headache: Differential diagnosis and management of three types. *Postgrad Med* 1992; 29(8): 21–29.

Dubose CD., Cutlip AC, Cutlip WD. Migraines and other headaches: An approach to diagnosis and classification. *Am Fam Phys* 1995; 54(6): 1498–1504.

Isselbacher KJ, Braunwald E, Wilson JD, Martin JB, Fauci AS, Kasper DL. *Harrison's Principles of Internal Medicine,* 13th ed. New York: McGraw-Hill; 1994.

Olsen J. Headache Classification Committee of the International Headache Society. Classification and diagnostic criteria for headache disorders, cranial neuralgia, and facial pain. *Cephalalgia* 1988; 8(suppl 7): 1–96.

Stevens MB. Tension-type headaches. *Am Fam Physician* 1993; 47(4): 799–805.

Weiss J. Assessment and management of the client with headaches. *Nurse Practitioner* 1993; 18(4): 44–57.

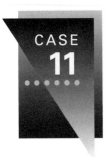

A 28-year-old woman
with cough and fatigue

SCENARIO

Barb Jones is a 28-year-old obese, Caucasian female who was seen 2 weeks ago for a cough productive of yellow sputum, dyspnea, and fatigue. She was treated for bronchitis and given a course of antibiotics. She presents today with progressive dyspnea, orthopnea, and paroxysmal nocturnal dyspnea. She continues with a cough productive of yellow sputum. She also complains of abdominal tightness, bloating, nausea, and worsening fatigue.

● TENTATIVE DIAGNOSES

Based on Barb's presentation and symptoms, what are the differential diagnoses? Include rationale for each.

● HISTORY

What further information from her history is necessary to assist in developing a diagnosis?

● PHYSICAL ASSESSMENT

Based on the subjective data, what parts of the physical examination should be performed and why?

● DIFFERENTIAL DIAGNOSES

What are the significant positive and negative data that support or refute the differential diagnoses for Barb Jones?

● DIAGNOSTIC TESTS

What additional data and/or diagnostics are needed to confirm the priority diagnosis? Include your rationale for the tests.

● DIAGNOSES

After combining subjective and objective data with test findings, what is the diagnosis? Identify data that support this diagnosis.

● THERAPEUTIC PLAN

1. *What type of CHF (systolic vs diastolic) should Barb be treated for?*
2. *What are the pharmacologic agents you should prescribe for Barb Jones?*
3. *What education should be presented and reviewed with Barb and her family?*
4. *What are the dietary restrictions you would recommend to Barb and her family?*

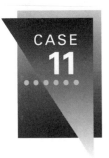

TUTORIAL

A 28-year-old woman with cough and fatigue

SCENARIO

Barb Jones is a 28-year-old obese, Caucasian female who was seen 2 weeks ago for a cough productive of yellow sputum, dyspnea, and fatigue. She was treated for bronchitis and given a course of antibiotics. She presents today with progressive dyspnea, orthopnea, and paroxysmal nocturnal dyspnea. She continues with a cough productive of yellow sputum. She also complains of abdominal tightness, bloating, nausea, and worsening fatigue.

● TENTATIVE DIAGNOSES

What are the potential diagnoses you have identified based on the preceding scenario?

DIAGNOSIS	RATIONALE
Bronchitis	Ms. Jones presents with a productive cough and dyspnea.
Congestive heart failure	Barb presents with shortness of breath, progressive dyspnea, orthopnea, nocturnal dyspnea, and fatigue. Her abdominal complaints are suspicious of signs for right heart failure.
Hypothryoidism	Progressive fatigue may be a symptom of a thyroid abnormality.
Anemia	Fatigue and dyspnea are symptoms of anemia. Anemia is a possibility since Barb is of menstruating age.
Peptic ulcer disease/GERD	Barb complains of abdominal tightness, bloating, and nausea. All are symptoms of a GI disorder.

● HISTORY

What further information from her history is necessary to assist in developing a diagnosis?

REQUESTED DATA	DATA ANSWER
Medication	Omeprozole (Prilosec) 20 mg BID.
	Clarithromycin (Biaxin) 500 mg BID.
	Albuterol (Proventil) MDI.
	Metoclopramide (Reglan) 10 mg QID.
Allergies	Sulfa.
Past medical history surgeries	S/P C-section × 2; 1988, 1990.
	S/P cholecystectomy, 1992.
	S/P tubal ligation, 1990.
OB/GYN history	LMP 2 weeks ago.
	G2P2A0.
Sleep pattern	Difficulty sleeping over last month secondary to dyspnea.
Social history	Married with 2 children (ages 5 and 7).
	Works full time as certified nurse assistant.
	Nonsmoker.
	Alcohol: None.
	No history of recreational drug use.
Family history	Father: deceased, age 49, CHF, COPD.
	Mother: living, age 51, history of CHF, HTN.
	2 siblings: ages 33 and 25, alive and well.
Weight change/appetite	Decreased appetite secondary to nausea.
	Weight gain of 7 pounds over last month.
	Caffeine: 6 Mountain Dew a day.

● PHYSICAL ASSESSMENT

Based on the subjective data, what parts of the physical examination should be performed?

SYSTEM	FINDINGS
Skin	Mucous membranes and nailbeds pink. No cyanosis. Skin cool and clammy.
Breath sounds	Few wheezes posteriorly. Bibasilar rales.
Heart sounds	No JVD. Carotid upstrokes full. +S_3 gallop; II/VI holosystolic murmur heard best at apex with radiation to L. axilla.
Vital signs	T: 98.9, B/P 124/62, Apical pulse: 114 and regular at rest, RR: 24 and shallow.
Abdominal	Morbidly obese. Abdomen distended with BS present. Epigastric tenderness. Liver span 14–16 cm by percussion.
Extremities	2+ Pitting pretibial edema bilaterally; 2+ peripheral pulses; no cyanosis or clubbing noted.

● DIFFERENTIAL DIAGNOSES

What are the significant positive and negative data that support or refute the differential diagnoses for Ms. Jones?

DIAGNOSIS	POSTIVE DATA	NEGATIVE FINDINGS
Bronchitis	Cough, wheezes, dyspnea, production of sputum.	Acute onset, fever, pleuritic pain.
CHF	Dyspnea, orthopnea/PND, rales, +S3, edema, weight gain, hepatomegaly.	JVD.
Hypothyroidism	Lethargy/fatigue, weight gain, edema, decreased appetite.	Dry skin, decreased bowel sounds.
Anemia	Fatigue, dyspnea, hepatomegaly, menstruation.	Pale mucous membranes, bruising, hematuria.
Peptic ulcer disease/ GERD	Nausea, abdominal bloating, epigastric tenderness, caffeine use.	Smoking history, alcohol use, epigastric burning, NSAIDs.

● DIAGNOSTIC TESTS

What additional data and/or diagnostics are needed to confirm the priority diagnosis? Include your rationale for the tests.

DIAGNOSTIC TEST	RATIONALE	RESULTS
CXR	Assess for cardiomegaly, pulmonary vasculature, pleural effusion.	Cardiomegaly, pulmonary vasculature.
Echocardiogram	Assess left ventricular function, ejection fraction, valvular abnormalities, heart chamber size.	Four-chamber dilation, LV ejection fraction 30%, presence of mitral regurgitation.
ECG	Assess heart rhythm. Rule out arrhythmia and ischemia.	Sinus tachycardia without ischemic changes.
Thyroid profile	Assess if thyroid disorder is present. An elevated TSH with a low T_4 supports primary hypothyroidism. Heart failure may be caused or aggravated by thyroid disorder.	TSH 12 µg/dL. T_4 2.5 µg/dL.
Hemoglobin and hematocrit	Assess hemoglobin and hematocrit. If these values are low, perform CBC.	Hgb: 12.0. HCT: 37.5.
Chemistry 20	Includes electrolytes, liver enzymes, and renal function. Elevated serum creatinine may indicate renal abnormality that causes volume overload.	K+ 4.3. BUN/creatinine: 13/1.1. LDH: 320. SGPT: 69. SGOT: 63.

● DIAGNOSES

After combining subjective and objective data with test findings, what is the diagnosis? Identify data that support this diagnosis.

Congestive Heart Failure

Evidence of right-side and left-side heart failure (biventricular). Secondary to dilated cardiomyopathy with a moderate-to-markedly decreased LV ejection fraction (? etiology, idiopathic vs viral).

Data Supporting the Diagnosis of Congestive Heart Failure

1. Progressive dyspnea with the presence of orthopnea.
2. Chest radiograph: Increase in pulmonary vasculature and cardiomegaly.
3. Echocardiogram: Markedly impaired systolic function with a decrease in the ejection fraction.
4. Physical findings:
   a. Bibasilar rales
   b. Peripheral edema
   c. Nausea, abdominal distension, and bloating with hepatomegaly. Elevated liver enzymes, secondary to portal congestion consistent with right-side heart failure.
   Weight gain with decreased appetite (Hoole et al., 1995).

Hypothyroidism

Decreased T_4, elevated TSH, chronic fatigue.

● THERAPEUTIC PLAN

1. What type of CHF (systolic vs diastolic) should Barb be treated for?

The plan of care for Barb Jones should address CHF secondary to systolic dysfunction.

2. What are the pharmacologic agents you should prescribe for Barb Jones?

Pharmacologic Treatment

A. ACE inhibitor/vasodilator

Assists with afterload reduction. Titrate to blood pressure response, dizziness, or other side effects.

Caution should be taken with concurrent use of potassium-sparing diuretics.

	STARTING DOSE, MG	MAXIMUM DOSE, MG
Enalapril (Vasotec)	2.5 BID	20 BID
Captopril (Capoten)	6.25–12.5 TID	50 TID
Lisinopril (Zesteril)	5 QD	20 QD

(continued)

	STARTING DOSE, MG	MAXIMUM DOSE, MG
Quinapril (Accupril)	5 BID	20 BID
Moexipril (Univasc)	7.5 QD	30 QD

Contraindications to use of ACE inhibitors include hyperkalemia (serum potassium >5.5 mEQ/L that is nonreducible), pre-renal azotemia, or history of adverse reaction to ACE inhibitors. In this case, consider hydralazine/isosorbide (Konstam, 1994).

B. Diuretics

Diuretics should be started if symptoms of volume overload are evident. Assessment of baseline potassium levels is important prior to initiation.

STARTING DOSE

Hydrochlorothiazide HydroDiuril	25 mg qd
Furosemide (Lasix)	20–40 mg QD

Follow-up monitoring of electrolytes and renal function necessary. Once serum potassium levels are stable, check every few months.

May need to use higher doses in renally impaired patients and lower doses in the elderly population.

C. Lanoxin

Lanoxin is indicated for use in patients with severe heart failure and symptomatic mild-to-moderate heart failure after treatment with ACE inhibitors and diuretics.

Initial dose: 0.25 mg QD

Use 0.125mg QD in the presence of reduced renal function and elderly and baseline conduction abnormality. A serum digoxin level test at 1 week after therapy is started is recommended. Titrate to a therapeutic response. Monitor for signs of digoxin toxicity with an elevated serum level (Konstam, 1994).

Refer to physician if difficulty develops in keeping a patient's condition compensated.

Barb Jones' medication profile:

DRUG	DOSE, QD
Lisinopril (Zestril)	5 mg
Furosemide (Lasix)	40 mg
KCl	10 mEq
Lanoxin	0.25 mg
Levothyroxine (Synthroid)	0.05 mg

3. *What education should be presented and reviewed with Barb and her family?*

   A. Educate the patient and family about medications, the disease process, importance of follow up, and medication compliance.
   B. Instruct the patient and family on early signs of recurrent or worsening heart failure. Modify activity as necessary. Regular exercise is encouraged to increase functional status and decrease symptoms.
   C. Smoking cessation should be strongly reinforced.
   D. Influenza and pneumonia vaccinations are recommended for heart failure patients unless there is a previous contraindication.
   E. A record of daily weights is important. A weight gain of 3–5+ pounds in 1 week should be reported to the health care provider (Smith et al., 1992).

4. *What are the dietary restrictions you would recommend to Barb and her family?*

   A. Dietary restrictions include:
      1. Low sodium diet (2 gms a day)
      2. Fluid restriction if indicated
      3. No more than one beer, mixed drink, or glass of wine should be consumed daily.

REFERENCES

Hoole A, Pickard C, Ouimette R, Lohr J, and Greenberg R. *Patient Care Guidelines for Nurse Practitioners* (4th ed.). Philadelphia: J.B. Lippincott; 1995.

Konstam M, Dracup K. *Heart Failure: Evaluation and Care of Patients with Left Ventricular Systolic Dysfunction, Clinical Practice Guideline* No. 11. AHCPR Publication 94-0613. Agency for Health Care Policy and Research, Public Health Service, U.S. Department of Health and Human Services: 1994.

Smith T, Brawnwald E, Kelly R. The management of heart failure. In *Heart Disease: A Textbook of Cardiovascular Medicine*. Philadelphia: W.B. Saunders; 1992: 464–509.

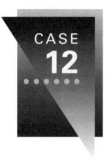

A 36-year-old woman with a breast lump

SCENARIO

Jeanie Stone is a 36-year-old Russian female who noticed a lump 2 days ago in her right breast. She is concerned it might be cancer.

● TENTATIVE DIAGNOSES

Based on the information provided so far, what are potential differential diagnoses?

● HISTORY

What are significant questions in Jeanie's history?

● PHYSICAL ASSESSMENT

What are the significant portions of the physical examination that should be completed for Jeanie?

● DIFFERENTIAL DIAGNOSES

What are the significant positive and negative data that support or refute your diagnoses for Jeanie?

● DIAGNOSTIC TESTS

Based on the history and physical examinations, what, if any, diagnostic tests would you do. Include your rationale for the tests.

● DIAGNOSIS

What diagnoses do you determine are appropriate for Jeanie?

● THERAPEUTIC PLAN

1. *What psychosocial interventions can you use for Jeanie concerning her anxiety?*

2. *What instructions will you give to Jeanie regarding the mammogram?*

3. *To whom should Jeanie be referred for a biopsy?*

4. *What suggestions would you make for Jeanie to control the discomfort of having fibrocystic disease?*

5. *What preventive measures would you recommend to Jeanie?*

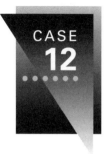

TUTORIAL

A 36-year-old woman with a breast lump

SCENARIO

Jeanie Stone is a 36-year-old Russian female who noticed a lump 2 days ago in her right breast. She is concerned it might be cancer.

● TENTATIVE DIAGNOSES

What are the potential diagnoses you have identified based on the preceding scenario?

DIAGNOSIS	RATIONALE
Fibrocystic breast disease	Jeanie has a breast lump.
Fibroadenoma	Jeanie has a breast lump. Fibroadenoma is the most common benign tumor in the female breast, occurring most often in 20- to 30-year-olds (Woolf et al., 1996).
Breast cancer	Risk of breast cancer in U.S. women is 1/9. A breast mass is the usual presenting symptom.

● HISTORY

1. What are significant questions in Jeanie's history?

REQUESTED DATA   DATA ANSWER

REQUESTED DATA	DATA ANSWER
Allergies	NKA.
Current medications	OCPs, vitamins. Takes ASA occasionally for headaches.
Surgery/transfusions	No surgery/no transfusions.
Past medical history and hospitalizations/fractures/injuries/accidents	Healthy, no hospitalizations other than for childbirth.
Present illness: How did she notice the mass, is it tender, describe the lump in terms of size, mobility, any enlarged lymph nodes, previous breast surgery, nipple discharge.	Noticed the lump while taking a shower. Not sure if she ever noticed it before. It feels like the tip of her finger, firm, and seems to move when she touches it. At times during her period her breasts seem very sore, and it is hard for her to exercise and run. Denies nipple discharge, enlarged lymph nodes, or previous breast surgery. Breastfed all her children for 5 months.
OB/GYN history	Menarche: 10. Cycle: Periods every 28–30 days, lasting 7 days. Periods are heavy intially, but then very scant bleeding. C/o some dysmenorrhea for first day, but it is controlled with ASA. LNMP: Due to start any day. Last pap/pelvic/breast exam: $1\frac{1}{2}$ years ago. Mammogram: Never had one. BSE: Not real regular. G 3 P 3 A 0
Social history	Tobacco: never smoked. Alcohol: Rare social, white wine. Drugs: Denies. Caffeine: Drinks decaffeinated sodas. Exercise: Bikes or runs regularly.
Diet/appetite/weight change	Eats a healthy diet. Husband competes in triathlons and is usually in training. Tries to eat low-fat diet, no or little added salt. Usually bakes meats. Weight has been stable for many years.
Family history	Father: 68, HTN. Mother: 67, frail, DM. Siblings: 7 siblings, 4 brothers, 2 with ETOH abuse, and 1 with MS; 3 sisters, 1 with non-Hodgkin's lymphoma. Husband: 45, healthy, runs, swims, bikes on regular basis. Children: 3 boys, 13, 11, 7, all healthy, all compete in sports.
Family history of breast cancer	No first-degree relatives with history of breast cancer.

● PHYSICAL ASSESSMENT

What are the significant portions of the physical examination that should be completed for Jeanie?

SYSTEM	RATIONALE	FINDINGS
Vital signs	Provides baseline data.	B/P 110/58 HR 56 R 20 T 98.2 Ht. 5'8" Wt. 130
General appearance/skin	Provides overall perspective of patient's status.	Healthy-looking female sitting on exam table. No skin lesions.
Lungs	Provides baseline data.	CTA.
Heart	Provides baseline data.	RRR, no MRG.
Breasts	Thorough evaluation because system involved.	Breasts symmetrical. Normal contour, no increased vascular pattern. No discolorations, retraction, dimpling or edema. No axillary, supraclavicular, or infraclavicular lymph nodes palpable. Breasts somewhat lumpy, primarily in outer quadrants. Small, firm, mobile, somewhat tender lesion, 1 cm in size located at 2 o'clock on rt. breast.

● DIFFERENTIAL DIAGNOSES

What are the significant positive and negative findings that support or refute your diagnoses for Jeanie?

DIAGNOSIS	POSITIVE DATA	NEGATIVE DATA
Fibrocystic breast disease	Tender breast lump, no FH of breast cancer, lump occurring premenstrually.	No c/o bilateral breast pain, menses occurring before age 11.

(continued)

DIAGNOSIS	POSITIVE DATA	NEGATIVE DATA
Fibroadenoma	Tender breast lump, no FH of breast cancer, single, firm, mobile breast mass.	Menses occurring before age 11, tender breast lump.
Breast cancer	Breast lump in rt. breast, menses occurring before age 11, occurs in women $\frac{1}{9}$; 95% of cases occur in women >35.	Tender breast lump, no FH of breast cancer, no nipple discharge.

● DIAGNOSTIC TESTS

Based on the history and physical examination, what, if any, diagnostic tests would you do?

DIAGNOSTIC TEST	RATIONALE	RESULTS
Mammogram	Initial test ordered to evaluate lump.	Fibrocystic breast disease.
Fine needle aspiration	Can be done when mass is easily palpable and cystlike.	Not done.
Open biopsy	Definitive step in diagnosing breast cancer.	Not done.

● DIAGNOSES

What diagnoses do you determine as being appropriate after a review of the subjective and objective data? Fibrocystic breast disease with cyst.

Data Supporting the Diagnosis

No + FH of breast cancer in first-degree relatives
Tender breast lump that occurred premenstrually
Firm, mobile lump, + mammogram for fibrocystic changes

● THERAPEUTIC PLAN

1. *What psychosocial interventions can you use for Jeanie concerning her anxiety?*

You can inform Jeanie about the frequency and generally benign nature of breast changes. Although women without a +FH also get breast cancer, you can reassure her that she does not have many risk factors for breast cancer. She does not have a +FH, she eats a healthy diet and exercises. You can also explain that 50% of women have fibrocystic disease. This disease causes small multiple cysts that respond to hormonal changes around the period. Mammography will help demonstrate the fibrocystic disease in Jeanie's breasts.

2. *What instructions will you give to Jeanie regarding the mammogram?*

Tell Jeanie that the mammogram may be uncomfortable owing to the compression of the breast. It is usually not painful. It might be less painful for Jeanie to wait until after her period to have the mammogram. ASA, ibuprofen, or acetaminophen may help decrease breast tenderness. Deodorant and powder may interfere with the accuracy of the X-ray, so Jeanie should be instructed not to wear them to the exam.

3. *To whom should Jeanie be referred for a biopsy?*

If Jeanie is still concerned or the mammogram is unequivical concerning diagnosis, she should be referred to a surgeon for an open biopsy. In many cities there are surgeons who specialize in diseases of the breast.

4. *What suggestions would you make for Jeanie to control the discomfort of having fibrocystic disease?*

- Oral contraceptives may slow or prevent the development of new fibrocystic changes. Symptoms are suppressed in 70%–90% of women with fibrocystic changes.
- Vitamin E (150–600 IU daily) may decrease the pain and tenderness associated with fibrocystic changes of the breast. Although controversial, vitamin E has proven effective in relieving the symptoms in some women. A trial should be used for 2–3 months.
- Danazol (Danocrine) also will reduce pain, tenderness, and nodularity caused by fibrocystic changes. This drug should only be used after other methods have failed.
- Caffeine consumption should be reduced, since this may reduce tenderness and nodularity. Jeanie should decrease her intake of cola, coffee, and chocolate from her diet.
- Other lifestyle changes that may be effective include: low-salt diet, warm compresses, support bra, and mild analgesics (Branch, 1994; Uphold & Graham, 1994).

5. *What preventive measures would you recommend to Jeanie?*

The NP should review with Jeanie the importance of doing regular BSE. This is particularly important since she has fibrocystic changes in her breasts. If done on a regular basis, Jeanie will become familiar with the nodules/cysts in her breasts, and the effect of the hormonal changes on them. The NP should demonstrate the recommended technique for BSE and have Jeanie return the demonstration. Using breast models with lump or masses may help in giving Jeanie the confidence to recognize what she is feeling for in the BSE.

Jeanie should have a mammogram once between 35 and 40, every 1–2 years between 40 and 50, and annually thereafer (Woolf, 1996).

REFERENCES

Branch L. Breast health, in Youngkin E, Davis M. (eds). *Women's Health: Primary Care Clinical Guide.* Norwalk, CT: Appleton Lange; 1994.

Uphold C, Graham M. *Clinical Guidelines in Family Practice,* 2nd ed. Gainesville, FL: Barmarrae Books; 1994.

Woolf S, Jonas S, Lawrence R. *Health Promotion and Disease Prevention in Clinical Practice.* Baltimore: Williams & Wilkins; 1996.

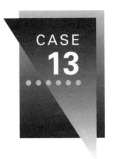

A 15-year-old boy requesting well physical and sports examination

SCENARIO:

John is a 15-year-old African-American male. He presents for a pre-participation physical exam for football. He has been in good health since his last physical exam 1 year ago. He lives with his mother and 12-year-old sister. John will be a sophomore in high school this Fall.

● TENTATIVE DIAGNOSES

Based on the information provided by John so far, what are potential differential diagnoses?

● HISTORY

What are significant questions in the history for an adolescent pre-participation physical exam?
What are the key points to cover on the review of systems?

● PHYSICAL ASSESSMENT

What are the significant portions of the physical examination that should be completed for John as an adolescent?
What are specific tests that should be part of the sports physical?

● DIFFERENTIAL DIAGNOSES

What are the significant positive and negative data that support or refute your diagnoses for John?

● DIAGNOSTIC TESTS

Based on the history and physical assessment, what, if any, diagnostic tests would you do for John? Include your rationale for the tests.

● DIAGNOSES

What diagnoses are appropriate for John?

● THERAPEUTIC PLAN

1. *What recommendations would you make for John's participation in football this season?*
2. *What health maintenance issues would you discuss with John today?*
3. *Of all the information obtained from John, which topics would you keep confidential?*
4. *What guidance would you provide for John's mother concerning his peer interactions and desire to spend more time with his peer group?*
5. *What recommendations would you make to John and his mother about his diagnoses?*
6. *What patient education needs does John have at this time, based on your diagnoses?*

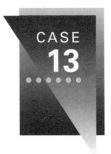

TUTORIAL

A 15-year-old boy requesting well physical and sports examination

SCENARIO

John is a 15-year-old African-American male. He presents for a pre-participation physical exam for football. He has been in good health since his last physical exam 1 year ago. He lives with his mother and 12-year-old sister. John will be a sophomore in high school this Fall.

● TENTATIVE DIAGNOSES

What are the potential diagnoses you have identified based on the preceding scenario?

DIAGNOSIS | RATIONALE

DIAGNOSIS	RATIONALE
Diagnosis not applicable at present.	Well visit. When reviewing this case, keep in mind that the preparticipation physical exam may be the only health maintenance visit for an adolescent.

● HISTORY

1. *What are significant questions in the history for an adolescent pre-participation physical exam?*

REQUESTED DATA | DATA ANSWER

REQUESTED DATA	DATA ANSWER
Allergies	No food, drug, or insect allergies.
Current medication	None.

(continued)

REQUESTED DATA	*DATA ANSWER*
Childhood illnesses	Chicken pox.
Infectious disease exposure	No known exposure to active tuberculosis, neighborhood not of high prevalence.
Immunizations	Childhood immunizations up to date; second MMR 7th grade; last tetanus, 13 years old.
Surgery	None.
Hospitalizations	None.
Injuries	Sprained ankle last Spring in basketball, no rehab, no pain now.
Family history major illnesses	Father: Died of heart attack at age 42 when John was 5 years old. Maternal grandmother: Adult onset diabetes, diet only. No other significant family history.
Nutrition/exercise	Typical day: Breakfast: none; Lunch: fast food hamburger, fries, milkshake; Dinner: meat, potato, milk; Snacks: chips, milk. Exercise: runs 2–3 miles 5 times a week, plus various sports practice.
Relationship with mother	Good relationship, able to talk about most things with her.
Relationship with sister	"Okay."
Peers	Many friends, makes friends easily, best friend for 5 years. Enjoys playing pickup basketball, "hanging out."
Sleep patterns	Sleeps 6–8 hours/night, falls asleep easily, feels rested.
Carry a weapon	Denies.
Juvenile justice system	No arrests.
Employment	Works odd jobs in the neighborhood: lawn care, house cleaning.
School	C student, enjoys social aspects of school, no suspensions. Plans to be pro football player or own his own business.
Sexuality	Heterosexual, no current girlfriend, sexually active since 14 years old, 2 lifetime partners, uses condoms sometimes, no sexually transmitted infections, no known children. Denies sexual abuse.
Substance use	Has tried marijuana three times this Summer with friends. Does not plan to use during football season. Drinks beer <1 time/month. Three 12-oz beers for intoxication. Denies any other drugs, tobacco, or steroids.

(continued)

REQUESTED DATA	DATA ANSWER
Interview with mother	No health concerns. Some concern that he spends more time with friends than at home. Mother knows and likes all of his friends.

2. *What are the key points on the review of systems?*

SYSTEM REVIEWED	DATA ANSWER
HEENT	No recent upper respiratory infection. No visual changes.
Respiratory	No cough or shortness of breath with exercise.
Cardiac	No history of chest pain, dizziness, or tachycardia with exercise.
Genital/urinary	Denies dysuria, penile discharge, or lesions on penis.
Muscular skeletal	Review of each joint reveals no pain, injury or decreased motion at any joint. Ankle injury: Twisted right ankle during basketball game, swollen for 1 week, no radiographs, no rehabilitation. Denies pain or swelling now.
Neurological	No history of head injury, no loss of consciousness, no syncope.
Skin	Concerned about acne on face, washes face with deodorant soap.

● PHYSICAL ASSESSMENT

What are the significant portions of the physical examination that should be completed for John as an adolescent?

SYSTEM	RATIONALE	FINDINGS
Height/weight	Provides baseline data needed to assess growth and development.	H: 68″ Wt: 135 lbs. Body Mass Index (BMI): 20; 50th%.

(continued)

SYSTEM	RATIONALE	FINDINGS
HEENT	Recommended for sports exam (Uphold, 1994).	Vision screen OD 20/100, OS 20/100. Shoddy lymph nodes, otherwise negative.
Chest	Assess for respiratory difficulty.	Palpable firm, rubbery breast nodule on left, below nipple, and extending beyond areolar perimeter. Exam otherwise negative.
Heart	Assess for irregular heart rate and abnormal sounds.	HR: 64. B/P: 104/70. Heart RRR, no clicks or murmurs.
Abdomen	Provides data related to possible organomegaly (Hergenroeder & Brecker, 1990).	No masses or tenderness, active bowel sounds.
Genitalia	Indicates growth and development; Tanner staging.	Tanner stage 4, testicular volume 15 cc. Both testicles descended, no masses, no hernia.
Muscular/skeletal	Important to assess for sports participation.	Increased ankle laxity bilaterally. Equal and normal flexibility, alignment, stability, and strength at all other joints. No muscular atrophy or hypertrophy.
Neurological	Needed for baseline neuro screening.	Cranial nerves II-XII intact. Reflexes 2+.
Skin		Papular acne forehead, chin, no erythema. Skin otherwise clear.

What are specific orthopedic tests that should be part of the sports physical?

ASSESSMENT	FINDINGS
Acromioclavicular joints, shoulder motion, and symmetry	AC joints with good ROM, full external rotation of arms. Shoulders symmetrical.

(continued)

ASSESSMENT	*FINDINGS*
Cervical spine motion	Able to look over both shoulders, touch ears to shoulders.
Trapezius strength	Able to shrug shoulders against resistance.
Deltoid strength	Able to abduct shoulders 90° against resistance.
Elbow and wrist motion	Able to flex and extend elbows, able to pronate and supinate wrists.
Hand or finger motion and deformities	Able to spread fingers, make a fist.
Knee symmetry and effusion	Able to tighten and relax quadriceps, no joint effusion.
Hip, knee, and ankle motion	Able to "duck" walk 4 steps (buttocks on heels).
Scoliosis, hip motion, hamstring tightness	Able to bend at waist with knees straight. No evidence of scoliosis.
Calf symmetry, leg strength	Able to raise up on toes and raise heels.

● DIFFERENTIAL DIAGNOSES

What are the significant positive and negative findings that support or refute your diagnoses for John?

DIAGNOSIS	*POSITIVE DATA*	*NEGATIVE DATA*
Decreased visual acuity	OS 20/100, OD 20/100.	
Acne	Papules present on forehead, chin.	
Ankle laxity	Increased ankle laxity bilaterally on exam.	
Substance abuse	Per history, admitted to using marijuana 3× in past. Also drinks 12-oz beer approximately 1×/month.	
Poor dietary habits	History revealed no breakfast, high-fat fast foods for lunch, with frequent snacks of high-fat foods.	

(continued)

DIAGNOSIS	POSITIVE DATA	NEGATIVE DATA
Sexually active adolescent without consistent condom use	History revealed inconsistent use of condoms with female partners.	No hx of STDs.
Gynecomastia	Physical examination revealed a firm, rubbery breast nodule on left breast.	

● DIAGNOSTIC TESTS

Based on the history and physical examination, what, if any, diagnostic tests would you do?

DIAGNOSTIC TEST	RATIONALE	RESULTS
Cholesterol screen	The National Cholesterol Education Program Expert Panel on blood cholesterol levels (NCEP) (1991) recommends screening all adolescents whose parent at age 55 or younger suffered a documented myocardial infarction.	180 mg/dL.
Urine leukocyte esterase	Asymptomatic males can be screened effectively for chlamydia and gonorrhea through the detection of pyuria using leukocyte esterase activity in urine (Biro, 1992).	Negative.
Hemoglobin/hematocrit	May or may not be done depending on the screening practices of the care provider. John is asymptomatic of anemia. There is little evidence to suggest any benefit to screening for or treating mild iron deficiency anemia (Report of US Preventive Services Task Force, 1996).	Not obtained.

(continued)

DIAGNOSTIC TEST	RATIONALE	RESULTS
Drug testing	John has reported experimentation with marijuana and alcohol. Based on his history there is no reason to suspect usage beyond the amount he reports. Drug testing should always be done with a clear plan of action in mind and with the adolescent's knowledge.	Not done.

● DIAGNOSES

What diagnoses do you determine as being appropriate after a review of the subjective and objective data?

1. Decreased visual acuity
2. Acne
3. Borderline hypercholesterolemia
4. Ankle laxity with increased risk for injury
5. Substance use
6. Poor dietary habits
7. Sexually active adolescent without consistent condom use
8. Gynecomastia

● THERAPEUTIC PLAN

1. *What recommedations would you make for John's participation in football this season?*

   No restrictions based on the results of today's exam (Committee on Sports, 1994).

2. *What health maintenance issues would you address with John today?*

   1. Offer hepatitis B vaccine. Rationale: Universal hepatitis B vaccination is recommended for all adolescents. The past decade has seen a 20% increase in hepatitis B infections among adolescents (Brookman et al., 1995).
   2. Teach testicular self-exam. Rationale: Testicular cancer is the most common solid tumor in young men (Wingo, Tong, and Bolden, 1995). Research has not demonstrated that men who have been taught the technique are more likely to perform it or detect early stage tumors (Westlake, 1987). John is not at high risk for a testicular tumor because he has no history of cryptorchidism, mumps orchitis, or a hydrocele. The provider could chose to spend teaching time addressing other behaviors.

3. Injury prevention education regarding seatbelts, safety equipment for football, including mouthguard. Rationale: The Guidelines for Adolescent Preventive Services (GAPS) (1994) recommends that all adolescents receive annual health guidance to promote the reduction of injuries.

4. Tuberculin skin testing would not be done. Rationale: The American Academy of Pediatrics (1994) recommends against annual skin testing of adolescents who live in low prevalence communities and lack risk factors for exposure to tuberculosis.

3. Of all the information obtained from John, which topics would you keep confidential?

Information regarding John's substance use and sexual activity would not be shared at this time. Rationale: The parameters of confidentiality should be discussed initially with John and his mother. The care provider must clearly state when confidentiality will be broken. The limits of confidentiality vary depending on the type of practice and current laws of the state. When breaking confidentiality, the adolescent must be notified first.

John has not demonstrated that he is involved in an organized pattern of behavior with substance use. John describes a low intensity experimental use versus a pattern of abuse and dependency. Care providers must determine their own level of comfort with this issue.

A decision to break confidentiality about John's sexual activity may prevent the development of a trusting relationship with John and the care provider. Research has demonstrated that a lack of confidentiality is a barrier to care for adolescents (Resnick, Blum, and Hedin, 1992). The care provider can encourage John to talk with his mother about substance use and sexuality issues.

4. What guidance would you provide for John's mother's concerning his peer interactions and desire to spend more time with his peer group?

A review of normal psychosocial development of the middle adolescent. Between the ages of 14–18, the adolescent moves away from the home and family and moves toward the peer group. The middle adolescent has an increased need for independence. Reinforce her efforts to get to know the people with whom John is spending his time. Remind his mother that she needs to continue to communicate with John about her expectations. Assist his mother in balancing supervision and the promotion of his independence.

5. What recommendations would you make to John and his mother about his diagnoses?

Refer to optometry/opthamology for eye exam and possible glasses.

6. *What patient education needs does John have at this time, based on your diagnoses?*

   1. Acne: Review skin care; instruct patient not to squeeze the acne lesions. Instruct John to wash with mild soap and water. Treatment: Topical therapy with benzoyl peroxide 10% gel should be effective because the acne is noninflammatory and confined to the face. Instruct John to apply a thin layer to his entire face nightly. Some discoloration of bedsheets and towels may occur from the gel. Reinforce that treatment is aimed at prevention of new lesions; therefore, it may require 2–3 months before maximum benefit is seen. If drying and scaling of the skin occurs, decrease the amount applied (Rothman and Lucky, 1993).

   2. Borderline hypercholesterolemia: The cholesterol level of 180 mg/dL is considered borderline. Following NCEP (1991) guidelines, a repeat total cholesterol should be obtained in 1 month. If the average of the two values is <170 mg/dL the level should be repeated in 5 years. If the average is ≥170, a fasting lipoprotein analysis should be obtained.

   3. Ankle laxity with potential for injury: Strengthening of the joint through range-of-motion exercises will assist in injury prevention. Range-of-motion exercises can increase the strength of the ankle joint. Teach John to "write the alphabet" in the air with the great toe, exercising the ankle joint through the complete range of motion (O'Nieal, 1996). The team trainer may be a source of additional strengthening exercises or a referral to physical therapy may be appropriate.

   4. Subtance abuse: Support John's decision to avoid substance use during the football season and encourage him to consider continuing to abstain. Provide accurate drug information regarding the health hazards and consequences of drug use. Emphasize the short-term negative effects of drugs and alcohol.

   5. Poor dietary habits: John's mother should be present for all nutrition education. Utilize the food guide pyramid to educate about a balanced diet. Stress sport's nutrition points:

      a. Food from the base of the pyramid—bread, cereal, rice, and pasta, will provide the best source of additional calories needed for an active adolescent.

      b. Water should be taken at regular intervals before, during, and after activity.

      c. 16 oz of water should be consumed for each pound of weight loss due to exercise.

      d. Salt tablets can be dangerous and are unnecessary (McKeag, 1986).

   6. Sexually active adolescent without consistent condom use: Review John's risk for sexually transmitted infections and pregnancy. Demonstrate with John the correct use of a condom and provide condom

samples. Role play with John communication strategies to discuss sexual history and contraception plans with a new partner.

7. Gynecomastia: Discuss with John and his mother that gynecomastia is a benign growth of breast tissue associated with puberty. Over half of all adolescent males will have some degree of gynecomastia, and in all but a small percentage of cases the gynecomastia will resolve in 12–18 months. No further work up is necessary (Neinstein, 1991).

REFERENCES

American Academy of Pediatrics Committee on Infectious Diseases. Screening for tuberculosis in infants and children. *Pediatrics* 1994; 93:131–34.

American Medical Association. *Guidelines for Adolescent Preventive Services (GAPS)*. Baltimore: Williams & Wilkins; 1994.

Biro FM. Adolescents and sexually transmitted diseases. Maternal and Child Health Technical Information Bulletin. National Center for Education in Maternal and Child Health; 1992.

Brookman RR, Koff RS, Schaffner W, Margolis HS, Collins M, Bloom BS, Coupey SM. Critical issues surrounding Hepatitis B vaccination for adolescents: a round table. *J Adol Health* 1995; 17:208–233.

Committee on Sports Medicine and Fitness. Medical conditions affecting sports participation. *Pediatrics* 1994; 5:757–760.

Hergenroeder AC, Brecker TJ. Preseason cardiovascular examination: A review. *J Adol Health Care* 1990; 11:379–386.

McKeag DB. Adolescents and exercise. *J Adol Health Care* 1986;7:1215–1295.

National Cholesterol Education Program. Report of the Expert Panel on Blood Cholesterol Levels in Children and Adolescents. NIH Publication No. 91-2732, USDHHS. Bethesda, MD; 1991.

Neinstein LS. *Adolescent Health Care A Practical Guide,* 2nd ed. Baltimore: Urban & Schwarzenberg; 1991.

O'Nieal ME. Common wrist and ankle injuries. *Adv Nurse Pract* 1996; 8:31–36.

Report of the US Preventive Services Task Force. *Guide to Clinical Preventive Services,* 2nd ed. Baltimore, Williams & Wilkins; 1996.

Resnick MD, Litman TJ, Blum RW. Physician attitudes toward confidentiality of treatment for adolescents: Findings from the upper midwest regional physician survey. *J Adol Health* 1992; 13:616–622.

Rothman KF, Lucky AW. Acne vulgaris. *Advances in Dermatology*. St. Louis: Mosby-Yearbook; 1993.

Uphold C, Graham M. *Clinical guidelines in family practice,* 2nd ed. Gainesville, FL: Barmarral Books; 1994.

Westlake SJ, Frank JW. Testicular self-examination: An argument against routine teaching. *Fam Pract* 1987; 4:143–148.

Wingo PA, Tong T, Bolden S. Cancer statistics 1995. *CA Cancer J Clin* 1995; 45:8–30.

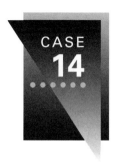

A 62-year-old man with a facial rash and a red eye

SCENARIO

Bill Hamilton is a 62-year-old African-American male who complains of a painful red eye. He first noticed the red eye on Sunday, with a few red bumps on his face 1 or 2 days later. Since then the rash has spread to the tip of his nose. Several of the spots under his eye look like blisters and are crusting over. His eye continues to hurt and he c/o blurry vision.

● TENTATIVE DIAGNOSES

Based on the information provided so far, what are potential differential diagnoses?

● HISTORY

What are significant questions in the history for Bill?
What are the key points to cover on the review of systems?

● PHYSICAL ASSESSMENT

What are the significant portions of the physical examination that should be completed for Bill?

● DIFFERENTIAL DIAGNOSES

What are the significant positive and negative data that support or refute your diagnoses for Bill?

● DIAGNOSTIC TESTS

Based on the history and physical assessment, what, if any, diagnostic tests would you do? Include your rationale for the tests.

● DIAGNOSIS

What diagnoses are appropriate for Bill?

● THERAPEUTIC PLAN

1. *What are the goals of management for HZ?*
2. *What treatment would you start Bill on immediately?*
3. *What referral should be made for Bill immediately?*
4. *What self-care measures can you recommend for Bill?*
5. *Bill complains of severe pain in his eye and face. What explanation would you give him regarding the pain, and what treatment would you recommend?*
6. *Bill's wife has heard that this rash is contagious. What explanation and instruction would you give her concerning this rash?*
7. *Are there any sequalae that may occur as a result of this rash?*

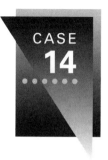

TUTORIAL

A 62-year-old man with a facial rash and a red eye

SCENARIO

Bill Hamilton is a 62-year-old African-American male who complains of a painful red eye. He first noticed the red eye on Sunday, with a few red bumps on his face 1 or 2 days later. Since then the rash has spread to the tip of his nose. Several of the spots under his eye look like blisters and are crusting over. His eye continues to hurt, and he c/o blurry vision.

● TENTATIVE DIAGNOSES

What are the potential diagnoses you have identified based on the above scenario?

DIAGNOSIS	RATIONALE
Contact dermatitis	Bill could have been exposed to a substance, having a subsequent dermatologic reaction to it.
Herpes simplex	Herpes simplex presents with vesicles, and can occur on the face.
Herpes zoster	Herpes zoster presents with painful vesicles.
Impetigo	A bacterial infection that can affect the face.
Conjunctivitis, uveitis	Bill's red eye could be caused by a viral or bacterial infection, based on his complaints of a painful red eye.
FB of the eye	Bill's complaint of a painful, red eye could be caused by a FB in the eye.

● HISTORY

1. What are significant questions in Bill's history?

REQUESTED DATA	DATA ANSWER
Allergies	NKDA
Current medications	Indapamide (Lozol) 2.5 mg day for HTN. Many types of vitamins. Albuterol (Proventil) MDI 2 puffs QID as needed. Beclomethasone (Beclovent) 2 puffs BID.
Surgery	Thoracotomy 8 years ago for lung cancer. Numerous bronchoscopies for radiation/evaluation of lung cancer.
Past medical history and hospitalizations/fractures/ injuries/accidents	Childhood: chicken pox, mumps, measles. HTN for 15 years, treated with diuretics, well controlled. Diagnosed with large-cell lung cancer in 1988.
Appetite	Good. Lost approximately 25 pounds after initial treatment of lung cancer, then started eating again—wanted to he was make sure not emaciated. Gained back about 40 pounds.
24-Hour diet recall	B: Eggs, bacon, toast. L: Sandwich, with coffee or soda. D: Meat, vegetable, bread, dessert. S: Popcorn, desserts.
Social history	Tobacco: Smoked $2\frac{1}{2}$ ppd for 40 years. Alcohol: Drinks approx 2–4 beers/day (12 oz). Drugs: Denies. Caffeine: Drinks 3–6 cups of coffee, rare soda. Exercise: No regular.
Family history	Father: Died at 48, DM. Mother: Died at 76, obesity, heart problems. Siblings: Sister, died at 58, had been in poor health for a long time. Children: 6 children, 3 girls (all smoke), 3 boys (2 smoke). All healthy except 1 boy with alcohol abuse, and vocal cord nodules. Spouse: 1st wife deceased of lung cancer, 2nd HTN, otherwise healthy.
Income/insurance/home	Works full-time at Ford assembly plant, 6 days/week. Insurance carried through employer. Owns home.
Present illness: Has he put anything on rash? What	Eye redness began on Sunday (now Wednesday). Then rash began 1–2 days later. Tried hydrocortisone, with lit-

(continued)

REQUESTED DATA   DATA ANSWER

makes it better or worse? Exposure to any chemical or irritant?	tle effect. No itching. Rash becoming more painful and irritating as the days go on. No previous rash like this in past. No exposure to chemicals or change in routine or medicines. Wife does not have a rash. Denies any prob- lems with eyes before rash began.

2. *What are the key points on the review of systems?*

SYSTEM REVIEWED   DATA ANSWER

General	Feels fatigued much of the time. Usually takes a nap after work.
Skin	Pale skin. No other lesions anywhere else, just on face.
HEENT	Has noticed blurry vision since rash. Has reading glasses for near vision.
Lungs	Coughs frequently. Takes antibiotics frequently for infec-tion. Some SOB with activity.
Cardiac	Unremarkable, denies chest pain or discomfort.
GI/GU	Unremarkable.

● PHYSICAL ASSESSMENT

What are the significant portions of the physical examination that should be completed for Bill?

SYSTEM	RATIONALE	FINDINGS
Vital signs	Provides baseline.	B/P: 138/84. HR: 96 R: 20 T: 99.2 Ht: 5'11" Wt: 214 lbs

(continued)

SYSTEM	RATIONALE	FINDINGS
General appearance/skin	Provides overall description of patient.	Pale, obese male sitting on exam table with red rash visible on tip of nose and below rt. eye. Papular/vesicular rash, erythematous bases with pustules and crusts of 1 or 2 lesions. No honey-colored discharge. No involvement of left eye or side of face. Rash in somewhat linear pattern around rt. side of face into hairline.
HEENT	Need to evaluate eye, lymph nodes.	VA: 20/60 OD, 20/30 OS Rt. eye with injected conjunctiva, tearing. Rt. upper eyelid edematous. Photophobia. No foreign body visible with lid eversion. Fluorescein revealed no corneal abrasions. Unable to complete fundus exam owing to light sensitivity.
Lungs	Given PMH of lung cancer, need to obtain check on pulmonary status.	Clear, with occasional expiratory wheezes in posterior chest.
Heart	Baseline data.	RRR, no MRG.

● DIFFERENTIAL DIAGNOSES

What are the significant positive and negative findings that support or refute your diagnoses for Bill?

DIAGNOSIS	POSITIVE DATA	NEGATIVE DATA
Contact dermatitis	Papular/vesicular erythematous rash on face.	No history of contact with chemical irritants, or change in medication or exposure.
Herpes simplex	Papular/vesicular erythematous rash on face.	No previous history of herpes simplex, no contact with

(continued)

DIAGNOSIS	POSITIVE DATA	NEGATIVE DATA
		anyone who had herpes simplex, no disseminated pattern of distribution.
Herpes zoster	Papular/vesicular erythematous rash on face, involving one side of face only; dermatome-ophthalmic branch of the trigeminal nerve, painful rash, involvement of eye: conjunctivitis, photophobia, over 50 years of age, history of chicken pox, depressed immunity secondary to lung cancer.	No prodromal symptoms.
Impetigo	Papular/vesicular rash on face.	No honey-colored discharge, not a child, no crowded living conditions, no poor hygiene.
Conjunctivitis, uveitis	Red, injected painful conjunctiva with photosensitivity.	Red eye was prodrome for rash, no exposure to viral or bacterial conjunctivitis.
FB of eye	Red, injected painful conjunctiva with photosensitivity.	No recollection of FB going into eye. No FB visible.

● DIAGNOSTIC TESTS

Based on the history and physical examination, what, if any, diagnostic testing would you obtain?

DIAGNOSTIC TEST	RATIONALE	RESULTS
Tzanck smear	Smear shows giant and or multinucleated epidermal cells.	Not done.
Varicella zoster virus (VZV) antigen detection	Direct fluorescent antibody (DFA) detects VZV antigen in smear of vesicle base or fluid. Specific and very sensitive.	Not done.
Viral culture	Isolation of VZV.	Not done.

(continued)

DIAGNOSTIC TEST	RATIONALE	RESULTS
Dermatopathology	Lesional skin biopsy that shows vesicle formation and giant or multinucleated keratinocytes.	Not done.

● DIAGNOSES

What diagnoses are appropriate after a review of the subjective and objective data?

Herpes zoster (shingles) of the opthalmic branch of the trigeminal nerve.

Data Supporting the Diagnosis

Progression of rash from papules/vesicles initially changing to crusts/pustules. Dermatome involvement of right side of face including eye, tip of nose, cheek, and into hairline (opthalmic branch of trigeminal nerve), decreased immunity owing to lung cancer, age >50, painful rash, eye symptoms.

● THERAPEUTIC PLAN

1. *What are the goals of management for HZ?*

   The goals of management include:
   • minimize pain
   • reduce viral shedding
   • speed crusting of lesions and healing
   • ease physical, psychological, and emotional discomfort
   • prevent viral dissemination or other complications
   • prevent or minimize postherpetic neuralgia (PHN)

2. *What treatment would you start Bill on immediately?*

   Use of antiviral agents within 72 hours helps decrease the duration of the acute pain, accelerates the healing of the lesions, and may decrease the incidence of PHN. Choices of antiviral agents include:

   Acyclovir (Zovirax) 800 mg 5× day for 7–10 days
   Valacyclovir (Valtrex) 1000 mg TID for 7 days
   Famciclovir (Famvir) 500 mg TID for 7 days
   The use of cortisone is controversial. It is felt by some that use of Prednisone early in the course of HZ may reduce the likelihood of PHN, however, this has not been shown in controlled studies (Fitzpatrick et al., 1997).
   Bill was started on acyclovir 800 5× day.

3. What referral should be made for Bill immediately?

Because Bill has eye involvement, referral to an opthalmologist is imperative. It is also a good idea to refer Bill back to his oncologist, because he
can be considered immunosuppressed and may need IV acyclovir and
recombinant interferon to prevent dissemination of the herpes zoster
(Brunton, 1995).

4. What self-care measures can you recommend for Bill?

Application of moist dressings (water, saline, Burow's solution) may be
soothing and alleviate pain. Topical antibacterial ointment promotes
healing and prevents secondary bacterial infection as the lesions begin to
crust (Barker, Burton, and Zieve, 1995).

*5. Bill complains of severe pain in his eye and face. What explanation would
you give him regarding the pain, and what treatment would you recommend?*

The HZ virus gains access to the body during an episode of chicken pox.
The HZ virus remains dormant in the sensory ganglia, until a person's
immunity decreases. The virus then replicates, and travels down the sensory nerve causing pain in the l ocation of the nerve, and then the
painful skin lesions follow. Pain is caused by nerve inflammation, nerve
infection during the acute reactivation, and then nerve inflammation
and scarring with post-herpetic neuralgia (PHN) (Fitzpatrick, 1997).

Early control of pain is indicated with narcotic analgesics. Failure to
manage pain can result in failure to sleep, fatigue, and depression.

*6. Bill's wife has heard that this rash is contagious. What explanation and
instruction would you give her concerning this rash?*

Herpes zoster itself does not cause HZ or shingles in exposed individuals.
However, since HZ is caused by the varicella virus, people who have not
had chicken pox are susceptible to transmission of the virus via the air-
borne route. Bill should avoid being around people who are immunosuppressed, such as those on chemotherapy or persons with +HIV status.

7. Are there any sequelae that may occur as a result of this rash?

HZ can cause chronic problems. This is also classified as PHN, characterized by burning, ice-burning, shooting, or lacinating pain that can last
weeks, months, and years after the skin involvement has resolved. Antidepressants may be helpful for chronic pain of HZ. Capsaicin cream also
may be helpful. Topical analgesics as well as nerve blocks may assist in
the reduction of pain.

If the eye is involved, as in Bill's case, there may be a permanent loss of
vision depending on the extent of the lesions. Ramsay Hunt syndrome is
HZ affecting the facial and auditory nerves so that facial palsy occurs,
usually within 2 weeks of the initial outbreak. Tinnitus, vertigo, or deaf-
ness may result (Barker, Burton, and Zieve, 1995).

REFERENCES

Barker R, Burton J, Zieve P. *Principles of Ambulatory Medicine,* 4th ed. Baltimore: Williams & Wilkins; 1995.

Brunton S. Herpes Zoster: A management update. *Fam Pract Recert* 1995; 17(9): 14–25.

Fitzpatrick T, Johnson R, Wolff K, Polano M, and Suurmond D. *Color Atlas and Synopsis of Clinical Dermatology,* 3rd ed. New York: McGraw-Hill; 1997.

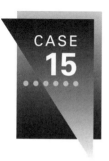

A 15-year-old boy with knee pain

SCENARIO

Roberto, a 15-year-old Hispanic male, presents to the primary care clinic c/o left knee pain for 3 days. He was kicked in the leg while playing soccer and has had pain and swelling ever since.

● TENTATIVE DIAGNOSES

Based on the information provided so far, what are potential differential diagnoses?

● HISTORY

What are significant questions in the history for a knee injury?

● PHYSICAL ASSESSMENT

What are the significant portions of the physical examination that should be completed for Roberto?

● DIFFERENTIAL DIAGNOSES

What are the significant positive and negative data that support or refute your diagnoses for Roberto?

● DIAGNOSTIC TESTS

Based on the history and physical assessment, what, if any, diagnostic tests would you obtain? Include your rationale for the tests.

● DIAGNOSIS

What diagnoses are appropriate for Roberto?

● THERAPEUTIC PLAN

1. *What is the initial management plan for a first-degree MCL sprain?*
2. *When should Roberto be seen again for this injury?*
3. *What evaluation should you do to determine if Roberto's injury is healing?*
4. *What should the plan of care for Roberto include at this point?*
5. *When should Roberto return for his final follow up?*
6. *What criteria will you use to determine he no longer needs follow up?*

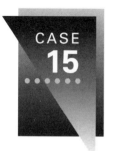

TUTORIAL

A 15-year-old boy with knee pain

SCENARIO

Roberto, a 15-year-old Hispanic male, presents to the primary care clinic c/o left knee pain for 3 days. He was kicked in the leg while playing soccer and has had pain and swelling ever since.

● TENTATIVE DIAGNOSES

What are the potential diagnoses you have identified based on the above scenario?

With all knee injuries the potential for multiple diagnoses exist. The symptoms of pain and swelling are common symptoms for all knee injuries. More details need to be obtained to help rule out any of these diagnoses.

DIAGNOSIS	RATIONALE
Meniscal injury	Twisting or rotational injuries may be associated with a variety of problems such as meniscal tears, ACL tears, patellar dislocation, and osteochondral fractures.
Anterior cruciate ligament (ACL) injury	Twisting or rotational injuries may be associated with a variety of problems such as meniscal tears, ACL tears, patellar dislocation, and osteochondral. Hyperextension knee injuries associated with an audible pop are associated with ACL tears (Mendelson & Paiemont, 1996).
Posterior cruciate ligament (PCL) injury	A direct blow to the front of the knee is associated with patellar injuries, ACL, and PCL problems (Mendelson & Paiemont, 1996).

(continued)

DIAGNOSIS	RATIONALE
Medial collateral ligament (MCL) injury	A direct blow to the lateral side of the knee can injure the medial collateral ligament.
Lateral collateral ligament (LCL) injury, left knee	A direct blow to the medial aspect of the knee can injure the lateral collateral ligament.
Osteochondral fracture	Twisting or rotational injuries may be associated with a variety of problems such as meniscal tears, ACL tears, patellar dislocation, and osteochondral fractures.
Disruption of left knee extensor mechanism	Popping sound at time of injury may be associated with disruption of the extensor mechanism, as would a decreased ROM.

● HISTORY

1. *What are significant questions in the history for a man with a knee injury?*

REQUESTED DATA	DATA ANSWER
Exact mechanism of injury	Roberto was trying to kick a soccer ball and was kicked by an opponent in the medial aspect of his lower leg. His left leg was fully extended when the injury occurred. Knowledge of the exact mechanism of injury is critical in developing an appropriate diagnosis for knee injuries. Certain mechanisms of injury are associated with likely diagnoses.
Did the knee swell after the injury? If so, was the swelling immediate or delayed?	Mild swelling began in Roberto's left knee the day after the injury. Swelling that occurs immediately after a knee injury is associated with hemarthrosis (effusion) and often indicates ACL tears (Sonzogni, 1996). Mild delayed swelling with absence of effusion is associated with less serious injuries.
Was an audible pop heard or felt at the time of the injury?	Roberto felt a pop but denies an audible pop when his left knee was injured. An audible pop is associated with ACL tears about half the time (Sonzogni, 1996).
Was Roberto able to finish the game?	Roberto was unable to finish the game and was taken to the sideline immediately after the injury. Those patients who develop severe pain, rapid effusion, and are unable to walk are likely to have suffered an ACL tear, an acute

(continued)

	patellar dislocation, or an osteochondral fracture (Rothenberg, 1993).
Has there been any locking, clicking, or catching of the knee post-injury?	Roberto denies any clicking, locking, or catching of his left knee post-injury. Clicking, locking, or catching of the knee is asociated with meniscal tears.
Allergies	None.
Current medications	None.
Surgery/transfusions	None.
Past medical history and hospitalizations/fractures/ injuries/accidents	None, healthy young male. No previous knee injuries.
Last complete PE	Prior to playing soccer.
Conditioning	Roberto is a well-conditioned athlete who is a starting player on the local high school soccer team. Occasional athletes lack adequate conditioning to prevent knee injuries. Most knee injuries suffered by the occasional athlete are overuse injuries (Moyer, 1996).

● PHYSICAL ASSESSMENT

What are the significant portions of the physical examination that should be completed for Roberto?

SYSTEM	RATIONALE	FINDINGS
Vital signs	Although not directly connected with Roberto's injury, taking VS provides a baseline of information and also can screen for problems such as HTN.	B/P: 110/60 P: 54 R: 18 T: 97.4 Ht: 5'11" Wt: 147 lbs
General appearance/skin	The general assessment gives an overall idea about the status of the patient.	Hispanic male, NAD, sitting on exam table.
Gait	Always note gait in any patient with a knee injury (Arendt, 1996).	Normal gait without limping or guarding.

(continued)

SYSTEM	RATIONALE	FINDINGS
Visual inspection of the knee	Note any effusion, contusions, or visible anatomic irregularities. Note symmetry of the knee as opposed to the opposite knee. Note the Q angle.	No swelling, no effusion, no contusions. No obvious anatomic irregularities.
ROM	Note active and passive ROM. Inability to actively extend the leg at the knee is associated with injury to the quadriceps extensor mechanism. The quadriceps extensor mechanism includes the patellar ligament, the patella, and the quadriceps tendon.	FROM—active and passive.
Assessing for effusion	Ballottment of the patella is present with an intra-articular effusion, whereas soft tissue swelling from contusion and collateral ligament injuries do not produce ballottment (Sonzogni, 1996). Large effusions are an indication for arthrocentesis.	No effusion noted with exam.
Palpation of the knee	Palpate the joint spaces, the patella, the collateral ligaments, the quadriceps tendon, the patellar ligament, and the bony structures.	Painful with palpation over the proximal medial collateral ligament.
Knee exam for ligament stability	Perform the Lachman test and the Drawer test to assess integrity of the ACL and PCL, respectively. Apply varus and valgus stress to the knee to assess medial and collateral ligament integrity. Always compare the injured knee with the opposing knee to ascertain any ligament laxity.	Lachman and Drawer tests neg. Positive medial knee pain with valgus stress, but no laxity noted.
Knee assessment for meniscal injury	Palpate the joint space for tenderness. Local tenderness is one of the cardinal signs	Painful with palpation to lt. medial knee joint line. McMurray test neg.

(continued)

SYSTEM	*RATIONALE*	*FINDINGS*
	of meniscal injury (Rothenberg and Graf, 1993). Perform the McMurray test to determine if meniscal injury exists.	
Assess adjacent joints for injury	Pain may be referred to the knee from the back and hip. Always assess adjacent bony and soft tissue areas for injury.	Lt. ankle, hip, with FROM and no tenderness.
Neurovascular	Always assess neurovascular function distal to the injury.	Lt. dorsalis pedis pulse + with quick capillary refill and + sensation to left toes.

● DIFFERENTIAL DIAGNOSES

What are the significant positive and negative findings that support or refute your diagnoses for Roberto?

DIAGNOSIS	*POSITIVE DATA*	*NEGATIVE DATA*
Meniscal injury to lt. knee	Pain with palpation to medial joint line; minimal swelling, moderate pain.	Mechanism of injury not consistent with meniscal injury. No history of popping, clicking, or locking of left knee. McMurray test negative.
ACL injury	Unable to continue playing soccer game.	Mechanism of injury not consistent with ACL tear. No effusion present; Lachman test neg, anterior drawer sign neg. Normal gait.
PCL injury	Minimal swelling left knee.	Mechanism of injury not consistent with PCL tear. Neg. posterior drawer sign.
MCL injury	Mechanism of injury consistent with MCL injury. Palpation along MCL elicits pain. Pain with valgus stress along MCL, no sign of insta-	

(continued)

DIAGNOSIS	POSITIVE DATA	NEGATIVE DATA
	bility or laxity. Minimal, if any, swelling noted; Mc-Murray test negative; Lachman test and Drawer test negative. FROM with full extensor mechanism intact.	
LCL injury	None.	Pain to medial aspect of knee. Mechanism of injury not consistent with LCL injury. No pain or laxity with varus stress; negative McMurray, Lachman, Drawer tests.
Osteochondral fracture left knee	Unable to bear weight post-injury left knee, unable to complete the soccer game postinjury; painful to bear weight postinjury.	Minimal swelling, no knee effusion, able to bear weight with exam. No varus/valgus stress left knee; negative Drawer, Lachman tests; extensor mechanism left knee intact. FROM lt. knee.
Disruption of lt. knee extensor mechanism	Roberto felt a pop to lt knee after injury; unable to complete the soccer game.	FROM of left knee with extensor mechanism intact. Able to actively extend lt. leg at home.

● DIAGNOSTIC TESTS

Based on the history and physical examination, what, if any, diagnostic tests would you obtain?

DIAGNOSTIC TEST	RATIONALE	RESULTS
Radiograph of left knee, AP, lateral, oblique and sunrise views	Knee radiographs post-injury may reveal avulsion fractures associated with ligamentous injuries, tibial plateau fractures, proximal fibula fractures, patellar fractures. Pure soft tissue injuries will not show up on radiographs, but effusions	WNL left knee radiographs.

(continued)

DIAGNOSTIC TEST   RATIONALE   RESULTS

and soft tissue swelling may
be obvious on radiograph
films. Stress views may re-
veal ligament laxity versus
epiphyseal injury in the
young skeleton.

● DIAGNOSES

What diagnoses do you determine as being appropriate after a review of the subjective andobjective data?

First-degree MCL sprain left knee

Data Supporting the Diagnosis

Mechanism of injury is consistent with a MCL injury. Roberto was kicked in the lower left leg, which thus caused valgus stress to the knee area. This resulted in pain and mildswelling with the MCL. First-degree MCL sprains are usually mild injuries. Patients with MCL sprains usually exhibit tenderness along the MCL with some swelling (Garth and Fagan, 1996).

● THERAPEUTIC PLAN

1. *What is the initial management plan for a first-degree MCL sprain?*

   - Rest: No weight bearing; crutches for 7 days. No sports for 2–4 weeks (Anderson,1995).
   - Ice: Apply ice to the medial knee joint area for 20 minutes every several hours.
   - Compression: A knee immobilizer is indicated.
   - Elevation: Keep the extremity elevated.
   - NSAIDS for pain: Start NSAIDS for pain; discuss potential side effects and recommend taking with food.
   - Patient education: Discuss anatomy and physiology of the knee with a description of injury and prognosis for return to full activities. Discuss potential medication side effects.

2. *When should Roberto be seen again for this injury?*

   Robert should be seen in 1 week; sooner with increased pain or swelling.

3. *What evaluation should you do to determine if Roberto's injury is healing at his 1 week follow up? (Write SOAP note.)*

S: Roberto returns 1 week later stating his left knee feels great now. He has used his knee immoblizer and avoided all sports. He admits, though, to not using his crutches the last 3–4 days because he felt so good. He is taking Advil 200 every 6 hours with food, and he used the ice until 2 days ago. He is ready to resume playing soccer, but his father is apprehensive about him returning so soon.

O: Hispanic male, NAD, normal gait. No knee immobilizer. Lt. knee: FROM, no swelling, or effusion. No tenderness with palpation over MCL. Negative varus/valgus stress. Neg. Drawer, McMurray, Lachman. Positive pedal pulse with quick refill and sensation to left toes.

A: Healing first-degree MCL sprain, lt. knee.

4. *What should the plan of care for Roberto include at this point?*

- Continue wearing neoprene knee brace.
- Begin rehabilitation: walking, straight leg raises, and use of stationary bike if available.
- Continue NSAIDS.
- No soccer yet.

5. *When should Roberto return for his final follow up?*

Roberto should return in 1 week.

6. *What criteria will you use to determine he no longer needs follow up?* *(Write a SOAP note.)*

S: Roberto returns for follow up 2 weeks after injury. He says his left knee feels perfect now, and he really wants to return to playing soccer. He admits to riding his bike some, and feels this helped strengthen his leg. He continues to take the Advil as directed, and has been wearing a light knee brace to his left knee.

O: NAD, normal gait. Lt. knee: FROM, no swelling, effusion noted. No pain to MCL. Negative varus/valgus stress.

A: Healing MCL sprain left knee.

P: Continue left knee brace.

Begin running, jogging, and conditioning this week, then return to full activity 3 weeks post-injury.

Recheck as needed in future.

REFERENCES:

Anderson B. *Office Orthopedics for Primary Care: Diagnosis and Treatment.* Philadephia: W.B. Saunders; 1995.

Arendt E. Common musculoskeletal injuries in women. *Phys Sports Med* 1996; 24(7): 39–47.

Garth W, Fagan K. Fractures and ligamentous injuries of the knee, in Masear V. (ed). *Primary Care Orthopedics.* Philadelphia: W.B. Saunders; 1996; 88–106.

Mendelson C, Paiemont G. Physical examination of the knee. *Prim Care Orthop* 1996; 23(2): 321–328.

Moyer R. Knee injuries in the occasional athlete: Diagnostic and therapeutic considerations. *Your Pat Fitness Int Med* 1996; 10(4): 21–26.

Rothenburg H, Graf B. Evaluation of acute knee injuries. *Postgrad Med* 1993; 93(3): 75–86.

Sonzogni J. Examining the injured knee. *Emerg Med* 1996; 28(7): 76–86.

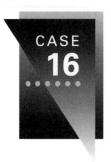

A 17-year-old woman
with abdominal pain

SCENARIO

Sheree Lang is a 17-year-old Native-American female complaining of abdominal pain for 2 weeks. She states she has pain with sexual intercourse, and it hurts to even walk.

● TENTATIVE DIAGNOSES

Based on the information provided so far, what are potential differential diagnoses?

● HISTORY

What are significant questions in Sheree's history?
What are the key points to cover on the review of systems?

● PHYSICAL ASSESSMENT

What are the significant portions of the physical examination that should be completed for Sheree?

● DIFFERENTIAL DIAGNOSES

What are the significant positive and negative data that support or refute your diagnoses for Sheree?

● DIAGNOSTIC TESTS

Based on the history and physical assessment, what, if any, diagnostic tests would you obtain? Include your rationale for the tests.

● DIAGNOSIS

What diagnoses are appropriate for Sheree?

THERAPEUTIC PLAN

1. *What are the indications for hospitalization to treat PID?*

2. *Discuss the complications about which Sheree needs to be warned.*

3. *What are the recommendations by the CDC for outpatient treatment?*

4. *What patient education does Sheree need to avoid getting PID again?*

5. *When should Sheree return for follow up?*

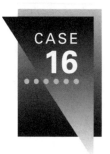

TUTORIAL

A 17-year-old woman with abdominal pain

SCENARIO

Sheree Lang is a 17-year-old Native-American female complaining of abdominal pain for 2 weeks. She states she has pain with sexual intercourse, and it hurts to even walk.

● TENTATIVE DIAGNOSES

What are the potential diagnoses you have identified based on the preceding scenario?

DIAGNOSIS	RATIONALE
PID: GC, chlamydia	Sheree is c/o abdominal pain × 2 weeks, pain with walking.
Ectopic pregnancy	Sheree is c/o abdominal pain × 2 weeks, pain with walking.
Endometriosis	Sheree is c/o abdominal pain × 2 weeks, pain with walking.
Appendicitis	Sheree is c/o abdominal pain × 2 weeks, pain with walking.

● HISTORY

1. What are significant questions in Sheree's history?

REQUESTED DATA	DATA ANSWER
Allergies	NKDA.
Current medications	Taking antidepressant paroxetine (Paxil) 20 mg QD and takes Axid OTC for stomach problems occasionally.
Surgery	Had C-section for daughter born 1 year ago, no transfusions.
Past medical history and hospitalizations/fractures/ injuries/accidents	No previous problems, except "nerves" and occasional stomach problems. Medications help. No injuries, fractures.
Adult illness	Frequent URIs each winter.
OB/GYN history	Menarche: Age 10, cycles are 26 days and last for 7 days. Heavy flow first day then moderate flow. Denies dysmenorrhea. LNMP: 2 weeks ago. Last pap/pelvic: during pregnancy >1 yr ago. BSE: No. Contraception: Uses DMPA. No barrier methods. G 1 P 1 A 0
STD risks	Number of sexual partners >5: Yes. Previous history of STDs: Had trich. once before. New partner within past 2 months: Yes. Drug abuse: Denies. Past hx PID: No.
Social history	Tobacco: smokes $\frac{1}{2}$ ppd × 3 years. Alcohol: Social only. Drugs: Denies. Exercise: No regular exercise.
Family history	Father: 37, healthy. Mother: 35, healthy, 1 episode depression 5 years ago. Siblings: 1 sister, 13, healthy. 2 brothers 11, 10, healthy. Children: 1 daughter, 13 months old.
Income/insurance/employment	Completing high school, senior. Attends special classes for girls with children at school. No income. Medicaid for self and daughter.

2. What are the key points to cover on the review of systems?

SYSTEM REVIEWED	DATA ANSWER
General	Doesn't feel well. Abdominal pain bothering her and interfering with activities.
Skin	Pale, no other problems.
Lungs	Denies SOB.
Cardiac	Denies problems.
GI/GU	Denies dysuria, frequency, urgency. States has a vaginal discharge—has noticed for past few months. Denies N/V.

● PHYSICAL ASSESSMENT

What are the significant portions of the physical examination that should be completed for Sheree?

SYSTEM	RATIONALE	FINDINGS
Vital signs	Provides baseline.	B/P 106/66 HR: 98 R 20 T 99.8 Ht: 5'6" Wt: 150 lbs
General appearance/skin	Provides overall impression of patient.	Pale, lying on exam table holding abdomen.
Lungs	Baseline information.	CTA.
Heart	Baseline information.	RRR, no MRG.
Abdomen	Important to conduct thorough exam of abdomen since c/o abdominal pain.	Abdomen protruberant, soft. No peristalsis visible. BS + all quadrants, tympany to percussion, guarding to palpation, no rebound tenderness. Tenderness of adnexae rt.> lt. No HSM.
Pelvic	Important to conduct to thoroughly evaluate ab-	External genitalia WNL, BUS glands without swelling, ten-

(continued)

SYSTEM	*RATIONALE*	*FINDINGS*
	dominal pain.	derness. +CMT, +adnexal tenderness. Mucopurulent d/c from os.
Rectal	Rectal exam assists in gathering data about abdominal pain.	Rectal sphincter intact. C/o pain with palpation/movement of cervix. Brown stool obtained.

● DIFFERENTIAL DIAGNOSES

What are the significant positive and negative findings that support or refute your diagnoses for Sheree?

DIAGNOSIS	*POSITIVE DATA*	*NEGATIVE DATA*
PID: GC, chlamydia	Abdominal pain which began around menses, history of new partner in past 2 months, no barrier methods of contraception, fever, >5 partners, adolescent, guarding of abdomen, mucopurulent d/c from os, +CMT, adnexal tenderness (Stone, 1996).	No previous history of PID.
Endometriosis	Abdominal pain increased with intercourse, early menarche.	Has been pregnant, negative FH, no dysmenorrhea, no irregular bleeding pattern, negative adnexal masses.
Ectopic pregnancy	Abdominal pain.	LNMP 2 weeks ago, uses DMPA contraception, last injection 9 weeks ago.
Appendicitis	Abdominal pain, rt. Adnexal pain >lt.	No n/v, no generalized abdominal pain, no rebound tenderness.

● DIAGNOSTIC TESTS

Based on the history and physical examination, what, if any, diagnostic tests would you obtain?

DIAGNOSTIC TEST	RATIONALE	RESULTS
CBC with diff. sed. rate	Helps to identify inflammatory process. Usually both WBC and Sed rate are elevated in PID.	Not done.
RPR	Rule out possible syphilis.	Negative.
U/A	Check for possible urinary infection.	WNL.
Pregnancy test, quantitative	Serum quantitative pregnancy tests assist in the diagnosis of ectopic pregnancy.	Negative.
C-reactive protein	Detects inflammation, sensitive for PID.	Not done.
Vaginal smear/cervical cultures	Helps to identify the causative organism.	Wet smear revealed no trichimoniasis, clue cells, or budding hyphae. DNA probe obtained for GC and chlamydia.
Ultrasound	Identifies fluid in the cul de sac, distended tubes or tubo-ovarian cyst.	Not done.
Laparoscopy	Most definitive diagnosis of PID and ectopic pregnancy. Invasive and expensive (DeCherney, 1994).	Not done.

● DIAGNOSES

What diagnoses do you determine as being appropriate after a review of the subjective and objective data?

Pelvic inflammatory disease (PID)

Data Supporting the Diagnosis

Abdominal pain that began around menses, history of new partner in past 2 months, no barrier methods of contraception, fever, >5 partners, adolescent, guarding of abdomen, mucopurulent d/c from os, +CMT, adnexal tenderness. Sheree's symptoms meet the minimum criteria as designated by the CDC, so no testing besides a wet smear and DNA probe was done (CDC, 1993).

● THERAPEUTIC PLAN

1. What are the indications for hospitalization to treat PID?

Pelvic abcess
Patient is toxic or noncompliant
Patient does not respond to treatment promptly (CDC, 1993)
Prepubertal client
Pregnant client (rare)
Patient with HIV (Forrest, 1994)

2. Discuss the complications about which Sheree needs to be warned.

Infertility
   One episode of PID will cause infertility in approximately 13% of women. After 3 or more episodes of PID, 75% of women become infertile (DeCherney, 1994).
Ectopic pregnancy
Chronic abdominal pain
Pelvic abcess
Pelvic adhesions
Premature hysterectomy
Depression (Youngkin, 1994)

3. What are the recommendations by the CDC for outpatient treatment?

Because the causative agents are usually GC or chlamydia, the CDC (1993) recommends the following:

Ceftriaxone (Rocephin) 250 mg IM stat plus
Doxycycline 100 mg PO BID for 14 days

4. What patient education does Sheree need to avoid getting PID again?

It is important to stress to Sheree the necessity of completing all the medications. Her partner should be evaluated and treated to prevent the risk of reinfection. Sheree should abstain from sexual intercourse during the course of treatment. The use of condoms in addition to the DMPA should be emphasized. Sheree should know that although the DMPA prevents pregnancy, it does not protect her against STDs, including HIV.

5. When should Sheree return for follow up?

It will be critical for Sheree to return in 48–72 hours for evaluation of her progress. If the NP has any concerns that Sheree will not return for follow up he/she should seriously consider hospitalization. Sheree should be aware that if her symptoms worsen during outpatient treatment, she should get in touch with her health care provider right away because hospitalization will probably be necessary. Sheree should be evaluated again in 7–10 days. It will be important to check for tenderness and masses. A microsopic re-examination should be done at this return visit 7–10 days after completing therapy. This return visit also gives the health care provider the opportunity to ask about and confirm the partner's treatment.

REFERENCES

Barker R, Burton J, Zieve P. *Principles of Ambulatory Medicine,* 4th ed. Baltimore: Williams & Wilkins; 1995.

CDC, 1993. Sexually transmitted disease treatment guidelines. *Nurse Pract* 1996; 7(1):47–50

DeCherney A, Pernoll M. *Current Obstetric & Gynecologic Diagnosis and Treatment* 8th ed. Norwalk, CT: Appleton, Lange; 1994.

Forrest D. Common gynceologic pelvic disorders, in Youngkin E. and Davis M. (eds). *Women's Health: A Primary Care Clinical Guide,* Norwalk, CT: Appleton, Lange; 1994.

Stone R. Primary care diagnosis of acute abdominal pain. *Nurse Pract* 1996; 21(12): 19–39.

Youngkin E, Davis M. *Women's health: A primary care clinical guide.* Norwalk, CT: Appleton & Lange, 1994.

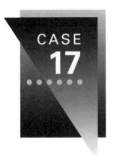

A 75-year-old woman with confusion and incontinence

SCENARIO

Mrs. Emmett is a 75-year-old Native-American female in to see you because of recent confusion. She is accompanied by her daughter. Mrs. Emmett is neatly dressed in her "Sunday best" dress. She is pleasant, talkative, and easily distracted. She relates she is not having much trouble with her HTN medicines, and says she believes it is important to take them. When engaged in small talk about current events, Mrs. Emmett states "I don't pay much attention to those things anymore." When asked who is the current president, she responds "there was no one like Ike. Those were the good old days." She states she doesn't get out much anymore. Stopped driving "because of the traffic" and got lost in town on more than one occasion. Her daughter reports that she used to play bridge, but had lost interest in that, in part because club members had complained about her not being able to keep up with the game. Admits to feeling lonely. Her daughter has helped with the shopping ("my arthritis really has been acting up") for the last few years and does the bills ("my eyes aren't as good as they used to be.") The daughter states that her mother usually has a great memory and can remember things way back, but has a tendency to repeat stories from years ago. The daughter adds lately her mother seemed more confused—for example, she has been calling her in the middle of the night talking about a long-lost relative. This morning, when her daughter went to check on her, she discovered that her mother was incontinent with soiled clothing and bed linens. This has not happened before.

● TENTATIVE DIAGNOSES

1. *Based on the information provided so far, what are potential diagnoses?*
2. *What are possible differential diagnoses for changes in cognitive status?*

● HISTORY

What are significant questions in Mrs. Emmett's and her daughter's history? What are the key points to cover on the review of systems?

● PHYSICAL ASSESSMENT

What are the significant portions of the physical examination that should be completed for Mrs. Emmett?

● DIFFERENTIAL DIAGNOSES

What are the significant positive and negative data that support or refute your diagnoses for Mrs. Emmett?

● DIAGNOSTIC TESTS

Based on the history and physical assessment, what, if any, diagnostic tests would you obtain? Include your rationale for the tests.

● DIAGNOSIS

What diagnoses are appropriate for Mrs. Emmett?

● THERAPEUTIC PLAN

1. *What might be the family's response to the diagnosis of Alzheimer's disease?*
2. *What treatments are available for dementia?*
3. *What are suggestions the NP could make in terms of family support for ongoing care?*
4. *What are home safety issues that will need to be discussed?*
5. *At what point will Mrs. Emmett's family know she is unable to care for herself?*
6. *What suggestions can you make so Mrs. Emmett does not feel so lonely?*
7. *What community resources might be helpful to the NP and Mrs. Emmett and her family?*
8. *Discuss how the plan of care might need to be readjusted and revised as the dementia progresses.*

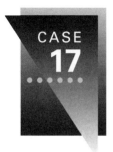

CASE
17

TUTORIAL

A 75-year-old woman with confusion and incontinence

SCENARIO

Mrs. Emmett is a 75-year-old Native-American female in to see you because of recent confusion. She is accompanied by her daughter. Mrs. Emmett is neatly dressed in her "Sunday best" dress. She is pleasant, talkative, and easily distracted. She relates she is not having much trouble with her HTN medicines, and says she believes it is important to take them. When engaged in small talk about current events, Mrs. Emmett states "I don't pay much attention to those things anymore." When asked who is the current president, she responds "there was no one like Ike. Those were the good old days." She states she doesn't get out much anymore. Stopped driving "because of the traffic" and got lost in town on more than one occasion. Her daughter reports that she used to play bridge, but had lost interest in that, in part because club members had complained about her not being able to keep up with the game. Admits to feeling lonely. Her daughter has helped with the shopping ("my arthritis really has been acting up") for the last few years and does the bills ("my eyes aren't as good as they used to be.") The daughter states her mother usually has a great memory and can remember things way back, but has a tendency to repeat stories from years ago. The daughter adds lately her mother seemed more confused—for example, she has been calling her in the middle of the night talking about a long-lost relative. This morning, when her daughter went to check on her, she discovered that her mother was incontinent with soiled clothing and bed linens. This has not happened before.

● TENTATIVE DIAGNOSES

Based on the information provided so far, what are potential diagnoses?

DIAGNOSIS	RATIONALE
Change in cognitive status: dementia	Dementia is a change in mental status characterized not only by declining memory but also declining functional capabilities, visual-spatial difficulties, or language impairment (AHCPR, 1996). Ms. Emmett presents a history of getting lost, vague answers, and dodges specific information, especially about recent events. Long-term memory can be preserved for some time as a dementing process continues. Note the change in level of functioning prior to this onset of acute confusion. Caregivers can be the best source of information about the functional and mental status of the patient. The transfer of ADLs can occur gradually, and the extent of this transfer may not be fully realized by the caregiver. The reason why this transfer has occurred can be blamed on arthritis, diminished vision, and so forth.
Change in cognitive status: delirium	Abrupt onset of change in mental status, abrupt onset of confusion, and urinary incontinence are clues to a delirium. By definition, delirium is an abrupt change in mental status characterized by inattention, disorganized thinking, an altered level of awareness, and a fluctuating course. Delirium has many causes or precipitating events, including: infections, cardiac events, TIA, medication side effects, electrolyte imbalance, alcohol intoxication, and other medical problems.
Change in cognitive status: depression	Loss of friends or loss of independence may be causes for a dysphoric or depressed state. Depression can present itself as a state of reduced alertness or apathy or even as a change in the mental status of an elder.
HTN	By history.

What are possible differential diagnoses for changes in cognitive status?

DIFFERENTIAL DIAGNOSES   RATIONALE

Dementia: Alzheimer vs non-Alzheimer type	Up to 70% of dementias are thought to be of the Alzheimer type, and about 10% are thought to be of a vascular type (Geldmacher & Whitehouse, 1996). The clinical presentations can be very similar, both having a progressive decline. Some types of dementia may be partially reversed, for example, those types caused by polypharmacy. Even in irreversible dementias, problematic symptoms such as wandering can be treated with some success (AHCPR, 1996).
Delirium: hyper/hypothyroidism	Hyper/hypothyroidism is a common finding in the elderly. This may present as a change in mental status or loss of interest in usual activities.
Delirium re: nutritional deficiencies	Eating alone and changes in the ability to taste and chew foods may result in inadequate nutrition. Prolonged nutritional deficiencies may affect cognition.
Delirium re: anemia	Changes in mental status may indicate anemia. Mrs. Emmett states she has arthritis. If she is taking OTC NSAIDS for her arthritis pain she may have an asymptomatic GI bleed.
Delirium re: electrolyte imbalance	Changes in mental status can be triggered by electrolyte imbalances. Her anti-HTN medicine may cause electrolyte imbalances.
Delirium re: UTI	Sudden changes in mental status may indicate an infectious process. UTIs are common in elderly women for a variety of reasons. The sudden incontinence may reflect a deteriorating mental status, but also may reflect the presence of a UTI. Certainly, dehydration, change in hormonal levels, and inattention to personal hygiene may contribute to the likelihood of a UTI.
Delirium re: cardiac event	Abrupt changes in mental status and functioning may indicate a cardiac event such as MI, CHF, or arrhythmia. The patient may be unable to describe events surrounding such an event.
Delirium re: neurological event	Abrupt changes in mental status and functioning may indicate a neurological event such as a TIA or CVA.

(continued)

DIFFERENTIAL DIAGNOSES   RATIONALE

Delirium re: medication side effects	Multiple medications, complicated dosing schedules, and continuing medications beyond therapeutic necessity all contribute to medication errors, drug interactions, and increased side effects.

● HISTORY

1. What are the significant questions in Mrs. Emmett's and her daughter's history?

REQUESTED DATA   DATA ANSWER

Allergies	Sulfa—breaks out in hives per daughter.
Current medications	HCTZ 25 mg QD. Ben-Gay analgesic rub. Centrum Silver MVI per daughter.
Surgery/transfusions	Cataract surgery 1992. Hysterectomy, 1950s reason unknown, no transfusions.
Past medical hstory and hospitalizations/fractures/injuries/accidents	Hospitalized for hyst. Pneumonia, 1960s; no fractures, injuries.
Adult illness	HTN, diverticulosis, cataracts.
OB/GYN history	G1P1A0. Never used hormones. Unknown last pap/pelvic. Never had mammogram, doesn't examine breasts.
Appetite	Usually about 140 lbs, wore size 12. Has lost 10 # over last 6 months. Appetite decreased—"food doesn't taste as good anymore."
24-hour diet recall	"Oh, you know—the usual."
Typical day	Up at 7, light breakfast, "putters around the house" rest of day.
Social history	Finished high school, had 1 year of secretarial school. Worked as housewife and mother. Now lives alone, daughter lives in town. Lives in single story home, five steps. Never used tobacco or alcohol. Three cups of coffee ("good strong coffee") a day.

(continued)

REQUESTED DATA DATA ANSWER

REQUESTED DATA	DATA ANSWER
Family history	Father: Died when she was young. Mother: Died of old age. Older brother: Fine (daughter states, in nursing home with Alzheimer's). Health of younger siblings is unknown. "I think they are in California." Daughter: Fine.
Relationship with spouse, children, lifelong friends	Widow "for a while now." Feels close to daughter and grandchildren. Doesn't see old friends as often as she used to.
Prevention immunizations, sigmoid, exercise, diet, eye, hearing, dentist	Can't state last physical, mammogram, pelvic. Not sure if she took the flu shot last year. Gets "plenty of exercise housecleaning." Had dentures and glasses for "a long time."
ADLs and IADLs	Set the stove on fire last week making coffee. Dresses, bathes, toilets self (usually, until the crises of yesterday). Ambulates independently. For the last several years, daughter helps with meal planning, shopping, paying the bills, and arranging transportation.

2. *What are the key points to cover on the review of systems?*

SYSTEM REVIEWED DATA ANSWER

SYSTEM REVIEWED	DATA ANSWER
General	Acute confusion, agitation noticed yesterday: did not know day. Agitated, reassurance helped, but essentially the same today.
Cardiac	No SOB, chest pain or pressure.
Neurological	"Memory pretty good for my age," no H/A, dizziness, LOC, or syncope. Tripped once and fell, no injury.
GU	Some burning, and frequency—started yesterday. Hasn't felt well for a while. Denies previous incontinence or UTIs.
Musculoskeletal	"Good days and bad days—doesn't everyone."
Sensory	Unable to further clarify.

● PHYSICAL ASSESSMENT

What are the significant portions of the physical examination that should be completed for Mrs. Emmett?

SYSTEM	RATIONALE	FINDINGS
Vital signs	Provide baseline data.	B/P 180/74 sitting. HR 80, R 20, T 98.8. Wt: 112 lbs. Ht: 5'4".
General appearance/skin	A complete exam is warranted for Mrs. Emmett due to the complexity of the symptoms, their interrelatedness, and the fact that patient is a poor historian.	Pale scattered keratosis, bruise left forearm, skin looks . fragile.
HEENT	Observe for neuro deficits, factors that would indicate nutritional deficiencies, factors indicating problems with eating, general state of hydration, and factors that can be addressed, ie, poor vision/cataracts so orientation can be facilitated.	Ear: TMs opalescent. Funduscopy: Unable to visualize due to cataracts. VA: Can read magazine. Peripheral vision via confrontation: Deferred, unable to follow instructions. Mouth: Mucosa dry, no lesions. Edentulous. Neck: No NVD, supple.
Lungs	Observe for presence of adventitious lung sounds that may indicate acute or chronic disease that may influence oxygenation and therefore delirium, ex. pneumonia.	CTA.
Heart	Observe for rhythm disturbance, rate abnormalities, cardiomegaly, and new murmurs. Recent changes may cause delirium, for ex. atrial fibrillation with slow rate may cause syncope, etc.	Regular rate and rhythm. S_1S_2 WNL. 2/6 systolic murmur at the sternal border radiating to the right, heard best sitting. No carotid bruits.
Breasts	Done as part of general survey. Breast cancers may metastasize to the brain, but	Symmetrical, no masses, no axillary nodes, no d/c.

(continued)

SYSTEM	*RATIONALE*	*FINDINGS*
	would most likely show as a focal neurological deficit rather than dementia/delirium seen here.	
Abdomen	New complaints of urinary incontinence, questionable hydration and food intake, unreliable historian mean a complete abdominal exam should be done.	BS+, soft, nondistended, slight suprapubic tenderness, no masses, no rebound tenderness, no HSM.
Pelvic	A complete exam is warranted for Mrs. Emmett because of the urinary incontinence.	Atrophic vaginal tissues, no d/c or urine leakage with exam. Urine strong-smelling. No lesions, pale cervix, stenosed os, no adnexal tenderness.
Rectal	Part of a general exam to observe for hydration, constipation, hemoccult for signs of GI bleeding (taking OTC NSAIDS).	Tight sphincter, hard stool in vault, no masses or hemorrhoidal tags.
Extremities	Observe for signs of impaired circulation, injury, ability to care for nails.	Pulses 2+, no edema, no varicosity.
Neurological	A complete exam is warranted to rule out focal neurological deficits, gait abnormalities, neuropathies related to circulatory or nutritional deficits.	CN I–XII intact, gait wide-based, small steps, decreased step height, hand grasp equal bilaterally. General muscle strength +3/5 upper and lower extremities. Unable to lift bag of groceries (approx. 10 lbs). Sensation intact, unable to determine joint position sense or vibratory sense. DTRs 3+ bilaterally. Babinski negative bilaterally.
Mental	A complete exam is warranted to identify mental status deficits (more than merely deficits in orientation) (Strub & Black, 1993).	Folstein mini-mental exam: 19/30. Deficits in short term memory, orientation, attention, and calculation.

● DIFFERENTIAL DIAGNOSES

What are the significant positive and negative findings that support or refute your diagnoses for Mrs. Emmett?

DIAGNOSIS	POSITIVE DATA	NEGATIVE DATA
Delirium	Sudden increase in confusion as exhibited by incontinence, inattention.	May be a progression of dementia.
Dementia	+FH of Alzheimers, progressive inability to do IADLs, vague answers, Folstein score.	None. UTI symptoms may exaggerate the presentation of cognitive deficits, but the presence of these deficits precedes the new complaint of urinary problems.
Depression	Loss of companionship, lack of interest in life and food.	Assessment colored by illness presentation.
UTI	Sudden incontinence, foul smelling urine, increased frequency and burning, suprapubic tenderness, constipated.	Afebrile.
HTN	Elevated systolic blood pressure, +FH of heart problems, unknown daily blood pressure control, SEM.	Unknown daily B/P, may have "white coat" HTN.
Cardiac event/failure	Long history HTN.	RRR, lungs clear, no SOB, no HSM, no NVD, no edema.
TIA	Sudden confusion, HTN, episode not directly observed, unreliable historian.	No focal deficits.
Nutritional deficiencies, dehydration	Dry skin and oral mucosa, unknown food and fluid intake patterns. HCTZ, unknown time frame for weight loss.	None.
Hyper/hypothyroidism	Dry skin, decreased appetite, age, female, agitation.	VS, DTRs normal.
Medication side effects	HCTZ prescribed, unknown compliance patterns.	Taking HCTZ for years.

● DIAGNOSTIC TESTS

Based on the history and physical examination, what, if any, diagnostic testing would you obtain?

It is unlikely that any laboratory result or other diagnostic procedure will identify correctable causes of dementia. So while these tests are generally to be ordered for demented persons, the likelihood of a positive result is less than 10% (Geldmacher and Whitehouse, 1996). Obviously, Mrs. Emmett has other physiological illnesses that make these tests advisable.

DIAGNOSTIC TEST	RATIONALE	RESULTS
U/A	Good choice to determine UTI. May consider C&S, but because this is not recurrent, may choose to empirically treat with non-sulfa drug.	Leukocytes: Large. Nitrites: +. Glucose: Neg. Blood: Mod.
Electrolytes, renal, liver (multichem analysis)	Because nutritional intake is essentially unknown, and because electrolyte imbalances can cause a change in mental status, a good choice. Mrs. Emmett is taking a K-depleting diuretic, although in unknown frequencies and amounts.	Na: 135. K+: 3.4. Cl: 108. CO2: 25. BUN: 25. Creat. 1.3. ALT: 35. AST: 27. Alk. phos.: 40. Glucose: 76.
CBC with differential	Good choice. Mrs. Emmett is pale and has some degree of peripheral neuropathy. This test would show anemia may be contributing to her present state. In addition, if an infection if present you might see changes in the WBC count.	RBC: 5.2 million. Hgb: 14 g/dL. MCV: 85 fl. MCH: 1.75 fmol. MCHC: 37%. WBC: 11,000. Segs: 60%. Basos: 0. Bands: 4%. Eos: 2%. Monos: 4%. Lymphs: 28%. Platelets: 220,000.

(continued)

DIAGNOSTIC TEST	*RATIONALE*	*RESULTS*
B12 and RBC folate	Good choice for determining nutritional status and the presence of pernicious anemia.	Folate: 320 ng/mL. B12: 500 pg/mL.
TSH, thyroid panel	Hypothyroidism in the elderly may present as a cloudiness of sensorium without the usual signs seen in younger people. Because TSH is the most sensitive test, the thyroid panel would only be ordered if the TSH is low.	TSH 4.0 mU/L. T4 8.0 g/dL. T3: 158 ng/dL. Free thyroxine index: 10.0.
CT or MRI of head	Expensive, but can show any lesions, areas of infarction, and presence of subdural hematoma that may explain the changes in mental status, especially if the changes are abrupt. The MRI may better identify areas of ischemia not detected by the CT. MRI may be used when the individual has a focal neuro deficit.	No areas of infarction, hematomas seen. No ischemia identified. Brain atrophy, no focal lesions.
Geriatric depression scale	Good choice to quantify and open discussion of feelings. Suggest to be done after mental status returns to baseline. Depression can make the dementia seem worse.	13/30 Mild depression. This test may be delayed until present delirium lifts.
Neurocognitive testing	May more precisely define areas of deficits, especially judgment, visual–spatial, construction, intelligence.	Not done at this time. Will plan to do once acute illness has improved. (Test shows decline in visual–spatial skills, judgment, and abstraction.)
CXR	Will help determine the size of her heart, presence of pulmonary lesions or tumors, CHF, or pneumonia	Slight cardiomegaly, atherosclerosis of aorta, osteoporosis, no masses, no acute disease.
RPR	Latent syphilis may present as dementia.	Nonreactive. This test may not be reimbursed by insurance carriers.

(continued)

DIAGNOSTIC TEST	RATIONALE	RESULTS
HIV	Dementia is not a common presenting symptom in HIV infection, but there is an HIV dementia. Mrs. Emmett does not have any known risk factors.	Not done.
EEG	Not routinely ordered for dementia, but may be helpful in identifying coexising seizure disorder.	Not done.
Genetic testing (apolipoprotein E4)	May be available, but because its value as a diagnostic or predictive test has not been established, do not recommend its use in general practice now (Geldmacher and Whitehouse, 1996).	Not done.

● DIAGNOSES

What diagnoses do you determine as being appropriate after a review of the subjective and objective data?

Delirium most likely related to UTI

Dementia, type not determined, but probable Alzheimer-type or multi-infarct

Data Supporting the Diagnosis

Delirium: The description of incontinence, suprapubic tenderness, foul smelling urine, in addition to positive U/A suggests an acute delirium related to UTI. Clearing the infection may return Mrs. Emmett to or near her baseline demented state.

Dementia: The Folstein mini-mental and ADL suggest a dementing process that has been progressing slowly over the years. Mrs. Emmett has a cognitive decline greater than merely memory loss. She is unable to care for herself, take care of financial obligations, or drive. The reasons given for stopping these activities should be carefully ascertained. +FH and gradual progression of the illness support the tentative diagnosis of Alzheimer's disease, but given Mrs. Emmett's long standing history of HTN, she may have a multi-infarct type of illness. Alzheimer's accounts for 70% of dementia with multi-infarct, or vascular dementia accounting for 10–20% of dementia (Geldmacher and Whitehouse,

1996). This diagnosis can only be made after other causes of dementia have been excluded, such as alcohol abuse, AIDS, neurosyphilis, previous head trauma, or other medical problems.

● THERAPEUTIC PLAN

1. *What might be the family's response to the diagnosis of Alzheimer's disease?*

At first the family may deny that the confusion seen is a continuation of an ongoing dementia. They may deny that this is true or cry at the loss of their mother as they knew her. It is frightening to project to the future knowing that their mother or grandmother may not recognize them and the real possibility of her inability to care for herself in the future.

2. *What treatments are available for dementia?*

The drugs tacrine (Cognex) and donepazil have shown some efficacy in treatment of mild to moderate Alzheimer's disease. These drugs do not change the fundamental brain deterioration that is taking place, but enhance cognitive function in a percentage of patients with Alzheimer's disease. Tacrine has been on the market for a longer period of time. It requires close monitoring of liver enzymes and QID dosing. Donepazil has recently been made available, requires no laboratory monitoring for adverse effects, and is dosed once a day. It must be understood that all patients are not a candidate for these medicines—for example patients with severe Alzheimer's—and that results will vary.

3. *What are suggestions the NP could make in terms of family support for ongoing care?*

Discuss the availability of support groups and home health care as well as respite services in the area. Suggest *The 36 Hour Day and Comforting the Confused* as resources for concrete tips on caring for someone with dementia.

4. *What are home safety issues that will need to be discussed?*

Issues such as cooking safety, firearm safety, environment modification, developing a fire plan, and calling for help should all be discussed with Mrs. Emmett and her family. Suggest telephone reassurances and life-call program if available (Reichel & Rabins, 1995).

5. *At what point will Mrs. Emmett's family know she is unable to care for herself?*

It is important to discuss planning for continued care, prior to needing a high level of care that can be provided in the home. Making arrangements for 24-hour in-home care or transfer to some type of institutional living can take time. Waiting for an emergency to begin planning can only lead to frustration.

6. *What suggestions can you make so Mrs. Emmett does not feel so lonely?*

Programs such as Meals on Wheels, adult day care, and supervised senior activities might be helpful to provide companionship and cognitive stimulation for Mrs. Emmett. Because she previously enjoyed people, she may enjoy getting out of the house.

7. *What community resources might be helpful to the NP and Mrs. Emmett and her family?*

Social Workers/Elder Services: Identification of community resources, financial and insurance resources, assistance with referral home care agencies, and help to obtain higher levels of care (nursing home placement) as the need arises.

Home health agencies: Provide in-home personal and nursing care, such as bathing assistance, medication setup, BP monitoring, and nursing observations.

Chaplain/Parish Nurse: Provide spiritual support for the patient and family. May be aware of volunteers who are able to visit or call.

Alzheimer Association and Support Group: Provides information and support from those whose families who have similar problems.

Geriatric Evaluation Team: Comprehensive evaluation of medical problems and mental status. Usually part of a medical school. Aware of new treatments or approaches that may be beneficial.

Area Office on Aging: Listing of governmental programs for the elderly available in the area.

Attorney: Assistance in legal matters such as assigning a power of attorney.

Alzheimer's Association
Chicago, IL
800 272-4380

Alzheimer's Disease Education and Referral Center
Silver Springs, MD
800 438-4380

Administration on Aging
Washington, DC
206 619-1006

Eldercare Locator
Washington, DC
800 677-1116

American Association of Retired Persons (AARP)
Washington, DC
800 424-3410

8. Discuss how the plan of care might need to be readjusted and revised as the dementia progresses.

This family will need ongoing care and support as they struggle with the demands of deterioration in cognitive abilities. The rate of progression can not be predicted for any individual. Periodic re-evaluation of mental and functional status is needed. Episodic illness may have prolonged effect—the patient may never quite return to baseline functioning. The needs of the Mrs. Emmett and family are likely to be dynamic. Families vary in their ability and willingness to care for a lived one with altered mental status. Some graciously accept the challenge, whereas for others it is an overwhelming situation. It is not unusual for one member of the family to be selected by the family to shoulder the greater share of the responsibility. The realignment of roles and responsibilities is stressful. The focus of care can then shift from the patient to the family, as they are educated and supported in this illness process.

REFERENCES

Clinical Practice Guideline: Recognizing and Initial Assessment of Alzheimer's and Related Dementias. Agency for Health Care Policy and Research. 1996. Publication Number 97-R123 (1-800-358-9295).

Geldmacher D, Whitehouse P. Evaluation of dementia. *N Eng J Med* 1996; 335(5):330–336.

Hoffman S, Platt C. *Comforting the Confused.* New York: Springer; 1991.

Mace N, Rabins P. *The 36 Hour Day.* Baltimore: Johns Hopkins University Press; 1981.

Reichel W, Rabins P. Evaluation and management of the confused, disoriented or demented elderly patient, in Reichel W. (ed). *Care of the Elderly,* 4th ed. Baltimore: Williams & Wilkins; 1995.

Strub R, Black, F. *The Mental Status Examination in Neurology.* Philadelphia: F.A. Davis; 1993.

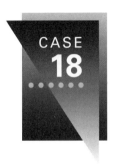

A 3-week-old infant well-child check

SCENARIO

June, an unmarried 18-year-old Hispanic female, brings her 23-day-old daughter (Amanda) to the office for the first well-child check. Amanda is June's first child. June states that Amanda's feedings and activity level have decreased over the last 2 weeks. Her mother notes that she seems to be more irritable and difficult to console.

● TENTATIVE DIAGNOSIS

Based on the information provided by Amanda's mother so far, what are potential differential diagnoses?

● HISTORY

What are significant questions in the history for a 3-week-old well-child physical? What are important developmental questions that need to be addressed? What are the key points to cover on the review of systems?

● PHYSICAL ASSESSMENT

What are the significant portions of the physical examination that should be completed for Amanda?

● DIFFERENTIAL DIAGNOSES

Examine all the data up to this point. Link the subjective and objective data to the appropriate differential diagnoses. Identify both positive and negative data that support or refute the possible diagnoses.

● DIAGNOSTIC TESTS

What additional data and diagnostic tests need to be collected or performed to confirm the diagnosis?

● DIAGNOSIS

What are your conclusive diagnoses? What information assisted you in your decision?

● THERAPEUTIC PLAN

1. *What are issues to consider when deciding on treatment for Amanda?*
2. *What are suggestions to improve the fat content of maternal breast milk?*
3. *What are resources of financial assistance for Amanda and her mother?*
4. *What referrals would be appropriate for Amanda and her mother?*
5. *What follow up would you plan for Amanda?*
6. *Based on the information given about Amanda, what impact do you think her birth had on her mother?*
7. *What community resources would be helpful for Amanda and her mother?*
8. *Amanda returns for a follow up 1 week later. Her weight is 2525 grams. She is more alert and active during the examination. What adjustments would you make in the therapeutic plan developed at the first visit?*
9. *What anticipatory guidance should be given to the mother related to Amanda's growth and development?*
10. *What information should be given to Amanda's mother related to immunizations?*

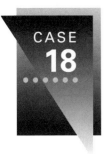

TUTORIAL

A 3-week-old infant well-child check

SCENARIO

June, an unmarried 18-year-old Hispanic female, brings her 23-day-old daughter (Amanda) to the office for the first well-child check. Amanda is June's first child. June states that Amanda's feedings and activity level have decreased over the last 2 weeks. Her mother notes that she seems to be more irritable and difficult to console.

● TENTATIVE DIAGNOSIS

Based on the information provided by Amanda's mother so far, what are potential differential diagnoses?

DIFFERENTIAL DIAGNOSES   RATIONALE

DIFFERENTIAL DIAGNOSES	RATIONALE
Congenital heart disease	Presents with decreased feedings, decreased activity level, and failure to thrive.
Sepsis-bacteremia	Many cases of neonatal sepsis present with non-specific symptoms of decreased organ profusion, such as decreased activity level, failure to thrive, and poor feedings. Group B streptococcus (GBS) is the most common neonatal Gram-positive pathogen (Klaus and Fanaroff, 1993). Although fever is the hallmark of adult bacteremia, infants may present with normal, low, or elevated temperatures.
Neurological/metabolic diseases: Increased intercranial pressure (IICP), Intraventricular hemorrhage (IVH), acidosis, inborn errors of	Amanda demonstrates a progressively decreased activity level that may be the result of poor cellular function of the neurological system and other metabolic disorders. This often results in

(continued)

DIFFERENTIAL DIAGNOSES   *RATIONALE*
••

metabolism	lethargy, poor feeding, failure to thrive (FTT), and developmental delay.
Pulmonary (sequestered lobe)	Decreased lung capacity may result in decreased oxygenation during times of stress such as feedings, leading to this increased work of breathing that results in excess energy use and poor weight gain. Patients may compensate by increasing respiratory rate.
GERD	Amanda demonstrates failure to thrive and irritability, which are frequently seen in GERD. Growth and weight gain are adversely affected in $\frac{2}{3}$ of patients (Behrman and Vaughn, 1987).
Toxins	Although toxin exposure in a 23-day-old infant is unusual, substances that increase energy requirements such as cocaine and methylamphetamines have been demonstrated to cross through breast milk. Toxins that make the infant more sleepy and somnolent such as opiates, barbiturates, alcohol, or benzodiazepines likewise are transmitted through breast milk and can affect patient behavior. Infants also may be exposed to toxins through medications and home remedies given by parents without provider knowledge.
Poor fat content in breast milk	Fats are the main energy source for newborns, providing 40–50% of the total calories in human milk (Tsang and Nichols, 1988). Fats are vital for normal growth and development. Fat content varies from mother to mother.
Poor feeder	Although found primarily in association with neurological injury, some infants have poor feeding mechanisms such as latching, suck, and swallow coordination. Poor feeding may also be the result of poor maternal technique and inexperience.
Failure to thrive (FTT)—inorganic	Psychosocial failure to thrive is the most common form of growth failure in infancy. It accounts for over 50% of cases (Zitelli and Davis, 1987).

● HISTORY

What are significant questions in the history for a 3-week-old well-child visit?
What are important developmental questions that need to be addressed?
What are the key points to cover in the review of systems?

REQUESTED DATA   DATA ANSWER

REQUESTED DATA	DATA ANSWER
Allergies	None known.
Medications	None.
Immunizations	Hepatitis B vaccine ×1.
Transfusion	None.
OBG history	No prenatal care until sixth month. G2P1A1. Rupture of membranes 18 hrs prior to delivery. GBS status: Culture negative at 34 weeks.
Birth history	Vaginal delivery and vacuum extraction. Apgars: 8/8 at 1 and 5 minutes. Weight of infant: 2465 grams. Length of stay in hospital: 24 hours.
Family history	Maternal GM: DM and HTN. Maternal GF: Chronic lung disease. Father: No information. Mother: Healthy.
Maternal diet: based on 24-hr recall	B: Dry bagel, juice. L: Rice, green beans, fat-free cheese, soda. D: Rice, orange, salad without dressing, soda. S: Apple.
Amanda's diet	Breast feeding 5–10 minutes per breast every 3–4 hours.
Sleeping pattern	Sleeping approximately 16 hours per night. Wakes at night for feedings.
Weight/height	Gained 1 oz and grew 0.5 in in 3 weeks.
Mother's education	Completed 11th grade.
Income	Unemployed. Recently applied for Medicaid.
Transportation	Requires use of public transportation.
Social habits	Tobacco: Smokes 1 ppd/5yr. Alcohol: Drinks socially with friends on weekly basis. Caffeinated beverages: Drinks 3–4 sodas/day. Recreational drugs: Denies use. Exercise: Exercises approximately 1 hour/day.
Ethnicity	Hispanic. No known cultural or religious practices.
Mother/infant relationship	Good bonding and eye contact.
Relationship with father of baby	Has not seen him since conception.

(continued)

REQUESTED DATA	DATA ANSWER
Relationship with parents	Parents divorced, good relationship with mother.
Amanda's development	Tracks well, able to lift head while prone, occasional smile.
Home	Lives with Amanda's grandmother at this time.
Social support	Has multiple friends. Grandmother and younger siblings supportive. No breast-feeding role models.
Review of systems	General: Denies fevers, but increased irritability noted. Resp: Denies tachypnea, SOB, choking, or cyanosis. CV: Denies sweating and SOB during feedings. GI: Occasional wet burps of 1–2 teaspoons, no vomiting. Denies diarrhea. GU: Urinary output sufficient. Wets 6 diapers/day. Neuro: Denies seizures, posturing, and lethargy.

● PHYSICAL ASSESSMENT

What are the significant portions of the physical examination that should be completed for Amanda? What is your rationale for the portions of the exam completed?

SYSTEM	RATIONALE	FINDINGS
General	Provides overall view of Amanda.	Irritable, but difficult to console. Nontoxic. Well-developed, well hydrated.
Vital signs	Provides baseline information.	HR: 160 RR: 56 Temp: 98.6°F Wt: 2465 grams Head circumference: 32.5 cm
Skin color and character	Well-baby check: need to do complete screen.	No cyanosis. Color pale, mucus membranes pink. Good capillary refill. No skin breakdown.
ENT	Well-baby check: need to do complete screen.	Normocephalic/atraumatic. Anterior fontanel soft and flat, 3+3 cm. PERRL, EOMI. No rhinnorhea. TMs yearly. Oro-

(continued)

SYSTEM	*RATIONALE*	*FINDINGS*
		pharynx nonerythematous, intact palate, tongue non-tettered. No macroglossia.
Neck	Well-baby check: need to do complete screen.	Full ROM. No thyromegaly.
Cardiovascular	Well-baby check: need to do complete screen.	Regular rate and rhythm. Normal S_1 and S_2. II/VI systolic murmur heard across entire precordium and back. Murmur also heard in both axillae without radiation. Nonbounding pulses present. No edema.
Chest	Well-baby check: need to do complete screen.	No grunting, retracting, or nasal flaring. Clear to auscultation.
Abdomen	Well-baby check: need to do complete screen.	Abdomen with good BS. Soft, full, nontender. No hepatosplenomegaly. Soft yellow stool in diaper.
Urogenital	Well-baby check: need to do complete screen.	Nonerythematous perineum. Tanner stage 1.
Extremities/hips	Well-baby check: need to do complete screen.	Good bulk and tone. Negative Ortolani and Barlow tests.
Back	Well-baby check: need to do complete screen.	No tracts or sinuses.
Neurologic	Well-baby check: need to do complete screen.	Mental status: Awake, alert, tracking. Reflexes: positive suck, rooting, and Moro reflexes. Step reflex present. No jitteriness. DTRs 2+ with four beats clonus in all four extremities.

● DIFFERENTIAL DIAGNOSIS

Examine all the data up to this point. Link the subjective and objective data to the appropriate differential diagnoses. Identify both positive and negative data that support or refute the possible diagnoses.

DIAGNOSIS	POSITIVE DATA	NEGATIVE DATA
Congenital heart disease	Systolic murmur, poor weight gain, decreased activity.	No edema, cyanosis; diaphoretic while feeding; no rales; deceased urine output; hepatosplenomegaly; no thready or bounding pulses.
Sepsis—bacteremia	Poor feeder, decreased activity, irritability.	No temperature instability; no respiratory distress; no lethargy; cyanosis; or decreased capillary refill.
Neurological/metabolic diseases	Irritability, poor feeding, and decreased activity.	No lethargy, seizures, posturing, change in reflexes; no abnormal tone or soft fontanel.
Pulmonary (sequestered lobe)	Poor weight gain.	No tachypnea, respiratory distress, or cyanosis.
GERD	Poor weight gain and irritable.	No vomiting, aspiration pneumonia; no apnea or bradycardia; no posturing or cyanosis.
Toxins	Irritability, decreased activity level, poor weight gain.	No jitteriness, no skin breakdown, no vomiting or diarrhea, no lethargy.
Poor fat content in breast milk	Poor weight gain, irritability.	None.
Poor feeder	Irritability, poor weight gain, decreased activity.	No problem with latching or rooting. No lethargy.
Failure to thrive (FTT)	Irritability, poor weight gain, inadequate social support.	No height and weight or head circumference abnormality. Amanda is not withdrawn, does not resist cuddling or have abnormal tone.

● DIAGNOSTIC TESTS

What additional data and diagnostic tests need to be collected or performed to confirm the diagnosis?

DIAGNOSTIC TEST	RATIONALE	RESULTS
CBC with differential and platelets	Good choice for intial evaluation for possible sepsis as well as inborn errors of metabolism. Although sepsis is not the most likely diagnosis in this infant, it has the greatest potential of causing severe morbidity and mortality. In an infant with FTT and irritability, **sepsis must always be considered.**	WBC: 9800. Hgb: 15/Hct 45. Polys: 60. Lymphs: 27. Monos: 9. Eos: 1. Bands: 1. NRBC: 2. Plat: 320,000. RBC: 5.1.
Cultures of blood, urine, and CSF	Diagnostic studies of choice to definitely rule out sepsis, meningitis, urosepsis, which all carry high risk of severe mortality and morbidity. In any infant under 1 month of age, subtle signs of bacterial infection such as FTT and irritability must be aggressively evaluated. Urine should always be obtained by catheterized specimen.	No growth seen.
Urinalysis	Good, cost-effective test to evaluate for possible urosepsis and major metabolic derangements. Should always be included in sepsis and FTT workup.	pH: 4.5. Specific gravity: 1.015. Gluose: neg. Ketones: 2+. RBCs: 10–20. No leuko, no crystals.
Urine for toxins	Good study as is the only way to evaluate an infant for longstanding toxin exposure. In the presence of FTT and irritability, toxin exposure is possible.	Negative.

(continued)

DIAGNOSTIC TEST	RATIONALE	RESULTS
Electrolytes, glucose, renal function, calcium (Ca), and magnesium (Mg)	Good screening exam to rule out some metabolic diseases which result in acidosis (low bicarbonate). Examples would include renal tubular acidosis, amino acidemia, and organic acidurea. Electrolyte, Ca, and Mg abnormalities can cause lethargy and cellular dysfunction.	Na: 144. K$^+$: 3.7. Cl: 116. CO2: 18. BUN: 30. Creat: 1.6. Ca: 8.5 (ionize 1.15). Mg: 1.4. Total protein: 4. Albumin: 2.6. Glucose: 68. Phosphorus: 3.2.
CXR	Test of debated significance, as this infant has no signs of respiratory distress. Is 3% falsely positive in children and adults without respiratory findings. May be useful in evaluating heart murmur or to rule out CHF and cardiomegaly.	WNL.
Head ultrasound (US)	Good, cost-effective study to rule out gross anatomic brain abnormalities and evidence of hydrocephalus. May be used to 6–9 months of age when anterior fontanel becomes too small for this study. US is less than $\frac{1}{3}$ cost of CT and $\frac{1}{5}$ cost of MRI. In infants with FTT and irritability, intracranial disease can play a significant role.	WNL.
EKG	Helpful, inexpensive evaluation of significant heart murmur to examine for conduction abnormalities and cardiomegaly. However, this infant has evidence of a classic flow murmur, and EKG may be reserved if all other diagnostic tests are negative.	Rt. axis deviation, mild rt. hypertrophy. Rate 170, NSR. Normal EKG.
pH probe /Tuttle test	Expensive, invasive evaluation of GERD. Would be war-	1% Reflux.

(continued)

DIAGNOSTIC TEST	RATIONALE	RESULTS
	ranted if the infant had more evidence of vomiting, choking, apnea, or cyanosis. Definitive study for GERD.	
Dietary diary for both mother and infant	Excellent, noninvasive, inexpensive study to determine nutritional status of both Amanda and her mother. With poor breast feeding and poor breast milk fat content as possible diagnoses for Amanda, this diary may provide important information.	Completes on a weekly basis. No water or formula supplement for Amanda.
Fractionization of breast milk for fat	Expensive test that provides necessary information if other components of FTT workup remain negative.	Not done.

● DIAGNOSIS

What are your conclusive diagnoses? What information assisted you in your decision?

A. Failure to thrive

Infants and children may be suspected or diagnosed as having failure to thrive by meeting any of four criteria:

1. Failure to re-achieve birth weight by 2 weeks of age.
2. Failure to gain 10–30 grams per day after 2 weeks (Klaus and Fanaroff, 1986).
3. Decline of growth that crosses two percentile lines (Rosenstein and Fosarelli, 1989).
4. Decline of growth that places the infant or child's weight two standard deviations below the mean for age (Klaus and Fanaroff, 1986).

Amanda meets the second of these criteria.

B. Poor fat content in maternal breast milk

Although an uncommon diagnosis, this may represent an underdiagnosed condition owing to the extensive workup required for an official diagnosis. All life-threatening disease states must be completely ruled out as possibilities before pursuing poor fat content in breast milk as the probable diagnosis. These life-threatening diagnosis states would include sepsis, increased ICP, hydrocephalus, some congenital infections, and most metabolic abnormalities. Predisposing factors for poor fat content in maternal breast milk in this mother include:

1. Poor dietary habits
2. Inexperience as a breast-feeding mother
3. Inadequate social support
4. Lack of breast-feeding role models
3. Peripheral pulmonic stenosis, innocent flow murmur

Murmurs represent turbulent blood flow through the heart and large vessels, and do not necessarily indicate a pathologic condition. In fact, more than 50% of all full-term infants have an innocent systolic mumur during the first week of life (Park, 1991). The most common of these murmurs is the peripheral pulmonic stenosis (PPS), which is caused by turbulent flow through the peripheral arteries and arterioles of the lungs. It is noted as a I-II/VI systolic murmur heard loudest at the left upper sternal border but is also noted across the entire precordium and back as well as in both axillae. As with other innocent flow murmurs, there should be normal pulses, capillary refill, and a lack of respiratory symptoms. Heart tones (S_1 and S_2) are always normal in flow murmurs and S_3 and S_4 are not heard.

Flow murmurs never inhibit activity or growth, nor do they have future consequences.

● THERAPEUTIC PLAN

1. What are issues to consider when deciding on treatment for Amanda?

Some issues to consider when deciding on the treatment for Amanda are:

1. Presentation of child: altered mental status and FTT
2. Lack of maternal experience: however, demonstrated appropriate choice to seek medical care at this time
3. Need for further education
4. Lack of financial resources
5. Must rely on bus for transportation

2. What are suggestions to improve the fat content of maternal breast milk?

Dietary intervention initially with general nutrition principles given by the nurse practitioner is appropriate. However, more in-depth intervention may be required by dietician if refractory to initial therapy. Emphasis should be placed on a better lifestyle through a balanced and healthy diet.

Specific suggestions would include:

1. Daily dietary diary: reviewed weekly
2. Increase meat content in diet, one meat/day: tuna, hamburger helper
3. Increase fat content of diet
4. Decrease amount of exercise
5. Try yogurt and peanut butter

The effectiveness of this therapy will be entirely dependent on the mother's compliance and close follow up. If the mother is encouraged to assume greater responsibility for her own nutritional needs, this should empower her to better care for both her own health as well as Amanda's.

Amanda's mother should be commended for choosing breast feeding as the method of feeding. The positive aspects of breast feeding should be emphasized.

3. What are resources of financial assistance for Amanda and her mother?

This mother should be referred to Women, Infants and Children (WIC), which will provide her with some financial supplies, such as food stamps, vouchers, and foodstuffs. The goal is to better balance her diet and to provide her with a means to succeed at breast feeding. When coupled with dietary instruction, this may be an effective way of enhancing self-image while also supplementing her diet. If the mother's diet is enhanced, Amanda's diet also will be improved.

4. What are referrals that would be appropriate for Amanda and her mother?

Referral to a lactation specialist may benefit this mother. There are many groups, such as La Lache League or Well-Start, that provide inexpensive instruction on breast-feeding techniques. In addition, most hospitals who provide delivery, postpartum, and nursery services have lactation consultants who can assist with the breast feeding process. These experts provide the experience and support for breast feeding that Amanda's mother lacks.

The NP should also involve social services in the care of this young family. Social services provide a route to obtain respite care, home health/public health visits, and access to support groups. They often have additional information on financial aid and other services that may benefit this family. The opportunity to assume greater control of her own life in a more financially sound environment gives this mother a greater chance for future success.

5. What follow up would you plan for Amanda?

Close follow up with the NP and other referred services is necessary to optimize success. Frequent follow ups allow the opportunity to provide needed postive feedback, encouragement, or redirection. Because the outcome of this treatment program depends on the mother's involvement with the system, the NP should monitor the mother's participation and the progress of this infant. The infant should be followed up in the hospital for 48 hours for possible sepsis, then weekly for 2 months for substantial weight gain or until the infant has returned to a normal growth curve. The frequency of visits then can be decreased to monthly.

6. *Based on the information given about Amanda, what impact do you think her birth had on her mother?*

Although the birth of a child can be a very joyous event, in Amanda's family, it will potentially be quite stressful. McCubbin and Patterson (1983) define a family stressor as "a life event or occurrence in or impacting upon the family unit which produces change in the family social system."

Some of the stresses that may be encountered by the birth of an unplanned infant would include:

1. Socioeconomic considerations
2. Child care
3. Altered communication and interaction patterns with peers
4. Altered roles and responsibilities
5. Altered time management
6. Altered social status

Appropriate interventions are:

1. Social service referral
2. Public health or home nursing visits
3. Support group for single mothers
4. Parenting classes
5. Self-fulfilling activities: respite care for mother
6. Family planning

7. *What community resources would be helpful for Amanda and her mother?*

- WIC federal/state/county funded: 800 825-5770
- Planned Parenthood: family planning: 800 752-6633
- La Lache League: breast feeding: 800 525-3243
- Early Start Parent Support Groups
- Parents Anonymous
- March of Dimes: education: 914 428-7100

    US Dept. of Education, TAPP Office of Special Education Programs
    Mary E. Shitzer Building, 330 C Street SW, Room 3072,
    Washington, DC, 20202-2651

8. *Amanda returns for a follow up 1 week later. Her weight is 2525 grams. She is more alert and active during the examination. What adjustments would you make in the therapeutic plan developed at the first visit?*

Failure to respond necessitates three steps:

1. Reassessment of the adequacy of diagnosis
2. Reassessment of the adequacy of treatment

3. Assessment of mother's involvement with referrals and her level of commitment

Common problems encountered would include undisclosed substance abuse and failure of compliance with therapy. Longstanding dietary habits are among the hardest lifestyle changes to make. Intervention by a dietitian and possibly more direct observation of the maternal diet and infant feedings are necessary at this time. Family stresses should again be addressed as they may contribute to the lack of success. The NP should again review involvement with all referrals and make sure the mother is keeping her appointments.

9. *What anticipatory guidance should be given to the mother, related to Amanda's growth and development?*

June should know that Amanda will be doing more reaching out in the next 2–8 weeks. She will also settle into a feeding and sleeping schedule. She will become more curious about her surroundings, and will be more responsive with eye contact and smiling. Amanda's stools will continue to be loose, and her urine will be light and colorless. She should continue to provide support and physical contact for Amanda. June should wrap Amanda snugly in blankets and provide body support for her. Amanda will like music, so playing lullabies will provide comfort for her. Suggested crib toys are things like a noisy clock, or a mobile close to Amanda's face.

Warn June that as Amanda becomes more active, it will be important to pay attention to safety issues. She should always hold on to Amanda while changing her diaper, and should not leave her unattended in high places. Joan should make sure she uses a car seat for transportation for Amanda, with the car seat placed in the back seat. June should have emergency phone numbers available so she can access them quickly in an emergency (Boyton, 1994).

10. *What information should be given to Amanda's mother related to immunizations?*

Amanda got the first of the hepatitis B series in the hospital. She will be getting the following immunizations at her 2-month check up: oral polio, DPT, Hib, hep B (2nd in series).

REFERENCES

Behrman R, Vaughan V. *Nelson Textbook of Pediatrics,* 13th ed., Philadelphia: W.B. Saunders; 1987.

Boyton R, Dunn E, Stephens G. *Manual of Ambulatory Pediatrics,* 3rd ed., Philadelphia: J.B. Lippincott; 1994.

Klaus M, Fanaroff A. *Yearbook of Neonatal and Perinatal Medicine.* St. Louis: Mosby; 1993.

Klaus M, Fanaroff A. *Care of the High Risk Neonate,* 3rd ed., Philadelphia: W.B. Sauders; 1986.

McCubbin H, Patterson J. *Family Stress Adaptation to Crises: A Double ABCX Model of Family Behavior.* Beverly Hills: Sage; 1983.

Park M. *Pediatric Cardiology Handbook.* St. Louis: Mosby; 1991.

Rosenstein B, Fosarelli P. *Pediatric Pearls: The Handbook of Practical Pediatrics.* St. Louis: Mosby; 1989.

Tsang R, Nichols B. *Nutrition During Infancy.* St. Louis: Mosby; 1988.

Zitelli B, Davis H. *Atlas of Pediatric Physical Diagnosis.* St. Louis: Mosby; 1987.

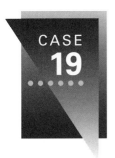

A 4-year-old boy with a sore throat and earache

SCENARIO

Cody Forrest is a 4-year-old African-American male who comes to the clinic today with his mother because he has had a sore throat for 3 days, and is now complaining about an earache.

● TENTATIVE DIAGNOSES

What potential diagnoses have you identified based on the preceding scenario?

● HISTORY

What are significant questions in Cody's history?
What are the key points to cover on the review of systems?

● PHYSICAL ASSESSMENT

What are the significant portions of the physical examination that should be completed for Cody?

● DIFFERENTIAL DIAGNOSES

What are the significant positive and negative data that support or refute your diagnoses for Cody?

● DIAGNOSTIC TESTS

Based on the history and physical assessment, what, if any, diagnostic tests would you obtain. Include your rationale for the tests.

● DIAGNOSIS

What diagnoses are appropriate for Cody?

● THERAPEUTIC PLAN

1. *Why do you presume that Cody has strep pharyngitis, even though the strep test was negative?*
2. *Based on your diagnosis, how will you treat Cody?*
3. *What are nonpharmacological therapies you would recommend to Cody's Mom?*
4. *When can Cody return to daycare?*
5. *What information would you give to Cody's mom concerning the incubation of strep throat and the likelihood that the rest of the family might get it?*
6. *What warning signs should you review with Cody's mom?*
7. *When should Cody return for follow up?*

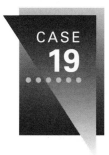

TUTORIAL

A 4-year-old boy with a sore throat and earache

SCENARIO

Cody Forrest is a 4-year-old African-American male who comes to the clinic today with his mother because he has had a sore throat for 3 days, and is now complaining about an earache.

● TENTATIVE DIAGNOSES

What potential diagnoses have you identified based on the preceding scenario?

DIAGNOSIS	RATIONALE
Pharyngitis, streptococcal	Cody complains of a sore throat for 3 days. This is a common symptom for pharyngitis.
Cold/viral syndrome	A sore throat is a common symptom seen with a cold.
Impacted cerumen in ear canal	An earache is a typical symptom when the ear canals are occluded with cerumen.
Otitis media	An earache is a common presentation for otitis media, along with a sore throat.
Otitis externa	A painful ear is a symptom of otitis externa.
Infectious mononucleosis	Complaint of a sore throat is frequently seen with mono.
Epiglottis	Complaints of a sore throat.
Sinusitis	A sore throat often accompanies sinusitis, as well as a feeling of ear fullness or pain.

● HISTORY

1. What are significant questions in Cody's history?

REQUESTED DATA	DATA ANSWER
Allergies	NKDA.
Current medications	None.
Childhood illnesses	Chicken pox.
Immunizations	Up to date.
Surgery	None.
Past medical history and hospitalizations/fractures/injuries/accidents	Frequent episodes of strep throat each winter.
Appetite	Not eating well for the past 3–4 days. He said it hurts his throat to eat.
24-Hour diet recall	B: Tried to eat oatmeal but threw it up. L: Dry toast and jello. D: Chicken soup/popsicle. S: Drinking sodas during the day.
Exposure to anyone who has strep throat/illness	Several children in daycare have had strep throat and have had colds with cough.
Birth history/growth and development	39 weeks' gestation, with no problems. Vaginal delivery, no problems. Normal growth and development, reached appropriate milestones at appropriate times.
Family history	Father: 32, healthy. Mother: 36, HTN. Siblings: 1 sister, age 7, healthy.

2. What are the key points to cover on the review of systems?

SYSTEM REVIEWED	DATA ANSWER
General	Mom states he is not as active as normal and that he is lying around on the couch.

(continued)

SYSTEM REVIEWED	DATA ANSWER
Skin	No problems.
HEENT	Runny nose with yellow drainage. No d/c from his ears. Mom thinks he does not hear as well as he normally does.
Lungs	Frequent cough, nonproductive. No wheezing.
Cardiac	No problems.
GI/GU	Had one episode of diarrhea on the first day, but none lately. Not urinating as often as normal.

● PHYSICAL ASSESSMENT

What are the significant portions of the physical examination that should be completed for Cody?

SYSTEM	RATIONALE	FINDINGS
Vital signs	Provides baseline data.	B/P: 90/60 HR: 120 R: 20 T: 101 Ht: 38″ Wt: 33 lbs
General appearance/skin	Provides an overall view of Cody.	Appears pale. Alert, lying on exam table.
HEENT	Provides signs of system most affected, able to identify inflammation.	Normocephalic, no sinus tenderness. Ear: Lt. TM dull, with erythema, rt. TM translucent. Dried d/c in nares. Pharynx, tonsils edematous, erythema with small amount exudate. No drooling. Neck supple, tender tonsillar and anterior cervical lymph nodes.
Lungs	Identify if there is lung involvement.	CTA.
Heart	Provide baseline information.	RRR, no MRG.

(continued)

SYSTEM	RATIONALE	FINDINGS
Abdomen	Important to evaluate abdomen in children with URI, especially because Cody had diarrhea (Dershewitz, 1993).	BS+, soft, no tenderness or masses. No HSM.

● DIFFERENTIAL DIAGNOSES

What are the significant positive and negative findings that support or refute your diagnoses for Cody?

DIAGNOSIS	POSITIVE DATA	NEGATIVE DATA
Streptococcal pharyngitis	Erythematous pharynx, enlarged tender lymph nodes, fever, vomiting, listless.	Unknown direct contact with someone with strep. No palatal petechiae, unknown incubation period.
Viral pharyngitis	Sore throat, many children at daycare ill, listless.	Fever, enlarged tender lymph nodes, vomiting.
Sinusitis	Yellow discharge from nares, temperature, listless.	No sinus tenderness.
Mononucleosis	Lymphadenopathy, fever, listless.	No rash.
Epiglottis	Erythematous pharynx.	Does not appear toxic, no abrupt onset of sore throat, no muffled voice sounds, no drooling.
Otitis externa	Ear pain.	No pain when auricle moved. Canal without erythema or exudate.
Otitis media	TM erythematous and dull, ear pain, fever, listless.	
Impacted cerumen in ear canals	Earache.	Ear canal open, able to see to TM.

● DIAGNOSTIC TESTS

Based on the history and physical examination, what, if any, diagnostic tests would you obtain?

DIAGNOSTIC TEST	RATIONALE	RESULTS
Rapid strep screen	Allows for in office confirmation of + strep. Depending on test, approx. 90% specific and sensitivity of 85–95% (Dershewitz, 1993).	Neg strep screen.
Throat culture	Most reliable identification of organisms. Some offices do a backup culture if the screen is negative.	Sent for culture—results return in 72 hours, not helpful for initial decision to treat.
Mono spot	Quick test that identifies the Epstein-Barr organism responsible for mono.	Sent for mono spot—not helpful for decision to treat.
CBC with differential	Identifies extent of infection.	Not done.
Hearing test	Identifies hearing loss.	Not done during acute period. More appropriate for follow up.

● DIAGNOSES

What diagnoses do you determine as being appropriate after a review of the subjective and objective data?

> Pharyngitis: Presumptive strep
> Otitis media

Data Supporting the Diagnosis

> Pharyngitis: Sore throat for 6 days, erythematous with exudate, swollen tonsils, fever, although strep screen negative, culture sent, exposure to kids at daycare, tender cervical lymph nodes.
> Otitis media: Painful ear, TM erythematous, dull, fever

● THERAPEUTIC PLAN

1. *Why do you presume that Cody has strep pharyngitis, even though the rapid strep screen was negative?*

   Cody's symptoms are such that he sounds as if he has strep throat. He has the triad of symptoms characteristic of strep: fever; enlarged, tender cervical lymph nodes; and erythematous pharynx with exudate.

2. *Based on your diagnosis, how will you treat Cody?*

   Cody and his mother will have the choice of oral antibiotic agents or an injection. Procaine PCN 600,000 units IM could be given in the office or Pen-Vee K 250 mg TID or amoxicillin (250/5 mL) 5 mL TID for 10 days are options, because Cody is not allergic to any medications. Cody likes the bubblegum-tasting medication and chooses the liquid antibiotic. The amoxicillin has the added advantage of being an effective treatment for his OM (Hoole et al., 1995).

3. *What are nonpharmacological therapies you would recommend to Cody's Mom?*

   Hard candy, lozenges, or warm salt water gargles may be used to help soothe his sore throat. Popsicles, sherbet, or jello might also be used to help his sore throat. Increasing Cody's intake of fluids will also be helpful in treatment of his symptoms.

4. *When can Cody return to daycare?*

   Cody should not return to daycare until his temperature is normal. Cody will not be contagious in approximately 24 hours when he starts taking the antibiotic.

5. *What information would you give to Cody's mom concerning the incubation of strep throat and the likelihood that the rest of the family might get it?*

   Strep throat is transmitted by close or direct contact. It is likely that the rest of the family has been exposed to the bacteria. The incubation period for strep throat is 1–3 days. If any member of the family has similar symptoms within the next day or so they should come in to the office for a strep test, and then will be treated accordingly.

6. *What warning signs should you review with Cody's mom?*

   The development of a rash, facial swelling, or throat tightness. These symptoms might indicate an allergic response to the medication. In addition, Cody's mom should be alert for increased pain, drooling, dyspnea, and an inability to fully open his mouth. These symptoms are indicative of peritonsillar abscess and she should seek medical care immediately.

Complications of strep throat include scarlet fever, peritonsillar abscess, glomerulonephritis, and rheumatic fever (Boynton et al., 1994).

7. *When should Cody return for follow up?*

Cody will not need to return for follow up unless his symptoms do not improve within 72 hours. Only patients who have immune problems or other medical conditions may need a follow up culture.

REFERENCES

Boynton R, Dunn E, Stephens G. *Manual of Ambulatory Pediatrics,* 3rd ed. Philadelphia: J.B. Lippincott; 1994.

Dershewitz R. *Ambulatory Pediatric Care,* 2nd ed. Philadelphia: J.B. Lippincott; 1993.

Hoole A, Pickard C, Ouimette R, Lohr J, Greenberg R. *Patient Care Guidelines for Nurse Practitioners,* 4th ed. Philadelphia: J.B. Lippincott; 1995.

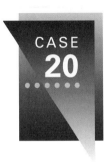

A 44-year-old man with chronic back pain

SCENARIO

Bill is a 44-year-old Caucasian male who comes to your office asking for a refill of Tylenol with Codeine for back pain. His severe pain began 8 months ago. The initial back injury was caused by an MVA 3 years ago. He reports obtaining his past two refills from different emergency departments. Since Bill has separated from his family he is staying in a friend's apartment. He says he is having trouble keeping his job and paying his bills. He has not seen his wife and three children for several months.

● TENTATIVE DIAGNOSES

Based on the information provided so far, what are potential differential diagnoses?

● HISTORY

What are significant questions in the history for a man complaining of chronic back pain?
What additional information do you need in terms of pain assessment?

● PHYSICAL ASSESSMENT

What are the significant portions of the physical examination that should be completed for Bill?

● DIFFERENTIAL DIAGNOSES

What are the significant positive and negative data that support or refute your diagnoses for Bill?

● DIAGNOSTIC TESTS

Based on the history and physical assessment, what, if any, diagnostic tests would you obtain? Include your rationale for the tests.

● DIAGNOSIS

What diagnoses are appropriate for Bill?

● THERAPEUTIC PLAN

1. *What are the issues to consider for Bill when deciding on treatment?*
2. *List short-term and long-term goals appropriate to include in a health care contract with Bill.*
3. *What are the necessary steps in treatment for Bill?*
4. *What other health care providers should be included on the interdisciplinary team to assess Bill and help manage the therapeutic plan?*
5. *If Bill did not have a substance dependence problem, how might the management of his pain differ?*
6. *Based on the information given so far about Bill, what impact do you think this situation has had on his family?*
7. *Bill returns in 6 weeks with reports of successful withdrawal from drugs, and participation in a recovery program. Bill says he is feeling better in general, but still needs help with pain relief. Lab work reveals no anemia and normal liver and renal function. What adjustments could you make to the therapeutic plan?*
8. *What are the principles of pain management?*
9. *Where can an NP obtain more information concerning substance abuse and pain management and/or additional resources for assisting affected clients?*

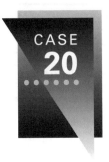

TUTORIAL

A 44-year-old man with chronic back pain

SCENARIO

Bill is a 44-year-old Caucasian male who comes to your office asking for a refill of Tylenol with Codeine for back pain. His severe pain began 8 months ago. The initial back injury was caused by an MVA 3 years ago. He reports obtaining his past two refills from different emergency departments. Since Bill has separated from his family he is staying in a friend's apartment. He says he is having trouble keeping his job and paying his bills. He has not seen his wife and three children for several months.

● TENTATIVE DIAGNOSES

Based on the information provided so far, what are the potential differential diagnoses?

DIAGNOSIS	RATIONALE
Chronic pain disorder	Bill complains of chronic back pain.
Opiate withdrawal	Bill has sought refills of pain medicine from the ED instead of a primary provider.
Opiate abuse	Bill has sought refills of pain medicine from the ED instead of a primary provider.
Opiate dependence	Bill has sought refills of pain medicine from the ED instead of a primary provider.
Malingering	Always a concern when a client seeks pain medicine from EDs for a problem such as back pain, especially when the accident occurred 3 years ago.
Back pain	C/o of back pain from MVA 3 years ago, but pain increased in past 8 months.

● HISTORY

1. What are significant questions in the history for a man complaining of chronic back pain?

REQUESTED DATA   DATA ANSWER

REQUESTED DATA	DATA ANSWER
Allergies	None.
Current medications	Tylenol with Codeine 2 tabs po prn for pain (admits to self-medication of 4–10 tabs/day. Laxative every week. Methocarbamol (Robaxin) 750 mg as needed for muscle spasms.
Immunizations	Td 1994 (sutures lt. arm from MVA). No hep B or pneumo-coccal vaccines.
Surgery/transfusions	Septoplasty 1991 s/p nasal fx. Concussion 1994 after MVA alcohol treatment program. 1994 after DUI arrest.
Past medical history and hospitalizations/fractures/injuries/accidents	Chicken pox as child. Lt. shoulder dislocation 1982. Rt. ankle sprain × 2, 1985, 1989. Rib fx from MVA 1994.
Adult illness	Chronic bronchitis × 5 years. PUD, asymptomatic. No history of GI bleed.
Last complete PE	1994 during alcohol treatment.
Appetite	Decreased × 3 months. Intermittent nausea, no vomiting. Lost 15 lbs in past 3 months after separating from wife.
24-Hour diet recall	B: 2 slices bacon, 1 fried egg, 1 piece toast, 3 c. coffee. L: None. D: Fried hamburger, french fries, 16 oz cola.
Sleeping	Back pain awakens him 2–3 times a night. Increased difficulty when runs out of medicine. Feels tired in morning. Muscle aches in back and legs all day.
Social history	Tobacco: Smokes 1 ppd/×25 yrs. Alcohol: Hx of problem drinking. Received treatment in 1994, no drinking × 1 yr. Now drinks when pain med is unavailable. Caffeinated beverages: 4 c. coffee, 2 colas/day. Drugs: None. Exercise: None currently. Ran 3× week until ankle sprain in 1989.

(continued)

REQUESTED DATA | DATA ANSWER

REQUESTED DATA	DATA ANSWER
Family history	Father: Died 62 y/o from GI bleed, alcoholism. Mother: Age 68, arthritis, H/A. Siblings: 1 brother, 46, HTN. 1 sister, 38, healthy. Children: 3: One male, 22; one female, 18; one male, 13, all healthy.
Social organizations	Veterans group (no hx of combat during service). AA for 6 months in 1994. Church activities until 1 yr ago. Coached son's baseball team until 3 years ago.
Relationship with wife	Expresses resentment about being "kicked out" of the house because of anger outbursts, spending habits, and withdrawal from family.
Relationship with children	Believes younger son and daughter miss him. Older son resents him for not taking better care of himself and family, as well as being intoxicated in front of his friends.
Relationship with mother/ siblings	Visits mother 2× each month, sister weekly. Both are supportive. Last saw brother during holidays.
Employment/insurance	$35,000/year earned in factory. 3rd job in past 5 years. Wife works in retail. Family coverage medical/dental through his work.
Length of symptoms	Pain for 2 years since MVA. Increased pain for 8 months.
How has pain affected your ADLs?	Misses work at least 2× month. Does not participate in family activities. "Always" going to health care providers. "They can't find a cause for my pain."
Losses in your life?	Separation from family. Father's death. Refinanced home due to spending problems.
Legal charges	DUI after MVA 1994. No ongoing litigation.
What do you do for the pain?	Take more medication and drink alcohol.
Do you ever think about hurting yourself?	No.
Do you ever think about hurting others?	No.

2. What additional information do you need in terms of pain assessment?

PAIN ASSESSMENT*	ANSWER	
On a scale of 1–10, with 0 being no pain and 10 being the worst pain you can imagine, rate your pain at its worst in the past 24 h.	8	
What number best describes the least pain you've felt in the past 24 h?	5	
Rate the amount of pain you have now.	7	
In the past 24 hrs, how much relief has medication given you? (0–100%).	50%	
Describe how your pain interferes with the following activities in the past 24 hours: (0: does not interfere. 10: completely interferes).	*General ability	7
	*Walking ability	6
	*Relation with	5
	other people	5
	* Enjoyment of life	8
	*Mood	6
	*Normal work	8
	*Sleep	9
What is the quality of the pain?	Sharp, constant.	
Onset of pain?	Always present.	
What makes it better?	Tylenol with Codeine.	
What makes it worse?	Walking, physical labor.	
What is an acceptable level of pain for you?	3.	
What was the pain like that made the MD put you on Tylenol with Codeine?	Constant severe pain.	

*Pain Assessment, AHCPR (1994).

● PHYSICAL ASSESSMENT

What are the significant portions of the physical examination that should be completed for Bill?

SYSTEM	RATIONALE	FINDINGS
Vital signs	Baseline data.	B/P: L 142/88 R 146/90 sitting P: 92 R: 20, T: 98.0° F Ht: 5'10" Wt: 190 lbs
General appearance/skin	Mental status and mood helps assess psychological status and stability. Status of skin helps assess presence/ absence of drug withdrawal, IVDA, liver disease, and bleeding disorder (Fleming & Barry, 1992).	Appears anxious with labile affect. Cooperative. Skin cool, mild diaphoresis on trunk, no needle marks (tracks), no jaundice or petechiae.
HEENT	Could defer VA and exam of ears. Condition of nasal mucosa helps assess drug use. Fundoscopy, thyroid, venous distention, and carotid exams are indicated when patient has HTN.	Eye: VA OD 20/40, OS 20/30, O/U 20/30 uncorrected. Fundoscopy: red reflex intact bil. No AV nicking, no lesions. Ear: Lt. cerumen occluding canal. Rt. canal clear. TM pearly gray, + cone of light. Nose: thin clear d/c bil. Mucosa pink. Septum deviated rt. No perforation. Mouth: Poor dentition, receding gums, no lesions. No erythema, lesions, or exudate. Neck: No carotid bruits, no JVD, thyroid non-palp, no masses, no enlargement.
Lungs	Bill smokes, so respiratory status should be evaluated.	CTA.
Heart	Assess CV status in middle-aged smoker with HTN.	S_1 S_2 WNL, no MRG.

(continued)

SYSTEM	RATIONALE	FINDINGS
Back	C/o severe back pain—assess for objective evidence.	Mild tenderness of paravertebral muscles to palpation. Neg SLR, and crossover SLR.
Abdomen	Bill c/o constipation. In addition, because Bill is hypertensive, the abdomen should be checked for bruits. Also, because he has a history of ETOH dependence, it is important to evaluate liver size.	Hyperactive BS, no bruit. Soft, with mild tenderness throughout. No rebound. No masses or HSM.
Rectal	C/o constipation. 44-year-old male at lower age range for BPH.	Anus without lesions, and with intact tone. Rectum without masses. Prostate firm, symmetric, not enlarged, no masses or tenderness.
Genital	May defer if Bill is asymptomatic.	Penis circumcised, no lesions or urethral d/c. Testes descended, nontender, no masses or lesions bil. No inguinal hernia palpated.
Neurological	Especially important to assess neuro status of lower extremities in patient with low back pain to establish baseline and determine objective evidence of deficits.	CN II–XII intact. Strength/sensation WNL. Steady gait, neg. Romberg. Intact tandem walk, heel/toe walk. DTRs 2+, alert, oriented ×3.
Extremities	Evaluate for edema because he has history of HTN. Important to assess musculoskeletal status of arms and legs, given history of MVA, shoulder injury, and low back pain.	Pulses 2+ bil. No edema or lesions. ROM: decreased neck extension, lt. shoulder abduction and external rotation. Otherwise full ROM neck, shoulders, elbows, wrist, trunk, hips, knees, and ankles. No deformity.

● DIFFERENTIAL DIAGNOSES

What are the significant positive and negative findings that support or refute your diagnoses for Bill? (In order to assist with the development of differential diagnoses in this case, it will be helpful to become familiar with definitions of terms found in substance abuse and pain literature.) (APA, 1994).

DIAGNOSIS	POSITIVE DATA	NEGATIVE DATA
Chronic pain disorder associated with psychological factors	Pain is the predominant focus of the clinical presentation, severe enough to warrant clinical attention. Pain causes significant distress or impairment in work and social relationships. Psychological factors present. Pain does not appear to be intentionally produced. Medical condition appears to play no role or minimal role in onset or maintenance of pain. For chronic pain, symptoms are present over 6 months (American Psychiatric Association [APA], 1994).	Pain may have a physiological basis not yet revealed on history and physical (H & P). History of MVA in 1994 with significant trauma.
Chronic pain disorder with both psychological factors and a general medical condition	Pain is the predominant focus of the clinical presentation, severe enough to warrant clinical attention. Pain causes significant distress or impairment in work and social relationships. Psychological factors present. Pain does not appear to be intentionally produced. Medical condition appears to play no role or minimal role in onset or maintenance of pain. For chronic pain, symptoms are present over 6 months (American Psychiatric Association [APA], 1994).	Physical exam did not reveal objective source of pain.

(continued)

DIAGNOSIS	*POSITIVE DATA*	*NEGATIVE DATA*
Chronic pain disorder associated with a general medical condition	History of MVA.	Physical exam did not reveal source of pain.
Opiate withdrawal	Decrease in use after prolonged (over several weeks) use. Symptoms of dysphoric mood, nausea, muscle aches, lacrimation, rhinorrhea, pupillary dilatation, diarrhea, insomnia (APA, 1994).	
Opiate abuse	Recurrent use leads to failure to fulfill major role obligation (APA, 1994).	Evidence of tolerance and withdrawal. Great deal of time involved in obtaining substance. Family, social and occupational activities given up (meeting criteria for dependence overrides diagnosis of abuse) (APA, 1994).
Opiate dependence	Evidence of tolerance and withdrawal. Substance taken in larger amounts over longer period of time than intended. Great deal of time spent in activities necessary to obtain substance (ED visits). Work, social activities reduced (American Psychiatric Association, 1994). History of problems with alcohol in past (Vallerand, 1991).	
Malingering	Bill states he wants Tylenol with Codeine for pain. Discrepancy between claimed degree of pain and lack of physical findings.	He cooperated during the history and exam. No ongoing litigation.
Back pain	MVA 3 years ago. Mild paravertebral tenderness to palpation.	Discrepancy between claimed degree of pain and lack of physical findings, -SLR, crossed SLR, DTRs 2+, able to heel-and-toe walk. WNL

(continued)

DIAGNOSIS	POSITIVE DATA	NEGATIVE DATA
		ROM. No bowel/bladder disfunction. Strength/sensation intact.
Constipation secondary to drug use and poor dietary habits	Takes laxative every week. Poor dietary habits.	
Alcohol abuse	History of alcohol abuse, received treatment for abuse in 1994, +DUI, + FH for alcohol abuse. Admits he drinks alcohol to combat pain when out of medication.	Consider criteria for dependence.

● DIAGNOSTIC TESTS

Based on the history and physical assessment, what, if any, diagnostic tests or additional data would you obtain?

DIAGNOSTIC TEST	RATIONALE	RESULTS
Stool for guaiac	Test for GI bleeding.	Negative.
Urine toxicology screening test	Identify the presence of current opioids. Identify other drugs which Bill may be using to cope with withdrawal or pain. In addition, he may be abusing. (Opioids may be present from 12 hrs to several days in urine.) (APA, 1994.)	+ For opioids.
Labs: CBC, LFT, electrolytes, renal	History of alcohol use puts Bill at increased risk for GI bleeding and liver dysfunction. Also, baseline liver and renal status help determine safety of and risks for alternative and possibly long-term medication regimens that may be indicated for pain management.	H/H: 15.1/45.2. RBC: 5.2. WBC: 7.1. Platelets: 250. AST: 27. ALT: 35. Alk. Phos: 70. BUN: 10. Creatinine: 1.0. NA: 142 CI: 110.

DIAGNOSTIC TEST	RATIONALE	RESULTS
		K:4.2. CO2: 26.0.
EMG, CT, MRI	Other tests to evaluate physiological source of pain as indicated by exam.	Not done. PE revealed no signs and symptoms that required further testing. All these tests were completed within 2 months of initial injury.
Clinical interview DSM-IV or CAGE to assess alcohol dependency	Assess current severity of alcohol use. History is suggestive of alcohol abuse/dependence with a period of remission. Alcoholics are at increased risk for use/dependence upon other substances, and individuals dependent on other substances are at increased risk for alcohol dependence (Savage, 1993).	3/4 Bill is struggling to **cut down** amount of alcohol, **annoyed** when wife asked him to decrease alcohol. Has felt **guilty** about drinking. Bill states he does not drink in AM.
Assess social supports	Family, 12-step recovery network, or church group may be available to help Bill. A recovery setting increases Bill's chances of success and is critical to pain management (Savage, 1993).	Bill identifies sister and mother as supportive. He is willing to call them today to discuss today's visit.
Seek information from family or friends	Confirm Bill's history of drug, medication, and alcohol use (Wesson, Ling, and Smith, 1993).	Bill gives written permission for NP to speak with sister.
Self-report and if indicated clinician-completed depression scale	Persons with chronic pain are at increased risk for suicide, especially if associated with severe depression or terminal illness, such as cancer (APA, 1994).	Bill says he has no thoughts or plans of harming himself and agrees to call sister if mood worsens.

● DIAGNOSES

What diagnoses are appropriate for Bill?

Opiate dependence
Alcohol abuse
Tobacco dependence

Constipation secondary to opiate use
Chronic pain disorder

Data Supporting the Diagnosis of Opiate Dependence:

- Evidence of tolerance and withdrawal
- Substance taken in larger amounts over longer period of time than intended
- Great deal of time spent in activities necessary to obtain substance (ED visits)
- Work, social activities reduced

● THERAPEUTIC PLAN

1. What are the issues to consider for Bill when deciding on treatment?

- Need to treat withdrawal symptoms without simply giving another prescription of same drug and telling client to "cut down."
- Explain that pain may very well improve, or at least not become worse, if the patient is taken off opiates.
- Being taken off opiates and all other substances of abuse or dependence, such as alcohol, is key to assessing pain and planning long-term treatment (Savage, 1993).
- Identify appropriate setting for withdrawal. Bill needs adequate support and monitoring, such as a supervised detoxification program on an inpatient or outpatient basis.
- Explain rationale for diagnosis of opiate dependence, while acknowledging the significance of pain and the need for pain treatment.

2. List short- and long-term goals appropriate to include in a health care contract with Bill.

Set short- and long-term goals with Bill for health care contract. Discuss realistic expectations for course of treatment and outcomes. Negotiate NP/client responsibilities in the treatment plan. There are no "quick fixes." Different therapies will be tried. Improvement of pain is expected, but cannot guarantee complete resolution of pain. Refer to pain-rating scales for perspective.

Short-term goals

Detoxify from opiates
Remain substance-free
Resume job responsibilities
Identify any life-threatening diseases

Long-term goals

Improve pain
Resolve family conflict

Identify physiologic contributors to pain
Maintain active support group
Be substance-free until alternatives have been systematically tried
Continue care with one provider/team

3. *What are the necessary steps in treatment for Bill?*

- Supervised detoxification program, inpatient or outpatient setting.
- Refer to a substance abuse treatment/rehab program, either inpatient or intensive outpatient setting.

4. *What other health care providers could be included on the interdisciplinary team to assess Bill and help manage the therapeutic plan?*

Addiction specialist to help assess the severity of the substance dependence and monitor response to treatment. **Physician** for consultation and referral as well as to aid in interpreting tests and ordering procedures to determine any physiological source of pain. May collaborate in supervising outpatient detox. **Psychiatrist/Psychologist** to see if Bill meets criteria for other mental disorders that may take precedence over the determination of chronic pain disorder. **Licensed clinical social worker, psychiatric nurse specialist** for referral/consultation regarding addiction assessment, mental disorder determination, family counseling, relaxation training, biofeedback. **Physical therapist** to support alternative pain management modalities such as transcutaneous electrical nerve stimulation (TENS), hot packs, muscle strengthening.

Pain specialty consultants/teams, which may consist of MDs, physical medicine and rehabilitation specialists, advanced practice nurses, psychologists, social workers, and others.

5. *If Bill did not have a substance dependence problem, how might management of his pain differ?*

Although physiological dependence on narcotics for pain is common if narcotics are used regularly, the overwhelming majority of people stop taking narcotics when the pain stops (McCaffery and Beebe, 1989). Unless a client has a prior substance dependence problem, chances are low for development of psychological dependence on narcotic analgesics (Vallerand, 1991). Opiates may be appropriate for a client with chronic pain without a history of substance dependence. Keep in mind that the pain-relieving effects of nonnarcotic analgesics are underestimated and underused (McCaffery and Beebe, 1989), and also consider alternative and adjuvant therapies.

6. *Based on the information given so far about Bill, what impact do you think this situation has had on his family?*

Bill was organizing his life around opiates (and probably alcohol), while his family was organizing itself around responses to his substance dependence (Janosik and Green, 1992), reacting to the moods and money problems he created. They, especially his wife, may have had difficulty developing individual identities separate from the troubled family (code-pendence). The unpredictable nature of life with a person dependent on substances creates fear of losing control of what normality exists in the family (Janosik and Green, 1992). The children often suffer neglect, if not abuse, and can be confused by the adults' denial of the severity of the family's problems (Janosik and Green, 1992).

What would be appropriate interventions for Bill's family?

Family counseling and involvement of the family in the client's treatment enhances the chances for successful recovery from substance dependence (Janosik and Green, 1992, Martin, 1989) and management of chronic pain (Vallerand, 1991).

7. *Bill returns in 6 weeks with reports of successful withdrawal from opiates, and participation in a recovery program. Bill says he is feeling better in general, but still needs help with pain relief. Lab work reveals no anemia and normal liver and renal function. What adjustments could you make to the therapeutic plan?*

- Review client/NP contract.
- Revise goals as appropriate.
- Explain that total relief of pain may not be a realistic goal (Vallerand, 1991).
- Strive for a level of pain the client can live with.

8. *What are principles of pain management?*

Principles:
> Cultivate sense of control in client.
> Encourage client activities that keep him active and
> > productive.
> Involve client's family and friends in the plan.

Pharmacology:
> Use the least potent analgesic with the fewest side effects.
> Give each medication an adequate time trial.
> Use a regular dosing schedule, not prn.
> Recognize side effects and avoid oversedation.

Medications:
> Acetaminophen
> Acetylsalicylic acid (ASA)
> Nonsteroidal anti-inflammatory drugs (NSAIDs)
> Adjuvant analgesics: Tricyclic antidepressants, caffeine,
> > phenothiazines, anticonvulsants
> Controlled drugs: In the case of a client with a history of substance de-
> > pendence, alternative modalities must be exhaustively tried before
> > a return to controlled drugs is indicated. In additions to opiates,

benzodiazepines have the potential for abuse and dependence and can trigger cross-addiction (Savage, 1993).

Nonpharmacologic treatments:

Nerve block, transcutaneous electical nerve stimulation (TENS), biofeedback, massage, local heat and/or cold application, activity scheduling, relaxation training (Savage, 1993; Sees and Clark, 1993; Uphold and Graham, 1994; Vallerand, 1991).

9. *Where can a nurse practitioner obtain more information concerning substance dependence and pain management and/or additional resources for assisting affected clients?*

- See local Yellow Pages for Alcoholics Anonymous (AA), Narcotics Anonymous (NA), Adult Children of Alcoholics (ACOA). These organizations provide meeting lists, literature, and support groups.
- Identify local referral sources for detoxification and chemical dependency treatment programs, and mental health counseling.

Write or call for information:

Alcoholics Anonymous, General Service Office
A.A. World Services, Inc.
P.O. Box 459, Grand Central Station
New York, NY 10163
212 870-3400

Narcotics Anonymous
World Service Office, Inc.
P.O. Box 9999
Van Nuys, CA 91409
818 780-3951

To order clinical practice guidelines for pain management:

AHCPR Publications Clearinghouse
P.O. Box 8547
Silver Spring, MD 20907
800 358-9295
(fax) 301 594-2800

Information and educational materials on chemical dependency and related topics:

Hazelden Education Materials
P.O. Box 176
Center City, MN 55012-0176
800 328-9000 (U.S., Canada and the Virgin Islands)
612 257-4010 (outside the U.S. and Canada)
612 257-1331 (24-hour fax)

Nursing practice guidelines for pain management:
McCaffery M, Beebe A. *Pain: Clinical Manual for Nursing Practice.* St. Louis: Mosby; 1989.

REFERENCES

American Psychiatric Association. *Diagnostic and Statistical Manual of Mental Disorders,* 4th ed. Washington, DC: Author; 1994.

Fleming M, Barry K. *Addictive Disorders.* St. Louis: Mosby; 1992.

Janosik E, Green E. *Family Life: Process and Practice.* Boston: Jones and Bartlett; 1992.

Martin JC Fr. *Chalk Talks on Alcohol.* San Francisco: Harper & Row; 1989.

McCaffery M, Beebe A. *Pain: Clinical Manual for Nursing Practice.* St. Louis: Mosby; 1989.

Savage SR. Addiction in the treatment of pain: Significance, recognition, and management. *J Pain Sympt Manage* 1993; 8(5): 265–278.

Sees KL, Clark W. Opioid use in the treatment of chronic pain: Assessment of addiction. *J Pain Sympt Manage* 1993; 8(5): 257–264.

Uphold CR, Graham MV. *Clinical Guidelines in Family Practice.* Gainesville, FL: Barmarrae Books; 1994.

U.S. Department of Health and Human Services. *Management of Cancer Pain: Clinical Practice Guideline Number 9* (AHCPR Publication No. 94-0592). Rockville, MD: Government Printing Office; 1994.

Vallerand AH. The use of narcotic analgesics in chronic nonmalignant pain. *Holistic Nurs Pract* 1991; 6(1): 17–23.

Wesson DR, Ling W, Smith DE. Prescription of opioids for treatment of pain in patients with addictive disease. *J Pain Sympt Manage* 1993; 8(5): 289–296.

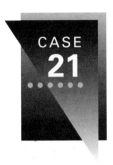

A 54-year-old man with blurred vision, polyuria, and fatigue

SCENARIO

Joe Hobbs is a 54-year-old obese, Caucasian male who presents to your clinic. Mr. Hobbs has not seen a health care provider in 6 years. He states that until 3 months ago he was feeling fine. Mr. Hobbs has slowly experienced a blurring of his vision. He also relates that he has been having polyuria, polydipsia, and fatigue. He currently takes no medications.

● TENTATIVE DIAGNOSES

Based on the information provided so far, what are potential differential diagnoses?

● HISTORY

What are significant questions in Joe's history?
What are the key points to cover on the review of systems?

● PHYSICAL ASSESSMENT

What are the significant portions of the physical examination that should be completed for Joe?

● DIFFERENTIAL DIAGNOSES

What are the significant positive and negative data that support or refute your diagnoses for Joe?

● DIAGNOSTIC TESTS

Based on the history and physical assessment, what, if any, diagnostic tests would you obtain? Include your rationale for the tests.

● DIAGNOSES

What diagnoses are appropriate for Joe?

● THERAPEUTIC PLAN

1. *Identify the risk factors that contributed to Mr. Hobbs' development of NIDDM.*

2. *Why did Mr. Hobbs exhibit the symptoms of polyuria, polydipsia, fatigue, and blurred vision?*

3. *What are the short-term management goals for Mr. Hobbs?*

4. *What patient education should Mr. Hobbs get related to his oral hypo-glycemic agent and management of his DM when ill?*

5. *What type of surveillance needs to be done in order to monitor the existence of chronic complications from diabetes?*

6. *When should Joe return for follow up?*

7. *What are support systems that are available to assist the NP, Joe, and Joe's wife in the management of NIDDM?*

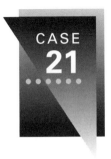

TUTORIAL

A 54-year-old man with blurred vision, polyuria, and fatigue

SCENARIO

Joe Hobbs is a 54 year-old obese, Caucasian male who presents to your clinic. Mr. Hobbs has not seen a health care provider in 6 years. He states that until 3 months ago he was feeling fine. Mr. Hobbs has slowly experienced a blurring of his vision. He also relates that he has been having polyuria, polydipsia, and fatigue. He currently takes no medications.

● TENTATIVE DIAGNOSES

Based on the information provided so far, what are potential diagnoses?

DIAGNOSIS	RATIONALE
Hypothyroidism	Mr. Hobbs is presenting with fatigue.
Eye problems such as presbyopia, cataract, glaucoma	Joe is c/o blurred vision, a common complaint of elderly people.
Anemia	Fatigue is a common presenting symptom of anemia.
Diabetes insipidus	Polyuria and polydipsia are symptoms of diabetes insipidus.
Diabetes mellitus	Polyuria, polydipsia, and fatigue are common symptoms seen with DM.

● HISTORY

1. What are significant questions in Joe's history?

REQUESTED DATA	DATA ANSWER
Allergies	NKDA.
Current medications	None.
Surgery/transfusions	Tonsillectomy at age 10.
Past medical history and hospitalizations/fractures/injuries/accidents	Unremarkable.
Sleeping pattern	Getting up recently to urinate three to four times a night.
Appetite/weight change	Has gained approximately 20 lbs in past year, but has lost 5 lbs in past 2 weeks without really trying. Has noticed that his thirst is tremendous, and he is unable to quench his thirst even with his usual soft drink.
24-hour diet recall	B: Sausage biscuit with gravy, coffee, and orange juice. L: Hamburger, french fries, soda. D: Meat, potato, gravy, vegetable, and salad. S: Potato chips or ice cream.
Social history	Tobacco: None. Alcohol: None. Drugs: Denies. Caffeine: Two cups coffee/day. Exercise: None.
Family history	Father: Died at age 55, HTN, DM. Mother: Age 74, Breast Ca. PGF: Deceased 49, MI. MGM: Deceased 65, CVA.
Employment	New job in past year as salesperson; does a lot of traveling.

2. What are the key points on the review of systems?

SYSTEM REVIEWED	DATA ANSWER
General	Feels fatigued after lunch. At times he does not feel he has enough energy to do his usual activities.
Skin	Dry, but no problems. Denies problems with healing.
HEENT	Vision change recently. He noticed his vision is blurry and has difficulty with reading. He does not wear corrective lenses. Denies loss of peripheral vision, or difficulty with glare.
Lungs	Denies problems breathing or SOB.
Cardiac	Denies chest pain or palpitations.
GI/GU	Denies dysuria, frequency or urgency, hesitancy in starting stream, no dribbling, retention.

● PHYSICAL ASSESSMENT

What are the significant portions of the physical examination that should be completed for Joe?

SYSTEM	RATIONALE	FINDINGS
Vital signs	Provides baseline data.	B/P 130/86, HR 78, R 22, T 98.2.
General appearance/skin	General overall picture of patient's status.	Alert, NAD.
Eyes	Look for changes in blood vessels of retina.	Optic disc margins well defined. No nicking or hemorrhages.
Neck	Check vascular status/thyroid.	Supple, no thyromegaly, bruits.
Lungs	Provides baseline data.	CTA.
Heart	Provides baseline data. Important to evaluate because he has a +FH.	RRR, No MRG.

(continued)

SYSTEM	*RATIONALE*	*FINDINGS*
Abdomen	Baseline data, check vascular status.	BS+, soft, no masses, tenderness, HSM, or bruits.
Extremities/feet	Assessment of peripheral vascular system (Kerstein, 1990).	Pulses 2+, skin warm and pink, no edema. Sensation intact. Feet dry, no callus.
Rectum	Assessment of prostate, check for blood loss.	Anal sphincter WNL, prostate firm, nonenlarged, no nodules, brown soft stool.

● DIFFERENTIAL DIAGNOSES

What are the significant positive and negative findings that support or refute your diagnoses for Joe?

DIAGNOSIS	*POSITIVE DATA*	*NEGATIVE DATA*
Hypothyroidism	Dry skin, fatigue.	No thyromegaly, intolerance to cold, alopecia, constipation.
Anemia	Fatigue.	No known blood loss.
BPH	Nocturia.	No hesitancy in starting stream, prostate WNL, no dribbling.
Diabetes insipidus	Polyuria, polydipsia.	No history of head trauma, does not take lithium, no sudden preference for iced water.
Eye problems such as presbyopia, cataract, glaucoma	Blurred vision.	Red reflex present, no tunnel vision, no peripheral vision loss, denies problems with glare.
Diabetes mellitus	Fatigue, polyuria, polydipsia, blurred vision, weight gain, and then weight loss without trying.	No peripheral neuropathy, no history of skin lesions or poor healing, or chronic fungal infections.

● DIAGNOSTIC TESTS

Based on the history and physical examination, what, if any, diagnostic testing would you obtain?

DIAGNOSTIC TEST	RATIONALE	RESULTS
CBC	Provide baseline information, r/o anemia.	WNL.
Lipid profile	Provide baseline information, particularly because Joe has a + FH.	Cholesterol: 260 mg/dL. Triglycerides: 330 mg/dL. HDC, 30. LDC, 193.
Chemistry	Provide baseline information.	FBS 350 mg/dL, otherwise WNL.
Thyroid profile	R/o thyroid dysfunction.	TSH 1.2. T4 WNL.
Hgb A1C	Provides indication of glucose levels for past 10–12 weeks. Not generally used for diagnostic purposes.	12%.
U/A	R/o UTI, check for ketones and glucose.	3+ glucose.
EKG	Document cardiac functions. Provide a baseline for future comparisons.	NSR.

● DIAGNOSES

What diagnoses do you determine as being appropriate after a review of the subjective and objective data?

Non-insulin dependent diabetes mellitus (NIDDM)

Data Supporting the Diagnosis

Elevated blood glucose, elevated HgbA1C, glycosuria, hypercholesterolemia, triglycerides, and hyperlipidemia all provide support for the diagnosis of NIDDM. In addition, his + FM of diabetes also lends support to this diagnosis, as does his recent weight gain and age > 40. Since Mr. Hobbs' blood sugar is considerably elevated (above 200 mg/dL), this is enough to make the diagnosis (Benso, 1988).

● THERAPEUTIC PLAN

1. Identify the risk factors that contributed to Mr. Hobbs' development of NIDDM.

Mr. Hobbs had the following risk factors that contributed to his development of NIDDM:

- sedentary lifestyle
- poor dietary history
- +FH of DM
- lack of medical care
- age > 40

All of these risk factors need to be addressed in his plan of care.

2. Why did Mr. Hobbs exhibit the symptoms of polyuria, polydipsia, fatigue, and blurred vision?

The elevated blood glucose levels that Mr. Hobbs experienced caused his body to increase urination and thirst owing to the osmotic diuresis that occurs with glycosuria. Fatigue is due to the lack of glucose for cells. All of the glucose is staying in the blood or being lost through urination. The blurring of his vision is caused by the change in the shape of the lens of the eye from the elevated glucose level. His vision will improve within 4–6 weeks after his blood sugar is normalized (Davidson, 1991).

3. What are the short-term management goals for Mr. Hobbs?

The short-term management of Mr. Hobbs will require immediate treatment of his hyperglycemia because his blood sugar was greater than 240 mg/dL. If his blood sugar had been less than 240 mg/dL, diet and exercise would have been the only therapy. To achieve good glycemic control, the nurse practitioner begins a second-generation oral hypoglycemic agent. The second-generation oral agents, Glipizide or Glyburide, can be started at low dosages. Since Joe's FBS was markedly elevated, he may need to be started on a slightly higher dose, such as 5 mg for Glipizide. Mr. Hobbs will have the dosage of his medication adjusted every one to 2 weeks, dependent on his home glucose monitoring.

Mr. Hobbs was also instructed by the nurse practitioner to start a low cholesterol and fat diet, with no concentrated sugar. He was given written instructions for this diet.

To address his sedentary lifestyle and aid in lowering his blood glucose, Mr. Hobbs agrees to begin a walking program. He will walk 20 minutes 4 days per week and gradually increase his walking time to between 30–45 minutes per day.

Mr. Hobbs was referred to a local diabetes education program for further information about diabetes, nutrition, exercise, foot care, home glucose monitoring, and long-term complications. A follow-up visit was scheduled in 2 weeks to review Mr. Hobb's glycemic control and further develop a management plan (Haire-Joshu, 1992).

4. *What patient education should Mr. Hobbs get related to his oral hypo-glycemic agent and management of his DM when ill?*

Mr. Hobbs should know that second-generation sulfonylureas have the slight potential to cause hypoglycemia. He should be aware of the symptoms of hypoglycemia, as should his wife. These symptoms are: shakiness, sweating, hunger, H/A, confusion.

People with NIDDM on an oral agent rarely develop hypoglycemia. To prevent hypoglycemia, Mr. Hobbs should eat regular meals. If hypoglycemia becomes a problem, the oral agent should be stopped to see if his hemoglobin A1C is normal. Joe should always carry a fast-acting carbohydrate in case of a hypoglycemic reaction.

Joe should carry medical identification concerning his DM.

In the event that Joe becomes ill, he should continue to take his Glipizide (Glucotrol). Joe should carefully monitor his blood sugar several times a day. He should get in touch with the health care provider if he can not take fluids, if his glucose is over 250 mg/dL for two blood sugar readings. If his blood sugar is less than 60 mg/dL for two readings, he should also call his health care provider (Cefalu et al., 1996).

5. *What type of surveillance needs to be done in order to monitor the existence of chronic complications from diabetes?*

Typically, long-term complications from diabetes do not occur until 10 to 15 years after diagnosis. However, in NIDDM, it is impossible to know how long the person has had diabetes. Prior to diagnosis, diabetes is usually present for a much longer time period than the person is symptomatic.

The main way to prevent the complications of diabetes is through improved glycemic control. A hemoglobin A1C of around 7% will maintain a blood sugar average of approximately 150 mg/dL. This level is sufficient to aid in the prevention of long-term complications from diabetes (ADA, 1995).

Retinopathy

To monitor for the long-term complications of diabetes, the nurse practitioner developed the next phase of the plan. An appointment was made with an ophthalmologist to monitor for retinopathy. Mr. Hobbs was advised that he would need an annual eye exam.

Nephropathy

Damage to the kidney is reflected by an increase in urinary protein. One of the first proteins to escape from glomerular filtration is microalbumin. Surveillance for kidney disease was obtained by measuring an overnight collection of urine for microalbumin. Mr. Hobbs was advised to void before retiring, and then collect any urine throughout the night and in the morning for the specimen. Optimally, this should be done annually. If cost is a factor, a random sample could be checked for microalbumin (Diabetes Control and Complications Trial Research Group, 1993).

Neuropathy

Vascular and neuropathic complications are monitored through symptoms evaluation, physical examination, and blood pressure evaluation. Persons with diabetes need to be questioned as to the existence of symptoms from the complications of diabetes, such as: 1) numbness or tingling of the feet; 2) impotence; 3) changes in bowel habits; or 4) dizziness associated with position changes.

The feet should be examined by the clinician at each visit. Careful attention by the clinician to the condition of the temperature of the feet, pulses of the lower extremities, deep tendon reflexes, sensation, and overall skin condition. Mr. Hobbs will need to be instructed on daily foot examination and skin care (Sammarco, 1991).

Cardiovascular Disease

DM is a major risk factor in the development of cardiac disease. Because Joe has NIDDM, and has a + FH for cardiovascular disease, it will be important for Joe to know the warning symptoms of cardiovascular disease. Each time he visits he should be asked about the following symptoms: chest pain, jaw pain, extreme fatigue, SOB, chest pressure, or arm numbness or pain. However, with diabetes, people often do not experience chest pain because the nerves to the heart can become damaged. If any of the symptoms occur, he should get in touch with his health provider right away, or call 911 (Watkins et al., 1990).

6. *When should Joe return for follow up?*

Joe should return initially in two weeks to evaluate his progress with oral hypoglycemia agent. If his blood sugars are within the goal set, he can return every 3 months for a repeat hemoglobin A1C. If this value is 7.0% he can then return every 6 months.

7. *What are support systems that are available to assist the NP, Joe, and Joe's wife in the management of NIDDM?*

Managing diabetes requires the client to work with the health care provider to develop a plan of care. The plan should require the input of dietitians, physical therapists, social workers, physicians, nurses, and nurse practitioners.

Most communities have diabetes education programs. These are usually run by certified diabetes educators. Support groups are beneficial to many clients. The American Diabetes Association and American Association of Diabetes Educators have programs in most cities.

REFERENCES

American Diabetes Association. Standards of Medical Care for Patients with Diabetes Mellitus. *Diabetes Care* 1995; 18: 8–15.

Benso W, Brown G, Tasman W. *Diabetes and Its Complications.* Philadelphia: W.B. Saunders; 1988.

Cefalu W, Colwell J, King G. What's new about the new oral diabetes drugs? *Patient Care* 1996; 30: 40–66.

Davidson MB. *Diabetes Mellitus: Diagnosis and Treatment.* New York: Churchill Livingstone; 1991.

Diabetes Control and Complications Trial Research Group. The Effect of Intensive Treatment of Diabetes on the Development and Progression of Long-Term Complications in Insulin-Dependent Diabetes Mellitus. *N Engl J Med* 1993; 329: 977–986.

Haire-Joshu D. *Management of Diabetes Mellitus: Perspectives of Care Across the Life Span.* St. Louis: Mosby; 1992.

Horrobin D. *Treatment of Diabetic Neuropathy: A New Approach.* New York: Churchill Livingstone; 1992.

Kerstein M. *Diabetes and Vascular Disease.* Philadephia: J.B. Lippincott; 1990.

Sammarco GJ. *The Foot in Diabetes.* Philadelphia: Lea & Febiger; 1991.

Watkins PJ, Drury PJ, Taylor KW. *Diabetes and Its Management.* Cambridge, MA: Blackwell Scientific; 1990.

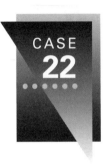

A 25-year-old woman with diarrhea and bloating

SCENARIO

Suzanne Wilson is a 25-year-old Asian female who complains of diarrhea and bloating. She has noticed that prior to the diarrhea she has abdominal pain that seems to be relieved by a bowel movement. She is finding it difficult to go to work having all these symptoms so frequently.

● TENTATIVE DIAGNOSES

Based on the information provided so far, what are potential differential diagnoses?

● HISTORY

What are significant questions in Suzanne's history?
What are the key points to cover on the review of systems?

● PHYSICAL ASSESSMENT

What are the significant portions of the physical examination that should be completed for Suzanne?

● DIFFERENTIAL DIAGNOSES

What are the significant positive and negative data that support or refute your diagnoses for Suzanne?

● DIAGNOSTIC TESTS

Based on the history and physical assessment, what, if any, diagnostic tests would you do. Include your rationale for the testing.

● DIAGNOSIS

What diagnoses are appropriate for Suzanne?

● THERAPEUTIC PLAN

1. *How would the NP test Suzanne for lactose intolerance?*
2. *What patient education should be shared with Suzanne regarding IBS?*
3. *What suggestions should be made regarding Suzanne's poor dietary habits, and to improve her IBS?*
4. *What medications might be useful for treating IBS?*
5. *What referrals would you make for Suzanne?*
6. *What are community resources for the NP and Suzanne related to IBS?*

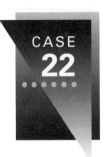

TUTORIAL

A 25-year-old woman with diarrhea and bloating

SCENARIO

Suzanne Wilson is a 25-year-old Asian female who complains of diarrhea and bloating. She has noticed that prior to the diarrhea she has abdominal pain that seems to be relieved by a bowel movement. She is finding it difficult to go to work having all these symptoms so frequently.

● TENTATIVE DIAGNOSES

Based on the information provided so far, what are potential diagnoses?

DIAGNOSIS	RATIONALE
Lactose intolerance	C/o diarrhea and bloating with abdominal pain.
Inflammatory bowel disease (IBD)	C/o diarrhea and bloating with abdominal pain.
Laxative abuse	Chronic diarrhea.
Colon cancer	C/o diarrhea, bloating, and abdominal pain.
Poor dietary habits	C/o diarrhea.
Intestinal infection (shigella, salmonellosis, giardia)	C/o diarrhea, bloating, and abdominal pain.
Diverticulosis	C/o diarrhea/abdominal pain.
Irritable bowel syndrome (IBS)	C/o diarrhea/abdominal pain for last 4 months.
Gastritis	C/o abdominal pain.
Hyperthyroidism	C/o diarrhea.

● HISTORY

1. What are significant questions in Suzanne's history?

REQUESTED DATA	DATA ANSWER
Allergies	NKA.
Current medications	Fluoxetine (Prozac) 20 mg QD for depression, Medroxy-progesterone (Depo Provera/DMPA) injection.
Surgery	Shoulder surgery 1995 for arthritic AC joint, no transfusions.
Past medical history and hospitalizations/fractures/injuries/accidents	Usually healthy, although she gets several URIs per season. Has been feeling blue for past 4 months. Started Fluoxetine, seems to be helping. Hospitalizations: childbirth.
Describe symptoms of diarrhea more in depth: onset, location of abdominal pain, how long does it last, what helps increases diarrhea and pain, relationship to diet.	Has noticed diarrhea off and on for years. Recently has been having diarrhea every other day. Seems to get a lot of gas, then abdominal pain, and ends up having diarrhea, which seems to get better for a short time after she has diarrhea. Has tried Tums and Pepto-Bismol with no relief. Finds when she is upset the diarrhea and abdominal pain seem to get worse. Has not noticed any particular foods that make the symptoms worse.
OB/GYN history	LNMP: 3 weeks ago. Last pap: 9 months ago. Mammogram: never had. G 3 P 2 A 1, spontaneous. Contraception now: DMPA.
Appetite/weight change/24-hr recall	Has good appetite, usually flucuates in weight ~5 lbs. No special diet. B: None except coffee (3–5 cups). L: 2 pieces of pizza, soda, sometimes piece of cake, candy bar. D: meat (fried chicken, hamburger), vegetable, drink. S: popcorn/pretzels.
Sleeping pattern	No problems with sleeping. Usually gets 6–7 hours sleep/night.
Social history	Tobacco: 1 ppd. Had smoked before for 5 years, just started smoking again owing to stress. Alcohol: Occasional, usually beer. Drugs: Denies.

(continued)

REQUESTED DATA	DATA ANSWER
	Caffeine: 3–5 cups coffee, and 1–3 sodas day.
	Exercise: Sporadic—usually in good weather.
Family history	Father: Died 51, MI, s/p CABG, smoked.
	Mother: 65, healthy.
	Brother: 45, smokes 1–2 ppd/possible alcohol abuse.
	Children: One daughter, 5; and son 3, healthy.
Relationship with husband	Has been having many arguments with husband for last 6 months. Disagrees with future plans, and level of communication with her and kids. Husband moved out approx. 1 month ago. She has the kids. Husband has not called or been to see children in last 3 weeks.
Relationship with family	Mother lives in another city 150 miles away. Mother is talking about moving down here to help, but Suzanne is not sure if she could handle having her mother live with her. Her brother lives in the same city, but she does not get along with her brother's wife. Does not feel her family is much of a support system.
Employment/insurance/income	Since Suzanne's husband left, money is very tight. Suzanne works as a salesperson at a local department store. It does not pay well, and she does not get any benefits because she works less than 36 hours/week. She does not qualify for Medicaid because she makes too much money.

2. *What are the key points on the review of systems?*

SYSTEM REVIEWED	DATA ANSWER
General	Suzanne admits to feeling fatigued and stressed. Denies jitters or intolerance to heat.
Skin	Pale, no problems.
Lungs	Denies SOB, although she does admit to a "smoker's cough."
Cardiac	Sometimes heart races but it goes away on its own.
GI/GU	Reports occasional constipation, no black, tarry, or bloody stools. No c/o of heartburn or waking at night with abdominal pain. No nausea or vomiting. Denies use of laxatives.

● PHYSICAL ASSESSMENT

What are the significant portions of the physical examination that should be completed for Suzanne?

SYSTEM	RATIONALE	FINDINGS
Vital signs	Provides baseline info.	B/P 122/80 HR 90 R 20 T 97.8 Ht. 5'3" Wt. 140 lbs
General appearance/skin	Provides overall picture of client.	Pale Asian female, NAD. Skin WNL, no lesions.
Thyroid	Assess thyroid gland.	Thyroid nonpalpable, no masses.
Lungs	Because Suzanne smokes it is important to screen.	CTA.
Heart	Suzanne c/o episodes of racing heart beat.	RRR, no MRG.
Abdomen	System of complaint.	Abdomen slightly protuberant, no peristalsis seen, BS+, no bruits, Increased tympany in LLQ. No HSM, tenderness to light palpation in LLQ. No CVA tenderness, no rebound tenderness, no masses.
Rectal	System of complaint.	Normal sphincter tone. No masses. Brown soft stool present in rectum.

● DIFFERENTIAL DIAGNOSES

What are the significant positive and negative data that support or refute your diagnoses for Suzanne?

DIAGNOSIS	POSITIVE DATA	NEGATIVE DATA
IBD	Diarrhea, abdominal pain.	No weight loss, blood in stool, low grade fever, tenesmus, sense of urgency, cramping, N/V.
Lactose intolerance	Diarrhea, abdominal pain.	No relationship to food or lactose products.
Intestinal infections	Diarrhea for 4 months, abdominal pain.	No one else in household has symptoms, recent travel, weight loss, fever, dehydration, or bloody or mucoid stools.
IBS	Continous symptoms for at least 3 months, abdominal pain relieved by defecation, change in frequency of stools, bloating, recent stress, no symptoms at night.	Rare constipation, no mucus in stools.
CA colon	Diarrhea, high-fat low-fiber diet.	Blood in stool, negative FH.
Diverticulosis	Abdominal pain, altered bowel habits, pain before BM, tender LLQ.	Age.
Hyperthyroidism	Diarrhea, episodes of heart racing.	Nonpalpable thyroid gland, no lid lag, no intolerance to heat, jitters, sleeping problems.
Laxative abuse	Diarrhea.	Denies use of laxatives.
Gastritis	Diarrhea, abdominal pain, bloating.	
Poor dietary habits	High-fat intake, increased diet of fast foods, decreased fiber intake.	No weight gain.

● DIAGNOSTIC TESTS

Based on the history and physical assessment, what, if any, diagnostic tests would you obtain?

DIAGNOSTIC TEST	RATIONALE	RESULTS
Flexible sigmoidoscopy	To exclude IBD and malignancy.	Not done. Suzanne refused because she had no insurance.
Colonoscopy	Rule out malignancy.	Not done because Suzanne is not >40.
CBC with diff	Rule out an infectious process.	WNL.
Chemistry	Provide baseline data regarding renal and liver function.	WNL except cholesterol 276, LDL 190, HDL 33.
TSH	To evaluate thyroid functioning.	2.0 mg/dL.
72-Hour stool collection for: fecal fat, amount of stool, osmolality, and electrolyte concentration.	Evaluate for metabolic defects.	Not done.
Stool studies/ova and parasite	R/O intestinal infections.	Blood: Negative. Fecal leukocytes: Negative. Negative for ova/parasites.
Barium enema	R/O IBD and malignancy.	Not done because Suzanne <40.
Hemoccult	R/O blood.	Negative.

● DIAGNOSES

What diagnoses are appropriate for Suzanne?

IBS
Poor dietary intake
R/O lactose intolerance

Data Supporting the Diagnosis

Suzanne's symptoms meet the Rome criteria for IBS:

- Continuous/recurrent symptoms >3 months
- Abdominal pain relieved with defecation associated with change in frequency and/or consistency of stool

- An irregular pattern of defecation at least 25% of time:
  - Altered stool frequency (>3 Bms/day or <3 Bms/day)
  - Altered stool form (hard/loose/watery)
  - Altered stool passage (straining or a feeling of incomplete emptying)
  - Passage of mucus
  - Bloating or feeling of abdominal distention (Barker et al., 1995)

She also reports increased stress recently, believed to play a role in IBS. Women are afflicted more frequently than men.

Because most people do not associate abdominal symptoms with milk intake, the NP should not r/o lactose intolerance without further testing.

● THERAPEUTIC PLAN

1. How would the NP test Suzanne for lactose intolerance?

The NP should recommend a lactose free trial for 3 weeks, eliminating all milk, and milk products, including butter, cottage cheese, yogurt, cheese, and ice cream. If symptoms disappear, than the association with lactose has been established. Suzanne may add items slowly until symptoms appear once again. This will establish the level of lactose the person can tolerate. Other, more specific tests for lactose intolerance are only indicated when nutritional status would be compromised by eliminating milk products unnecessarily. The hydrogen breath test is the easiest to perform and the most accurate.

Obviously, if the lactose tolerance test is positive, then Suzanne should avoid milk and milk products that produce the diarrhea and other symptoms. Use of lactase (Lactaid) may be helpful in reducing the symptoms of lactose intolerance.

2. What patient education should be shared with Suzanne regarding IBS?

Suzanne will need to be reassured that there is nothing wrong with her colon. It will be important to discuss with her the causes of IBS, and its relationship to increased stress. A positive provider–patient relationship also appears to be helpful in maintaining a more normal clinical course (Owens, 1995).

Lifestyle changes are an important part of treating IBS. Suggestions about eating regular meals, chewing thoroughly and slowly, drinking plenty of fluids, and exercising daily will help Suzanne in feeling better. It will also be important for her to respond to the urge to empty her bowels.

3. What suggestions should be made regarding Suzanne's poor dietary habits, and to improve her IBS?

Suzanne should avoid foods that seem to cause or increase her symptoms. Suzanne should add more fiber to her diet. The fiber adds bulk to help the colon function normally again (Dancey & Blackhouse, 1993).

Suzanne should eat 20–35 grams of fiber daily. She should replace foods high in fat and calories with high fiber foods, such as fruits, and vegetables. She can substitute whole grain breads for white bread and rolls. Brown rice instead of white rice will also add fiber. She could also substitute bran for bread crumbs in casseroles (Lynn & Friedman, 1995).

4. What medications might be useful for treating IBS?

- Adding a bulk forming fiber therapy to Suzanne's diet may help with restoring regularity. Medications such as Psyllium seeds (Metamucil, Konsyl) taken 1–2 tablespoons BID or TID for a 2-week trial may prove to help decrease her diarrhea.
- Antispasmodics such as Dicyclomine (Bentyl) 10–20 BID.
- Antidiarrheal agents:
  - Diphenoxylate-atropine (Lomotil), one to two tablets every 6 hours.
  - Loperamide (Imodium) one to two tabs every 8 hours.
- Antiflatulence:
  - Simethicone (Gaviscon, Mylicon) two to four tablets with meals.
  - Activated charcoal (Beano) before meals and HS (Tally, 1996).

5. What referrals would you make for Suzanne?

A counseling referral might prove to be helpful for Suzanne in terms of reducing her stress. Most health departments have low-cost counseling available on a short-term basis. Modifying situational factors and teaching relaxation techniques can sometimes decrease stress. Make sure to evaluate whether Suzanne is depressed because IBS patients as a whole have more depression, anxiety, and somatization of affect (Procter & Gamble, 1990).

6. What are community resources for the NP and Suzanne related to IBS?

In most communities there is a local support group for Crohn's and Colitis. These groups maintain a variety of educational materials, including information on IBS and IBD. Look in your local phone book.

> National Digestive Disease Information Clearing House
> Bethesda, MD
> (301) 654-3810

7. When should Suzanne be instructed to return for follow up?

Initially, Suzanne should return in 2 weeks to determine her response to the bulk forming agents. When there is a positive response, she can return every month for 1–2 months, and then every 6 months as needed.

REFERENCES

Barker L, Burton J, Zieve P. (eds.). *Principles of Ambulatory Medicine*, 4th Ed. Philadelphia: Williams & Wilkins; 1995.

Dancey C, Blackhouse S. Toward a better understanding of patients with irritable bowel syndrome. *J Adv Nurs* 1993; 18: 1443–1450.

Lynn R, Friedman L. Irritable bowel syndrome: Managing the patient with abdominal pain and altered bowel habits. *Med Clin North Am* 1995; 79(2): 373–390.

Owens D, Nelson D, Tally N. Irritable bowel syndrome: Long-term prognosis and the physician-patient interaction. *Annals Intern Med* 1995; 122(2): 107–112

Procter & Gamble. *What You Can Do About Irritable Bowel Syndrome.* Cincinnati: Procter and Gamble; 1990.

Tally N. Irritable bowel syndrome. *Res Staff Phys* 1996; 42(1): 11–16.

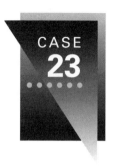

A 67-year-old man requesting a well physical

SCENARIO

Robert Gill is a 67-year-old Caucasian male coming to your office for the first time to become established as a patient. He is generally in good health with no acute problems.

● TENTATIVE DIAGNOSES

Based on the information provided so far, what are potential diagnoses?

● HISTORY

What are significant questions in Robert's history?

● PHYSICAL ASSESSMENT

What are the significant portions of the physical examination that should be completed for Robert?

● DIFFERENTIAL DIAGNOSES

What are the significant positive and negative data that support or refute your diagnoses for Robert?

● DIAGNOSTIC TESTS

Based on the history and physical assessment, what, if any, diagnostic tests would you obtain? Include your rationale for the tests.

● DIAGNOSIS

What diagnoses are appropriate for Robert?

● THERAPEUTIC PLAN

1. *How is melanoma classified?*
2. *What is the plan you will develop for Robert related to his skin lesion?*
3. *What is the plan you will develop for Robert related to his hypercholesterolemia?*
4. *What is the plan you will develop for Robert related to his enlarged prostate?*
5. *What is your goal LDL?*
6. *What health promotion/projection suggestions would you make to Robert?*
7. *How often should Robert return for follow up?*
8. *How do you think the diagnosis of skin lesion with possible malignancy might impact Robert and his family?*
9. *What community resources might be of assistance for Robert and his family?*

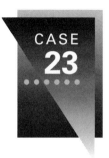

TUTORIAL

A 67-year-old man requesting a well physical

SCENARIO

Robert Gill is a 67-year-old Caucasian male coming to your office for the first time to become established as a patient. He is generally in good health with no acute problems.

● TENTATIVE DIAGNOSES

Based on the information provided so far, what are the potential diagnoses?

DIAGNOSIS	RATIONALE
Not applicable at this point.	Well physical and wanting to get established with a new health provider.

● HISTORY

1. What are significant questions in Robert's history?

REQUESTED DATA	DATA ANSWER
Allergies	Sulfa—reports hives and SOB 1–2 hours after taking Sulfa.
Current medications	Funisolide (Aerobid) 2 puffs BID prn.
	Simvastatin (Zocor) 10 mg po QD.
	Baby ASA I PO QD.
	OTC Tylenol or ibuprofen for occasional aches, pains, H/A.

(continued)

REQUESTED DATA	*DATA ANSWER*
Surgery	Cataracts × 2, last one 10 years ago. Double hernia repair 2 years ago. Total knee (rt) last year, good recovery.
Immunizations	Has had all childhood immunizations. Unsure of last tetanus. Has not had influenza or pneumococcal vaccines.
Past medical history and hospitalizations/fractures/injuries/accidents	All childhood illnesses, no accidents/fractures. No transfusions.
Adult illness	History elevated cholesterol—takes Zocor × 6 months. Asthma controlled with Aerobid. Only uses as needed, approximately 1–2 times/mo.
Appetite	Good, no weight changes in over 10 years.
24-Hour diet history	B: 3 cereals mixed with banana, berries, 2% milk, sugar, grapefruit juice and 1 c. coffee. L: Low-fat hot dog on bun, low-fat potato chips, and diet soda. D: Salad with radishes, carrots, celery, cauliflower, and broccoli, pork chop, steamed rice, and green beans. S: Chiffon cake with low-fat ice cream.
Sleeping pattern	No problems. Sleeps 7 hours/night. Gets up 1–2 times per night to urinate.
Social history	Tobacco: quit 32 years ago. Started age 15, 20 year history of 1–2 ppd, nonfiltered cigarettes. Alcohol: 3–4 beers on weekend. Caffeinated beverages: 2 c coffee in AM. 2–3 diet colas during day. Minimal chocolate intake. Drugs: None. Exercise: Daily: treadmill 2 miles, rowing machine/15 minutes, weight lifting 15 minutes, and 50 situps.
Family history	Father: Died age 25, aneurysm or MI. Mother: Died age 63, MI. Brother: Died age 47, ruptured aneurysm. Sister: One, 65, good health. Daughter: One, 42, good health.
Relationship with spouse	Married for 44 years. Loving relationship, no problems with sexual activity.
Relationship with child	Daughter moved here 4 years ago with husband. No grandchildren. Both daughter and spouse professional people with good jobs, wanted her parents close.
Social organizations	Church weekly. Active on several church committees.

(continued)

REQUESTED DATA	*DATA ANSWER*
Income	Social security and pension from a company where he worked for 40 years. Worked as an engineer outside most of the time. Wife also has a pension from her employment.
Insurance	Medicare and supplemental.
Home	Bought a new home near daughter.
Do you every have chest pain, discomfort, jaw aching, arm numbness, SOB, diaphoresis?	Denies any cardiac symptoms. Monitors B/P at home: B/P is usually normal.
Have you been having any urinary problems such as urgency, frequency, or pain with urinating?	Sometimes has difficulty starting stream. I was seeing a urologist in Michigan. I have not had other problems.
What losses have you had in your life?	Death of parents, brother, parents-in-law, and nephew.
How do you handle stress?	Prayer, speaks with wife, daughter, and friends. Also finds that exercise helps. "You just go on."
When were your last dental and eye exams?	4 years ago. Denies having problems with either.
Safety in house?	Smoke alarms: Yes. Guns: None. Hot water heater: Set at 140.
Any other problems I should know about?	Sometimes cannot hear well. I have noticed especially when there is a lot of noise around me, sometimes I have difficulty hearing women talk.

● PHYSICAL ASSESSMENT

What are the significant portions of the physical examination that should be completed for Robert?

SYSTEM	*RATIONALE*	*FINDINGS*
Vital signs	Provides baseline data.	B/P: 140/80; HR 86 regular. R: 22, T 98.9 F. Ht. 68". Wt. 160 lbs.

(continued)

SYSTEM	*RATIONALE*	*FINDINGS*
General appearance/skin	Provides a general view of how the patient presents. Because skin cancer risk increases with age or sun exposure, body surfaces should be evaluated for suspicious lesions.	Alert, NAD; Skin warm and dry. Color natural except for 10 cm lesion on Rt. clavicle, stains of brown and black with irregular border, non-tender. Two symmetrical scars on lower abd and scar on knee.
HEENT	Provides baseline data, especially because he c/o decreased hearing ability.	Normocephalic. Ears: ext. canals clear, TMs WNL, Rinne and Weber WNL. Eyes: PERRLA, EOM intact. Mouth: good repair. Neck: No carotid bruit, supple, no LA, thyroid nonpalpable.
Lungs	Important because he c/o intermittent asthma.	CTA.
Heart	Important system to assess given his age and +FH.	S_1S_2 WNL, no MRG.
Abdomen	Important system to assess given his age and potential for vascular problems. Also important to check for liver enlargement caused by Zocar.	BS +, soft, no HSM, no tenderness or masses. No bruits.
GU	Important to screen given his urinary complaints.	Circumcised male. No lesions noted, scrotum without lesions or masses.
Rectum	Need to assess for prostate enlargement and rectal bleeding.	Anal sphincter WNL. No masses, brown soft stool. Prostate smooth, symmetrical without nodules, slightly enlarged.
Neurological	Brief screening for baseline.	Strength/sensation intact. Normal gait. FROM. DTRs 2+; Alert and oriented.
Extremities	Check for lesions, cardiovascular status.	Peripheral pulses 2+. No edema.

● DIFFERENTIAL DIAGNOSES

What are the significant positive and negative findings that support or refute your diagnoses for Robert?

DIAGNOSIS	POSITIVE DATA	NEGATIVE DATA
Probably lentigo maligna melanoma	10-cm skin lesion with multiple colors, irregular border. Matches characteristics of lentigo melanoma: large, flat, irregular stain. Usually occurs in 6–7th decade. Worked outside most of his career.	No +FH of melanoma, not fair-haired or fair-skinned. Unsure of previous sunburns or use of sunscreen.
Bronchial asthma by history	Uses MDI with relief.	No adventitious lung sounds, no SOB.
BPH	Difficulty in starting streams, nocturia. Enlarged prostate on exam.	Urinary retention, nondistended bladder.
Hyperlipidemia	By history.	None.

● DIAGNOSTIC TESTS

Based on the history and physical assessment, what, if any, diagnostic tests would you obtain?

DIAGNOSTIC TEST	RATIONALE	RESULTS
Lipid profile	Re-evaluate his cholesterol levels because he is taking Zocor.	Tot. Cholesterol: 220. LDL: 170. HDL: 32. Trigylceride: 235.
EKG	Important to do if no EKG records can be obtained because he has a +FH.	NSR.

(continued)

DIAGNOSTIC TEST	RATIONALE	RESULTS
Hearing screen	Should do a baseline screen if audiology equipment is available.	Not able to do in office.
PEFR	Peak flow is inexpensive and noninvasive. Provides baseline data of FEV_1 abilities. Can help determine personal best.	PEFR: 440.
U/A	Because Robert reports hesitancy and nocturia as a problem, should do a u/a to r/o a UTI.	WNL.
Stool for guaiac	Information for cancer of the colon.	Negative.
Baseline labs if it has been at least a year: electrolytes, renal panel, liver function panel, TSH	Obtain baseline data. Important to evaluate because he is taking medications.	All WNL.
AHCPR Guidelines for BPH-UAU Symptom Index for initial assessment BPH problems	Rated on scale 0 (not at all) to 5 (almost always) on questions related to urination in past month.	Score 6.
PSA	Optional test: PSA may be done to help evaluate the presence of malignancy.	Robert refused.
Urinary flowrate, postvoid residual urine, pressure-flow urodynamic or cystoscopy studies	May consider these as second line tests or if BPH is moderate–severe. Not considered first line tests.	Not done at this time.

● DIAGNOSES

What diagnoses are appropriate for Robert?

Probable lentigo maligna melanoma
Intermittent asthma—stable
Hypercholesterolemia—improving
BPH

Data Supporting the Diagnosis

The diagnosis of melanoma is supported by the following data:

Irregular, large (10-cm) flat lesion of several colors. Robert worked outside as an engineer for many years.

BPH: Enlarged prostate gland, nocturia, hesitancy, male >65.

Hypercholesterolemia: Elevated labs, taking Zocor, +FH for cardiac events.

● THERAPEUTIC PLAN

1. How is melanoma classified?

TYPE	GENDER	AGE	SIZE	APPEARANCE
Superficial spreading	F > M	Median 5th decade	2 cm	Irregular plaque with variegate color (blue, black, gray, white, pink) scaly, crusty, notched borders, may raise or ulcerate
Nodular	M > F	Median 50	1–2 cm	Blister/dome shaped, symmetrical, blue-black lesion, may be amelanotic, may bleed or ulcerate
Lentigo maligna	F > M	Median 6th–7th decade	10 cm	Large, flat, irregular stain (brown, tan, dark areas), notched borders, may have raised nodules
Acral lentiginous	F = M	Median 5th–6th decade	3 cm	Haphazard staining, may be raised or ulcerated

Adapted from Lawler, 1991

2. What is the plan you will develop for Robert related to his skin lesion?

Excisional biopsy is the treatment of choice for the lentigo maligna, allowing for complete histologic examination and microstaging. Incisional or punch biopsy can result in cosmetic defects. Robert should be referred to a dermatologist/surgeon, depending on the result of the biopsy.

3. *What is the plan you will develop for Robert related to his hypercholesterolemia?*

It is important to acknowledge the success Robert has already had in the dietary control of his hypercholesterolemia, his exercise routine and drinking in moderation. Discuss the link between elevated cholesterol and coronary heart disease.

Based on HDL/LDL levels, monitoring should be every 1 to 2 years. Because Robert is taking an antilipemic drug, he should be monitored every 4 weeks for the first 15 months and periodically thereafter. Monitoring at least every 6 months is a sound plan of care. Robert could decrease fat content further by using skim milk instead of 2%, and by maintaining minimal meat intake. It will be important to evaluate the HDL/LDL ratio for Robert (Sloane & Hicks, 1993).

The aggressive treatment of hyperlipidemia in the elderly is a controversial issue. High cholesterol is a less powerful risk for CAD in the elderly. Previous studies did not include large numbers of older patients (Uphold and Graham, 1994).

4. *What is the plan you will develop for Robert related to his enlarged prostate?*

Using the AUA score as a guideline, Robert's score is less than 7, so he should be followed with the strategy of watchful waiting. His symptoms and clinical course should be followed annually.

Behavioral techniques to reduce symptoms:
- limit fluid intake after dinner
- avoid decongestants, anticholinergics, tranquilizers, or alcohol
- void frequently
- consider an alpha adrenergic blocker if his symptoms worsen. These agents frequently are helpful in terms of nocturia and symptom control, but no evidence exists that show long-term effectiveness. Caution if these drugs are used since they cause postural hypotension. Give at HS to help reduce these side effects.
- If symptoms increase or there are complications, refer to urologist (McConnell et al., 1994).

5. *What is your goal LDL?*

Because Robert has two risk factors for CAD other than his LDL cholesterol (male >45, +FH), but does not actually have CAD himself, the goal LDL should be <130 mg/dL (National Cholesterol Education Program, 1993).

6. *What health promotion/prevention suggestions would you make to Robert?*
- Use of seat belts
- Smoke detectors
- Avoid use of space heaters

- Immunizations:
  - Tetanus booster
  - Influenza vaccine every year
  - Pneumococcal vaccine once (Goldstein, 1993)

Teaching regarding skin protection:

- decrease future sun exposure
- avoid sun exposure between 10 AM and 2 PM
- use protective measures: hat, long sleeves, sunscreen SPF 15 or greater
- conduct annual skin surface examinations; have spouse help (Hicks, 1993).

7. *How often should Robert return for follow up?*

Robert should return for follow up initially every 3–4 months, depending on the results of his skin biopsy and other labs. He will need periodic labs to monitor for his Zocor therapy.

8. *How do you think the diagnosis of skin lesion with possible malignancy might impact Robert and his family?*

The family impact of a general physical exam is usually a comforting one. In this case, with the potential of a diagnosis of melanoma, one needs to realize the time between now and seeing the dermatologist or surgeon can be very tense. Be sure that Robert has an open door to you for support. Provide enough information to assist in allaying apprehension as much as possible. Explore the strength of the current support systems, call the wife/daughter if Robert wishes. Making the dermatologist/surgeon appointment for Robert is reassuring. You may also want to call Robert between the time he sees you and the surgeon, and/or between the time he sees the surgeon and gets the results of the tests and procedures.

9. *What community resources might be of assistance for Robert and his family?*

American Heart Association
National Center (check phone book for local resources)
7320 Greenville Ave.
Dallas, TX 75231

If appropriate:

American Cancer Society (local)

American Cancer Society (National) 800 1CS-2345

REFERENCES

Goldstein A. Health promotion, in Sloane P, Slatt L, Curtis P (eds). *Essentials of Family Medicine.* Baltimore: Williams & Wilkins; 1993; 163–173.

Hicks M. Well adult care, in Sloane P, Slatt L, Curtis P (eds). *Essentials of Family Medicine.* Baltimore: Williams & Wilkins; 1993; 145–153.

Lawler P. Cutaneous malignant melanoma, in Yarbro C (eds). *Seminars in Oncology Nursing.* Philadelphia: W.B. Saunders; 1991; 26–35.

McConnell J, Barry M, Bruskewitz R, et al. *Benign Prostatic Hyperplasia: Diagnosis and Treatment. Quick Reference for Clinicians.* AHCPR Publication No. 94-0583. Rockville, MD: Agency for Health Care Policy and Research, Public Health Service, U.S. Department of Health and Human Services. February 1994.

National Cholesterol Education Program. *Report of the expert panel on detection, evaluation, and treatment of high blood cholesterol in adults.* NIH Publication No. 89-2925. Bethesda, MD: U.S. Department of Health and Human Services, Public Health Service, National Institute of Health, National Heart, Lung, and Blood Institute. January 1993.

Sloane P, Hicks M. Preventive care: An overview, in Sloane P, Slatt L, Curtis P (eds). *Essentials of Family Medicine.* Baltimore: Williams & Wilkins; 1993; 113–117.

Uphold C, Graham M. Periodic health evaluation for adults. *Clinical Guidelines in Family Practice,* 2nd ed. Gainesville, FL: Barmarrae Books; 1994; 30–41.

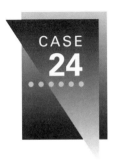

A 3-year-old girl with a rash

SCENARIO

Marsha Smith has brought her daughter Katie to your office. Katie is a 3 y/o Taiwanese female. She presents with a rash and a fever of 103°F for 2 days.

● TENTATIVE DIAGNOSES

Based on the information provided so far, what are potential differential diagnoses?

● HISTORY

What questions would you ask Marsha and Katie that would assist in developing a diagnosis?

● PHYSICAL ASSESSMENT

Is a complete physical exam necessary?
What parts of the exam would you include and why?

● DIFFERENTIAL DIAGNOSES

List and prioritize the four most probable differential diagnoses. With each diagnosis, list the positive and negative data that validate or refute the diagnoses.

● DIAGNOSTIC TESTS

Based on the history and physical assessment, what, if any, diagnostic tests would you obtain. Include your rationale for the testing.

● DIAGNOSIS

What is your conclusive diagnosis for Katie?
What positive and negative data assisted you in arriving at your decision?

● THERAPEUTIC PLAN

1. *What is the goal of care for Katie?*
2. *What referrals/consultation would you initiate prior to instituting the plan of care for Katie?*
3. *What is your rationale for this action?*
4. *What education does Marsha need related to Katie's illness?*
5. *What other preventive interventions should be included for Katie?*
6. *What follow-up care will Katie need?*

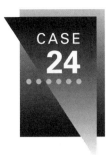

TUTORIAL

A 3-year-old girl with a rash

SCENARIO

Marsha Smith has brought her daughter Katie to your office. Katie is a 3 y/o Taiwanese female. She presents with a rash and a fever of 103°F for 2 days.

● TENTATIVE DIAGNOSES

What are the potential diagnoses you have identified based on the above scenario?

DIAGNOSIS	*RATIONALE*
Viral illness	Katie presented with a rash and fever × 2 days. Both of these symptoms are seen with a viral illness.
Roseola	Kate presented with rash and fever. Roseaola usually presents with high fever. After abrupt resolution of fever, rash develops.
Scarlet fever	Katie presents with rash and fever. With scarlet fever you would expect c/o a sore throat.
Bacterial meningitis	Katie presents with rash and fever. With meningitis you would expect a history of headache, N/V, nuchal rigidity, and irritability as well as rash and fever.
Kawasaki disease	Katie presents with rash and fever. Both of these complaints are seen with Kawasaki disease.

● HISTORY

1. What questions would you ask Marsha and Katie that would assist in developing a diagnosis?

REQUESTED DATA	DATA ANSWER
Allergies	NKA.
Current medications	Acetominophen (Tylenol) every 4 hours as needed for fever.
Recent changes in health	No problems until present complaint. Last check up 1 year ago.
Chief complaint	Rash and fever of 103°F for 2 days.
History of present illness	Fever, which has remained at 103°F for 2 days. Marsha reports that Katie's eyes are red, but no drainage has been noted. The rash is very red and all over. Her lips are also very dry.
Associated manifestations	No history of recent or concurrent respiratory infection.
Associated symptoms	Katie tells you her neck hurts.
History of exposure	No one else is sick at home. Katie is an only child.
Sleeping	Sleeps about 10–12 hours a night. Has awakened for past few nights crying.
Diet	Taking fluids only. Not hungry.
Elimination	Urinating QS, no diarrhea/constipation. BM QOD.
Birth history	Normal term pregnancy, with vaginal delivery. No problems.
PMH	Normally healthy. No hospitalizations or surgeries.
Growth and development	Normal, appropriate for age.
Family history	Father: 24, healthy. Mother: 22, healthy.
Immunizations	Up to date.

● PHYSICAL ASSESSMENT

Is a complete exam necessary? What parts of the exam would you include and why?

SYSTEM	RATIONALE	FINDINGS
Vital signs	Baseline data, gives indication of infection.	B/P: 88/56. HR: 100, R 22 T 103.
General appearance/skin	Gives overall view of how Katie looks. A thorough skin exam can provide clues related to diagnosis.	Erythematous macular papular rash over entire body.
HEENT	Valuable information related to type of infection is present as well as evaluating for dehydration and nuchal rigidity.	Injected bulbar conjunctiva bilaterally, no exudate. EOMs intact. VA os 20/40 od 20/40. Strawberry tongue, chelitis. Unilateral cervical LA, tender and eythematous. −Kernig's and Brudzinski signs.
Lungs	Provides information to determine if there is respiratory involvement.	CTA.
Heart	Baseline information.	RRR, no MRG.
Abdomen	Check for organomegaly/tenderness.	Abdomen soft, BS +, no tenderness or masses. No HSM.
Musculoskeletal	Provides clues for diagnosis. Helps to r/o arthritis.	Tender palms and soles.

● DIFFERENTIAL DIAGNOSES

List and prioritize the four most probable differential diagnoses. With each diagnosis, list the positive and negative data that validate or refute your diagnoses.

DIAGNOSIS	POSITIVE DATA	NEGATIVE DATA
Viral illness	Fever and rash present.	Chelitis, conjunctivitis.
Roseola	Fever and rash present. Fever has remained 103°F.	Chelitis, conjunctivitis, tender palms and soles.
Scarlet fever	Rash and fever.	No history of sore throat, rash does not feel like "sand-paper."
Strep pharyngitis	Fever, rash, tender anterior cervical lymph nodes.	No c/o pharyngitis, pharynx not erythematous.
Bacterial meningitis	Rash and fever present, neck hurts.	No excessive irritability, nuchal rigidity, no known exposure.
Kawasaki disease	Bilateral conjunctival injection, strawberry tongue, chelitis, fever, rash, cervical adeno-pathy, <5 y/o, Asian an-cestry.	No conjunctival exudate, no desquamation of skin, no edema, no noted behavioral changes, and no cardiac dysfunction, over 2 years of age.

● DIAGNOSTIC TESTS

Based on the history and physical examination, what, if any, diagnostic tests would you obtain?

DIAGNOSTIC TEST	RATIONALE	RESULTS
Rapid strep test	R/O strep throat.	Negative.
CBC with diff	Indicates an infection.	WBC: 16,000 Shift to the left >5% bands (neutrophils).

(continued)

DIAGNOSTIC TEST	RATIONALE	RESULTS
ESR	Elevated with an inflammatory process and in KD for first 2 weeks (Crain & Gershel, 1997).	ESR: > 20 mg/dL.
C reactive protein	Indicates the presence of an inflammatory process.	C reactive protein: >20 mg/dL.
Echo cardiogram	Need to evaluate for inflammation of the myocardium and the coronary artery wall with KD.	WNL (done as baseline, and 3 and 8 weeks later).

● DIAGNOSIS

What is your condusive diagnosis for Katie? What positive and negative data assisted you in arriving at your decision?

Kawasaki disease

Data Supporting the Diagnosis

The diagnosis of KD (mucocutaneous lymph node syndrome) is a clinical diagnosis and a diagnosis of exclusion. The acute phase lasts from 1 to 10 days and is characterized by fever, conjunctivitis, oropharyngeal changes, erythematous rash, lymph node enlargement, and behavioral changes. KD needs to be considered in any child with a fever and some (3/5) of the major manifestations:

- Fever of at least 5 days (some believe can diagnose before 5 days)
- Presence of 4 of principal features:
  - changes in extremities (swollen, indurated, erythematous, and tender palms and soles; desquamation of fingers and toes occurs later)
  - polymorphous exanthem (entire body; accentuated in perineal region)
  - bilateral conjunctivitis injection
  - changes in the lips and oral cavity
  - cervical lymphadenopathy (usually unilateral; one node >1.5 cm) (Uphold and Graham, 1994)

● THERAPEUTIC PLAN

1. What is the goal of care for KD?

The initial goal of therapy for KD is to reduce inflammation. The later goal is aimed at preventing coronary thrombosis by inhibiting platelet aggregation.

2. *What referrals/consultation would you initiate prior to instituting the plan of care for Katie?*

The NP needs to consult with his/her collaborating physician prior to treatment.

3. *What is your rationale for this action?*

Because treatment consists of high-dose IV immune globulin therapy, within 10 days of the onset of fever. This therapy, along with the use of ASA, decreases the prevalence of coronary artery dilation and aneurysms. Patients are usually followed up by a cardiologist.

4. *What education does Marsha need related to Katie's illness?*

For most patients, KD is a self-limiting disease and does not recur. The long term prognosis is unclear, although in the US the mortality rate is less than 0.5% (Behrman, 1993). Marsha should be taught the manifestations of possible complications, such as arthralgias, chest pain, and palpitations. Marsha should also know that KD is not spread person to person, and so no preventive measures need to be taken with the family.

5. *What other preventive interventions should be included for Katie?*

All Katie's immunizations should be given at the normal time. To reduce the risks of Reye's syndrome, Katie should get an influenza immunization. No parenteral live vaccines (measles, mumps, rubella) should be given for at least 5 months after the gammaglobulin therapy (Uphold and Graham, 1994).

6. *What follow up care will Katie need?*

Katie will need to be examined frequently during the next 2 months to detect arrhythmias, CHF, myocarditis, and valvular insufficiency. Echocardiograms will need to be done at 3 and 8 weeks after the onset of symptoms to screen for cardiac manifestations.

REFERENCES

Behrman R. (ed). *Nelson Textbook of Pediatrics*. Philadelphia: W.B. Saunders; 1993.

Crain E, Gershel J. *Clinical Manual of Emergency Pediatrics*, 3rd ed. New York: McGraw-Hill; 1997.

Uphold C, Graham M. *Clinical Guidelines in Family Practice*, 2nd ed. Gainesville, FL: Barmarrae Books; 1994.

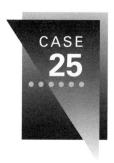

A 40-year-old woman with abdominal pain

SCENARIO

Tanya Steele, a 40-year-old Asian female, complains of a sudden onset of severe epigastric pain that started 2 weeks ago. She denies any abdominal trauma. The pain is very severe and generalized, with diffuse abdominal tenderness. She admits to a history of "heartburn" that she has treated with OTC antacids for the past few years. She also complains of cramping, epigastric pain, and shoulder pain for the past month.

● TENTATIVE DIAGNOSES

Based on the information provided so far, what are potential differential diagnoses?

● HISTORY

What are significant questions in Tanya's history?
What are the key points to cover on the review of systems?

● PHYSICAL ASSESSMENT

What are the significant portions of the physical examination that should be completed for Tanya?

● DIFFERENTIAL DIAGNOSES

What are the significant positive and negative data that support or refute your diagnoses for Tanya?

● DIAGNOSTIC TESTS

Based on the history and physical assessment, what, if any, diagnostic tests would you obtain? Include your rationale for the tests.

● DIAGNOSIS

What diagnoses are appropriate for Tanya?

● THERAPEUTIC PLAN

1. *What would be your initial treatment for cholecystitis?*
2. *What would be your plan for severe pain and vomiting?*
3. *What test might you order at this point if not done previously?*
4. *What referrals would you make for Tanya?*
5. *What follow up would you do for Tanya's elevated blood pressure?*
6. *How would you address Tanya's excessive alcohol intake?*
7. *How in-depth would you explore the issue of family violence? What is your rationale for this decision?*
8. *What are community resources for Tanya?*
9. *What other health maintenance recommendations would you make for Tanya?*
10. *When should Tanya return for follow up for her abdominal pain?*
11. *What patient education do you need to discuss with Tanya?*

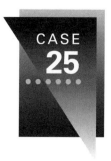

TUTORIAL

A 40-year-old woman with abdominal pain

SCENARIO

Tanya Steele, a 40-year-old Asian female, complains of an onset of severe epigastric pain that started 2 weeks ago. She denies any abdominal trauma. The pain is severe and generalized, with diffuse abdominal tenderness. She admits to a history of "heartburn" that she has treated with OTC antacids for the past few years. She also complains of cramping, epigastric pain, and shoulder pain for the past month.

● TENTATIVE DIAGNOSES

Based on the information provided so far, what are the potential diagnoses?

DIAGNOSIS	RATIONALE
Peptic ulcer disease	Tanya c/o of epigastric pain that has been relieved by antacids.
Cholesystitis, choledocholithiasis	She also c/o of cramping, epigastric pain that radiates to her shoulder.
GERD	Tanya c/o of heartburn relieved by antacids: This is a symptom of GERD.
Myocardial infarction	Tanya presents with heartburn, and radiation of pain up to her shoulder. MI must be considered in the differential until it is ruled out.
AAA	Although Tanya is somewhat young for an abdominal aneurysm, it must be a consideration given her symptoms of severe generalized epigastric pain.

(continued)

DIAGNOSIS	*RATIONALE*
Pancreatitis	Consider this as a diagnosis because the pain is located in the epigastric area.
IBD	Irritable bowel disease should be considered because Tanya's pain is crampy.
Renal colic	Renal colic can also produce crampy severe pain.
PID	With severe pain and cramping, you should consider PID as a possibility for Tanya because she is female.
Peritonitis: perforated viscus	Tanya is c/o of severe diffuse pain in her abdomen.

Because abdominal pain is so complicated there are many possible diagnoses. It would be important to determine if Tanya had a stable B/P, did not have involuntary guarding, a tense boardlike abdomen, or a pulsatile mass before proceeding with any questions. It it critical to determine if there is a surgical abdomen requiring immediate surgical consultation (Trott et al., 1995).

● HISTORY

1. What are significant questions in Tanya's history?

REQUESTED DATA	*DATA ANSWER*
Allergies	NKDA.
Current medications	OTC antacids and ibuprofen.
Surgery	C section × 3, 1981, 1983, 1984, one blood transfusion with last child.
Past medical history and hospitalizations/fractures/ injuries/accidents	Fx clavicle: 5 yrs ago. Fx ribs: 6 yrs ago.
Adult illness	Bronchitis and bilateral OM 4× per year. No back pain.
OB/GYN history	LNMP: 2 weeks ago.
Appetite	Decreased appetite. Has lost 10 lbs in past month without trying. No pain after eating.
Sexuality	Not sexually active × 2 years. Heterosexual.

(continued)

REQUESTED DATA DATA ANSWER

REQUESTED DATA	DATA ANSWER
Elimination	No N/V, no dark tarry stools. No history PUD.
Social history	Employment: Elementary school teacher. Tobacco: 25 Pack years. Alcohol: 1–2 40 oz beer every day, 1 pint gin/weekend. Caffeine: 6–8 cups caffeinated coffee/day. Drugs: Denies. Significant Other: None. Exercise: None.
Family history	Father: Deceased at 60, bilateral PE, HTN. Mother: 65 y/o ETOH abuse × 30 yrs. 10 yrs sobriety. Breast Ca: s/p rt. modified mastectomy.
CAGE questionnaire	1. Yes. 2. Yes. 3. Sometimes. 4. No.

2. *What are the key points on the review of systems?*

SYSTEM REVIEWED DATA ANSWER

SYSTEM REVIEWED	DATA ANSWER
General	Weight loss and fatigue.
Skin	Dry skin and hair.
HEENT	Frequent am H/As, frequent ear infections and colds, c/o bleeding gums, AM productive mucoid cough, denies neck stiffness or LA.
Lungs	C/o frequent bronchitis, PPD neg 7 mos ago.
Cardiac	C/o midsternal chest pain associated with meals.
GI/GU	No bowel/bladder problems. Cannot tolerate spicy or fatty foods.

● PHYSICAL ASSESSMENT

What are the significant portions of the physical examination that should be completed for Tanya? The initial quick assessment to rule out acute surgical abdomen will be indicated by **bold type.**

SYSTEM	RATIONALE	FINDINGS
Vital signs	Orthostatic blood pressure indicates volemic status. Temperature provides clues to possible infection, whereas an elevated HR indicates compensation to a change in status.	**B/P: 150/90 sitting; 142/88 standing. HR: 90** R: 20 T: 98.8 Ht: 5'4" Wt: 160 lbs
General appearance/skin	Indicates overall view of patient; helps rule out toxic appearance. Also observing for diaphoresis/cool clammy skin.	Appears pale. Skin warm and dry. Does not appear toxic.
Lungs	Provides a quick indicator of how well person is exchanging air.	CTA.
Heart	Need to evaluate to check for arrhythmias, MRG.	S_1S_2 normal. No MRG.
Abdomen	Helps provide information about abdominal status/ location of pain, and so on.	BS+, epigastric and RUQ tenderness. Liver enlarged, 16 cm MCL. No CVA tenderness. **No guarding, or tense board-like abdomen. No pulsative masses** (Burkhart, 1992).
Pelvic	Helps to r/o PID and STDs.	Vulva WNL, no erythema or d/c BUS WNL, uterus AV, normal size. No cervical motion tenderness, no adnexal tenderness.
Rectal	Helps identify melena and any masses.	Good sphincter tone, no masses, no tenderness, brown stool.

● DIFFERENTIAL DIAGNOSES

What are the significant positive and negative data that support or refute your diagnoses for Tanya?

DIAGNOSIS	POSITIVE DATA	NEGATIVE DATA
Peptic ulcer disease: Rule out perforation	Epigastric pain, history of heartburn, relieved by ant-acids, steady pain, anorexia.	No N/V, no dark tarry stools, no history of PUD.
Cholecystitis, choledo-cholithiasis	Cramping, epigastric pain, heartburn/intolerance for fatty/spicy foods, anorexia, pain in shoulder, RUQ ten-derness.	No spasmodic pain after eating.
GERD	Heartburn x 3 yrs relieved with antacids, mild epigastric tenderness.	No increase in heartburn with supine position, denies wak-ing at night with heartburn or cough.
MI	Heartburn, epigastric pain.	Denies substernal pain, N/V, diaphoresis, SOB.
AAA	Severe epigastric pain.	Female, no back pain, no hypotension/shock signs/symptoms, no abdominal bruit, no masses palpated.
IBD	Crampy pain, diffuse pain.	No hx prior attacks/ no consti-pation/diarrhea with blood or mucus, no fever.
Renal colic	Crampy severe pain.	No flank tenderness, no N/V, no hematuria, no CVA tender-ness.
PID	Severe abdominal pain and cramping.	Not sexually active, no fever, no cervical motional tender-ness, no adnexal tenderness.
Peritonitis: Perforated viscus	Severe diffuse pain in abdomen.	No fever, tense boardlike abdomen, no guarding, no N/V.
Pancreatitis	Epigastric pain, anorexia.	No boring epigastric pain, no N/V.
Hepatitis	+ ETOH history, enlarged liver, diffuse abdominal pain, RUQ pain.	No jaundice or abdominal tenderness.

● DIAGNOSTIC TESTS

Based on the history and physical assessment, what, if any, diagnostic tests would you obtain?

DIAGNOSTIC TEST	RATIONALE	RESULTS
CBC with differential	Good choice, assess blood loss, look for alteration in clotting factors as an indicator of liver disease, WBCs as indication of infection.	Hgb: 13.9. HCT: 40.0. RBCs: 4.0. WBCs: 12.5. Platelets: 200,000.
Amylase	Due to ETOH use—helpful to r/o pancreatitis, also may be elevated with acute cholecytitis.	Amylase: 200 U/dL.
Renal panel	Check kidney function. Low K+ can be assoc. with fatigue.	All WNL.
LFT	AST and ALT are liver enzymes released into the blood after liver injury. Helps identify hepatitis cause. Also helps identify bleeding disorders. Alkaline phosphatase is an indicator of obstruction to bile flow.	AST: 60. ALT: 60. Alk. Phos: 140. PT: 10.
CXR	Helps to rule out pneumonia.	WNL.
Abdominal: flat and upright	Helps to r/o obstruction/ assess bowel for free air for perforation, gas pattern, and organomegaly. HSM occurs in 25% of patients with acute cholecystitis.	WNL.
U/A	Identification of hematuria, elevated bilirubin, and possible stones (Mindelzun & McCort, 1996).	WNL.
Pregnancy test	Although patient claims not sexually active, pregnancy must be excluded in all women of childbearing age. Recommend serum pregnancy.	Negative.

(continued)

DIAGNOSTIC TEST	RATIONALE	RESULTS
Hemoccult	Identifcation of blood in stool.	Negative.
Pelvic/gallbladder ultrasound	Allows for visualization of gall-stones and possible aneur-ysm (Gill & Jenkins, 1996).	No acute disease.

● DIAGNOSES

What diagnoses do you determine as being appropriate after a review of the subjective and objective data?

Cholecystitis
Alcohol abuse
Tobacco abuse
Elevated B/P
Increased risk of breast cancer

Data Supporting the Diagnosis

Cholecystitis: episodic crampy pain, overweight, female, >40, elevated WBC

● THERAPEUTIC PLAN

1. *What would be your initial treatment for cholecystitis?*

   Minimally symptomatic patients may be managed initially with bed rest, clear liquids, and analgesics (after surgical consultation). Watchful waiting can be safely recommended to most patients with a first uncomplicated episode of biliar colic.

2. *What would be your plan for severe pain and vomiting?*

   Therapy for moderate to severe pain and vomiting includes IV fluids, nasogastric suction, and correction of any electrolyte imbalance. Antibiotics should be considered if the patient has fever or longer duration of symptoms.

3. *What test might you order at this time if not done previously?*

   A RUQ ultrasound would be helpful after the patient has NPO for 12 hours to rule out cholithiasis and obstruction.

4. *What referrals would you make for Tanya?*

   Primary care provider for HTN, cholecystitis, family violence, and tobacco abuse (assuming Tanya was seen in ED; if not, primary care provider would address above, and then refer). Mental Health counselor referral for alcohol abuse.

5. *What follow up would you do for her elevated blood pressure?*

Advise Tanya to return in 1 week for blood pressure check. At this time reduction in sodium intake would be recommended. (See elsewhere in this book for more in-depth discussion of HTN.)

6. *How would you address Tanya's alcohol dependence?*

Discuss with Tanya your concern that her intake of alcohol is excessive, and that her CAGE test indicates difficulty with controlling intake of alcohol. Determine what her feelings are on the issue of alcohol use. Recommend referral to mental health counselor and community resources. (See elsewhere in this book for substance abuse.)

7. *How in-depth would you explore the issue of family violence? What is your rationale for this decision?*

Often domestic violence is missed with professional encounters. This opportunity should be maximized because you have evidence of X-rays and substance abuse that increase Tanya's risk factors for family violence. She also admits to previous episodes of violence. Determine if her signficant other still makes contact with her, and if other partners are following the same patterns of interaction. Reassure her it is not her fault and make sure she is currently in a safe environment. Make referrals to family violence resources (see the following).

8. *What are community resources for Tanya?*

Women Helping Women (domestic violence)
Local crisis center
Local substance abuse and mental health offices
Local health departments (smoking cessation)
American Lung Association (smoking cessation)
American Cancer Association (smoking cessation)

> National Clearinghouse for Alcohol and Drug Abuse Information
> Office for Substance Abuse Prevention
> PO Box 2345
> Rockville, MD 20852
> 301 468-2600

> Drug Abuse and Alcoholism Newsletter (free)
> Vista Hill Foundation
> 3420 Camino del Rio North, Suite 100
> San Diego, CA 92108
> 619 563-1770

9. *What other health maintenance recommendations would you make for Tanya?*

Have her return for CBE; plan to review BSE when she returns; find out if she has had a mammogram.

Also recommend that she stop smoking. Tips:

Hide all ashtrays, matches, and so on.

Have on hand a supply of sugarless gum, carrot sticks, and so on.

Drink lots of liquid. Avoid coffee and alcohol.

Tell everyone you're quitting for the day.

When the urge to smoke hits, take a deep breath, hold it for 10 seconds, and release it slowly.

Exercise to relieve the tension.

Try the buddy system and ask a friend to quit too (Glynn & Manley, 1991).

10. When should Tanya return for follow up for her abdominal pain?

Tanya should return for follow up on her abdominal pain in 1 week, sooner if she experiences fever or severe pain. If she has no problems in 1 week, then follow up in 1 month, then 6 months.

11. What patient education do you need to discuss with Tanya?

Advise Tanya to avoid high fat spicy foods or anything she's noticed in the past that aggravates her stomach. A histamine antagonist might also be helpful, for example, cimetidine (400 mg QD) or famotidine (20 mg QD).

REFERENCES

American College of Emergency Physicians. Clinical policy for the initial approach to patients with a chief complaint of nontraumatic acute abdominal pain. *Ann Emerg Med* 1994; 23(4): 906–922.

Burkhart C. Guidelines for the rapid assessment of abdominal pain indicative of acute surgical abdomen. *Nurse Pract* 1992; 17(6): 43–46.

Gill B, Jenkins S. Cost effective evaluation and management of the acute abdomen. *Surg Clin N Am* 1996; 76(1): 71–82.

Glynn T, Manley M. *How to help your patients stop smoking: A National Cancer Institute manual for physicians.* Bethesda, MD: NIH; 1991.

Mindelzun R, McCort J. What radiographic views constitue acute abdominal series? *Am J Roentgen* 1996; 166(3): 716–717.

Trott A, Trunkey D, Wilson S. Acute abdominal pain: A guide to crisis management. *Patient Care* 1995; 29(13): 104–116.

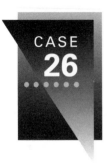

A 25-year-old-woman requesting birth control

SCENARIO

Sue Lang is a 25-year-old Caucasian female who presents today for an annual pelvic exam. She is requesting a method of birth control. Sue has used oral contraceptives (OC) in the past, and became pregnant while taking them. She does not particularly want to use OCs again.

● TENTATIVE DIAGNOSES

Based on the information provided so far, what are potential diagnoses?

● HISTORY

1. *What are significant questions in the history for Sue?*
2. *What are the key points to cover on the review of systems?*

● PHYSICAL ASSESSMENT

What are the significant portions of the physical examination that should be completed for Sue?

● DIFFERENTIAL DIAGNOSES

What are the significant positive and negative data that support or refute your diagnoses for Sue?

● DIAGNOSTIC TESTS

Based on the history and physical assessment, what, if any, diagnostic testing would you obtain? Include your rationale for the tests.

● DIAGNOSIS

What diagnoses are appropriate for Sue?

● THERAPEUTIC PLAN

1. *What are issues to consider when deciding on a contraceptive method for Sue?*
2. *What are the possible contraceptives to choose from?*
3. *What are factors that should be considered when Sue decides on a contraceptive?*
4. *What are the pros and cons of using Depo Provera as the contraceptive choice?*
5. *What are the side effects you need to discuss with Sue?*
6. *When should Sue return for follow up?*
7. *What recommendations can you make to Sue regarding her other diagnoses?*
8. *What patient education needs does Sue have at this time?*

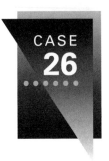

TUTORIAL

A 25-year-old woman requesting birth control

SCENARIO

Sue Lang is a 25-year-old Caucasian female who presents today for an annual pelvic exam. She is requesting a method of birth control. Sue has used oral contraceptives (OC) in the past, and became pregnant while taking them. She does not particularly want to use OCs again.

● TENTATIVE DIAGNOSES

Based on the information provided so far, what are the potential diagnoses?

DIAGNOSIS	RATIONALE
Annual pelvic exam	Well exam. When reviewing this case, keep in mind that the gynecology well exam may be the only health maintenance visit for a well female.
Family planning	Sue wants to begin birth control. Based on her past experience with OCs she will need a presentation of various types of family planning.

● HISTORY

1. What are significant questions in the history for Sue?

REQUESTED DATA **DATA ANSWER**

Allergies

Sulfa.

Current medications

Carbamazine (Tegretol) 200 mg BID, 400 mg HS.
Ibuprofen (Advil) PRN for H/A.
Vitamins.

Childhood illnesses/immuni-
zations

Chicken pox. All childhood immunizations, last measles
shot at 12 y/o.

Surgery

PE tubes, age 3.
Elective abortion, 1993.

Past medical history/hospitali-
zations/fractures/injuries/
accidents

No transfusions. Hospitalized for vaginal birth 1990, 1992,
1994: MVA, concussion. Takes Tegretol for seizures that
occurred as a result of the accident. Depression, 1994.
Resolved with counseling and no medications. Gestational diabetes during both pregnancies, controlled by
diet.

Adult illness

Has bronchitis ×1/year.

Last complete PE

1994; MVA workup.

OB/GYN history

Menarche: Age 12, periods usually last 5–6 days, cycles of
approx. 30 days, moderate flow, no cramping.
LNMP: 7/28/96 normal, skipped one cycle; anxious about
contraception.
Last pelvic: 1993.
Mammogram: never.
GPA: G3P2A1.
Contraception: Uses condoms when they think it is neces-
sary. No other contraception for 2 years.

Appetite

Small appetite, junk food. Decreased time to eat.

24-Hour diet recall

B: Coffee.
L: Mountain Dew, ham sandwich.
D: Fast food: Hamburger, fries, soda, 1 beer after.

Sleeping

5 hours per night. Usually tired.

Sexuality

Relationship with husband strained. Husband does not
mind the idea of another child. She is not interested in
having another child. This has decreased her sexual
interest.

(continued)

REQUESTED DATA	*DATA ANSWER*
Social history	Smoking: Smokes about 2 ppd × 10 yrs. Alcohol: Approximately 1 beer/day (12 oz)/6 pack/wk. Caffeinated beverages: 1 cup coffee/day, 4 sodas/day. Recreational drugs: Rare marijuana use. Exercise: Sporadic. Social organizations: None.
Family history	Mother: 45, perimenopausal, hormone therapy. Father: 46, HTN. Brother: 26, Good health, smokes. Husband: 28, well. Daughters: 6, 4, good health.
Work/finances	Both Sue and her husband are employed full-time as factory workers. Her husband works first shift at a book bindery. She works first shift at a gasket assembly. Her husband carries the insurance for the family, but no dental insurance.
Home	Lives in condominium, 30 minutes from work.
Relationship with husband/children	Argues frequently with husband about money, children, household chores, and sexual habits. Having intercourse approx. 2×/wk. Good relationship with daughters. Frustrated by trying to meet their needs and work full time.
Relationship with family	Sue's mother and siblings live approximately 250 miles away. Parents divorced when she was very young. Does not see family except at holidays. Her husband's family is located nearby, and they see them approximately 2–3×/month.
Losses in life	Concerned about loss of free time and relationship with husband. Felt similar to this when started Tegretol 3 years ago.
What do you do when you are stressed? How do you manage stress? Medications for stress?	Sometimes, all I want to do is cry and I find myself yelling at the kids. My husband does not understand. Smoke, talk on phone, have a beer. Have never taken medications for stress.
Do you ever think about hurting yourself?	No.
Do you ever think about leaving your husband?	Yes, but have never gone any farther than thinking about it.
Where do you see yourself in 10 years?	Here, alone with my children.

(continued)

REQUESTED DATA	DATA ANSWER
What are your thoughts on a birth control method?	I do not want to become pregnant. My husband does not seem to care. I don't want to use anything I may get pregnant on. I have heard good things about the shot and would consider that.

2. *What are the key points to cover on the review of systems?*

SYSTEM REVIEWED	DATA ANSWER
General	Feels healthy but tired most of the time.
Abdomen	Denies problems with constipation, diarrhea, or heartburn.
Gynecology/GU	Denies abdominal pain or tenderness. Denies vaginal discharge, odor, or itching. Denies breast tenderness or discharge. Denies pain on intercourse. Also denies symptoms of UTI.
Endocrine	Denies dysphagia, urinary frequency, thirst, poor healing of skin lesions, loss of weight.
Neurological	Denies frequent H/As, seizures, confusion or other problems.

● PHYSICAL ASSESSMENT

What are the significant portions of the physical examination that should be completed for Sue?

SYSTEM	RATIONALE	FINDINGS
Vital signs	Provides baseline information.	B/P: 130/72, P: 78, R: 22, T: 98^2
General appearance/skin	Overall view of patient.	Appears thin, and stated age. Skin pale, warm, and dry. Yellowing of skin around nail beds, unclean nails.

(continued)

SYSTEM	RATIONALE	FINDINGS
HEENT	Need to check for thyroid enlargement.	No thyromegaly.
Lungs	Baseline information, need on annual basis.	CTA.
Heart	Baseline information, need on annual basis.	S_1S_2 normal, no murmur.
Breasts	Needed as part of annual gynecological exam.	Soft, equal, no masses or nipple discharge. Bilateral fibrocystic changes. Does not do BSE.
Abdomen	Needed as part of annual gynecological exam.	BS +, soft without masses, no LA, no HSM.
Pelvic	Needed as part of annual gynecological exam.	Uterus: small AV, normal size and shape. Cervix: Parous, round, no lesions, no CMT. Discharge: WNL. Adnexa: Negative. Normal vulva, rectal deferred.
Neurological	Not a normal part of gynecological exam—would just need if concerned about depression.	Alert, moving frequently, poor eye contact. Screening neuro: strength/sensation intact, reflexes 2+.
Extremities	Baseline screening.	No edema.

● DIFFERENTIAL DIAGNOSES

What are the significant positive and negative data that support or refute your diagnoses for Sue?

DIAGNOSIS	POSITIVE DATA	NEGATIVE DATA
Family planning	Interested in contraception. Currently uses condoms, but is not confident of their protection.	None.

(continued)

DIAGNOSIS	*POSITIVE DATA*	*NEGATIVE DATA*
Altered health maintenance	Sue has not had an annual exam in 3 years. She does not do BSE. No regular exercise.	
Poor dietary habits	History revealed no breakfast, high-fat fast foods, increased caffeine intake.	
Altered family processes	History revealed that Sue's relationship with her husband is unstable, with frequent arguing, and increased stress on her part, decreased coping skills, role confusion.	No abuse, neglect, or desire to end relationship.
Depression	Frequent crying, feels stressed, depressed mood, sleep disturbance, irregular menses, decreased activity with organizations and parenting, PMH of depression.	No psychomotor retardation, denies suicidal ideation, no impaired concentration, WNL Beck Depression Scale.
Hypothyroid	Fatigue, female.	No edema, bradycardia, decreased BS, decreased appetite, hyperreflexia, hypotension, slurred speech, or hoarseness.
Anemia	Fatigue, female with irregular menses.	No bruising, hematuria, melena, HSM, murmur, no menorrhagia.

● DIAGNOSTIC TESTS

Based on the history and physical assessment, what, if any, diagnostic tests would you obtain?

DIAGNOSTIC TEST	RATIONALE	RESULTS
Pap smear	Yearly pap indicated (USPSTF, 1993). Sue has not had an exam in 3 yrs. Also needed as baseline prior to initiation of contraception.	WNL pap.
Pregnancy test	Missed one cycle. Inconsistent use of condoms. Important to know prior to beginning of new contraception method.	Negative.
Beck Self-Report Depression Scale	Good choice. Can help identify depression. Sue can complete while waiting for pelvic exam.	WNL.
Electrolytes, LFT, renal function, cholesterol	Baseline labs for general health status. Important to know prior to initiation of contraception method.	Not done, only if >30–40 for baseline.
H/H	Helpful to rule out anemia as cause of fatigue.	Not done, no complaints of heavy bleeding.
TSH	Will help discriminate a thyroid disorder as a cause of her fatigue.	No problems with amenorrhea or excessive fatigue.

● DIAGNOSES

What diagnoses are appropriate for Sue?

1. Potential for unplanned pregnancy
2. Family planning
3. Altered health maintenance
4. Poor dietary habits
5. Tobacco dependence
6. Altered family processes
7. Potential for depression

● THERAPEUTIC PLAN

1. What are issues to consider when deciding on a contraceptive method for Sue?

A. Privacy: Sue desires personal control.

B. Cost: Sue wants a reasonable contraceptive, one she could afford if she had no insurance coverage.

C. Availability: Must be able to obtain from current provider.

D. Efficacy: Desires a very reliable method.

E. Return to fertility: No desire for fertility for at least 2 years.

F. Interaction with other medications: Sue also takes Tegretol.

G. Lifestyle: Works full-time, two children, husband. Wants something that will not add stress by having to remember to take it.

H. Social habits: Smokes 2 ppd and moderate alcohol.

 I. Health care beliefs: Believes in contraception, ambivalent about abortion, feels comfortable with current provider.

J. Family issues: Role stress, turmoil in relationship with husband (Dickey, 1994).

2. What are the possible contraceptives to choose from?

TYPE	INSURANCE COVERAGE	FAILURE RATE	TEGRETOL INTER-ACTION	OFFICE USE	PRIVATE	APPROX. COST/YR
Cervical cap	Yes	18%	No	Yes	No	$50
Condom	No	12%	No	No	No	$50
Diaph-ragm	Yes	18%	No	Yes	No	$130
DMPA (Depo-Provera)	Yes	3%	No	Yes	Yes	$160
IUD	No	1–3%	No	Yes	Yes	$300
Norplant	Yes	2%	Yes	No	Yes	$600 initial fee
OC	Yes	3%	Yes	Yes	No	$300

Speroff & Darney, 1996.

3. *What are factors that should be considered when Sue decides on a contraceptive?*

When considering a method for Sue, her history, family, medications, health beliefs, insurance status, and ultimately her choice mandates the method. Sue is not interested in a barrier method. She cannot use OC or Norplant because of Tegretol use, and is uncomfortable with an IUD. Sue is interested in is Depo-Provera or DMPA. Because Sue has not been on any medication for depression, and now feels stable, this option can be considered after discussing the risks, benefits, side effects, and efficacy.

4. *What are the pros and cons of using Depo-Provera as the contraceptive choice?*

PROS	CONS
No effects with Tegretol. Although high progestin levels raise the seizure threshold, Depo-Provera does not raise the progestin level.	Return to fertility may be up to 6 months to a year.
Continuous method, given every 12 weeks.	Menstrual bleeding patterns are substantially disorganized, including vaginal spotting or bleeding, usually progressing to amenorrhea by 6 months in 50% of women.
Contains no estrogen, therefore less risk with smoking.	Needs to get injection within 5 days of next menstrual period.
Private method, not coitus dependent, does not require daily motivation/memory.	Urine pregnancy tests should be done before the initiation of the first injection.
	Hair breakage may be possible.
	A consent is usually required with each injection.

5. *What are the side effects you need to discuss with Sue?*

   A. Weight gain, ~ 2 lbs/yr, although some women experience very large weight gain, enough to want to discontinue method.
   B. Other side effects of nervousness, stomach pain or cramps, dizziness, weakness or fatigue, and decreased sex drive may occur. Many who experience these side effects report that these decrease over time.

C. If any problem is suspected, Sue should be seen at the earliest opportunity:
   1. Very heavy vaginal bleeding, or bleeding that lasts longer than 14 days.
   2. Irregular bleeding: If it becomes a problem, the bleeding can be treated with exogenous estrogen, 1.25 mg conjugated estrogen, or 2 mg estradiol, given daily for 7 days. An NSAID product can also be effective (Goldzieher, 1994).
   3. Concern about possible pregnancy.
   4. Onset or worsening of migraine or severe H/As.
   5. Decision to discontinue method.
   6. Onset of depression.

6. *When should Sue return for follow up?*

Sue will return every 12 weeks for injection of Depo-Provera. Each visit will include weight, B/P, and in some agencies a urine pregnancy test. It will be important to note and record Sue's emotional state, satisfaction with method, and bleeding patterns. The need to return regularly prior to the 13th week must be emphasized. Sue will need to know that if she returns later than the 13th week, a serum pregnancy will need to be drawn with a negative result before the injection can be given.

Sue's choice of method will affect her family. Their response should be obtained from Sue. Is she more relaxed now that she has a reliable method? Does her family respond in a positive way? Does she feel more empowered and less anxious? There are important factors to determine on the follow up visits.

7. *What recommendations can you make to Sue regarding her other diagnoses?*

Altered Health Maintenance

The annual Pap/pelvic exam should be reinforced at each of Sue's visits. At least every 3 months the provider can reinforce BSE and encourage Sue to complete the exam monthly. Sue would also benefit from regular exercise. Discussion of a variety of exercise options might be a way to entice Sue to begin. Regular exercise also makes a person feel more energetic and less fatigued (U. S. Preventative Services Task Force, 1996).

Poor Dietary Habits

Review the food pyramid with Sue to educate about a balanced diet. Encourage Sue to incorporate more fruits, vegetables, and fiber into her diet. It might be helpful to stress the importance of a balanced diet for her children as a reason to make lifestyle changes. Suggest that she involve the whole family in planning the menu and sharing the responsibility of food preparation.

Tobacco Dependence

It will be important to determine if Sue is interested in smoking cessation. If not, continue to ask her about it at each visit. Consider it one of the "vital signs" to obtain each time. This may not be the best time to consider smoking cessation because she identified it as a stress reliever for her. Let her know that you are available to discuss the specifics of smoking cessation when she is ready.

Components of a three-step procedure for advising smokers consists of the following (Barker, Burton, and Zieve, 1995):

Personalize and provide instructions.
Promote confidence.
Contract for specific behavior.
(Negotiating a specific quit date is very important also.)

Available materials to assist Sue can be obtained from the American Heart Association and the National Cancer Institute's *Quit for Good* Kit.

Altered Family Processes

It might be appropriate at this point to discuss the option of counseling for Sue and her husband. If he is not interested, at least the counselor could assist Sue in developing better coping skills, and assist her in better communication in the relationship. Consider mentioning to Sue the effectiveness of having family meetings to better negotiate family activites and responsiblities. Even the children can contribute to the work of the household.

Documentation of Sue's emotional state is important. Suggestions for improving her communication skills include:

A. Role playing situations that frequently occur at home (ie, who is responsible for meal preparation and cleanup, getting children ready for bed, helping with homework, or initiating intimacy, etc.).
B. Encouraging interaction with family or neighbors.

Potential for Depression

Most communities have resources that could be of help to Sue and her family. These resources are discussed in-depth in another chapter. Make sure that you at least provide Sue with crisis line phone numbers in case she needs assistance quickly. Sue may need referral to a psychologist/psychiatrist for further workup of her symptoms of depression.

  8. *What patient education needs does Sue have at this time?*

It is important that advance counseling be done prior to initiation of the method. Successful use depends on Sue being fully informed of the mechanism of action, mode of administration, effectiveness, adverse effects, and costs, as well as the pros and cons of the method. Other patient education points are discussed earlier under each diagnosis. Sue should be aware that other resources in the community related to family planning exist in the event her insurance ends, or she needs other options.

REFERENCES

Barker L, Burton J, Zieve P. *Principles of Ambulatory Medicine*, 4th ed. Baltimore: Williams & Wilkins; 1995.

Dickey R. *Managing Contraceptive Pill Patients*, 8th ed. Durant, OK: Essential Medical Information Systems, Inc.; 1994.

Goldzieher J. *Hormonal Contraception*, 3rd ed. Vancouver, BC: Essential Medical Information Systems, Inc.; 1994.

Speroff L, Darney P. *A Clinical Guide for Contraception*, 2nd ed. Baltimore: Williams & Wilkins; 1996.

U.S. Preventative Services Task Force. *Guide to clinical preventative services. Report of the U.S. Preventative Services Task Force.* Baltimore: Williams & Wilkins; 1996.

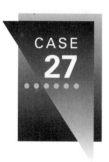

A 20-year-old woman with burning during urination

SCENARIO:

Marie is a 20-year-old Caucasian female. She presents with complaints of frequency, urgency, and burning on urination. She has been in good health since her last physical exam 6 months ago. She lives with her boyfriend and works as a dancer in a local ballet company. She was fitted for a diaphragm and instructed in the use of a diaphragm and spermicide as a birth control method during her last exam. She chose a diaphragm and spermicide over other methods of birth control in order to avoid any hormonally induced weight gain from the other methods.

● TENTATIVE DIAGNOSES

Based on the information provided so far, what are potential diagnoses?

● HISTORY

1. *What are significant questions in the history for a woman with dysuria?*
2. *What are the key points to cover on the review of systems?*

● PHYSICAL ASSESSMENT

What are the significant portions of the physical examination that should be completed for Marie?

● DIFFERENTIAL DIAGNOSES

What are the significant positive and negative data that support or refute your diagnoses for Marie?

● DIAGNOSTIC TESTS

Based on the history and physical assessment, what, if any, diagnostic testing would you do for Marie. Include your rationale for the testing.

● DIAGNOSES

What diagnoses are appropriate for Marie?

● THERAPEUTIC PLAN

1. *How can urinary tract infections be classified?*
2. *Why are these classifications important when developing a therapeutic plan?*
3. *What type of urinary tract infection does Marie have?*
4. *What criteria should be considered when developing a therapeutic plan for Marie?*
5. *What pharmacotherapy choices would you make for Marie?*
6. *What is the rationale for a 3-day treatment plan?*
7. *What can Marie do to prevent future urinary tract infections?*
8. *What therapeutic options are available for young women with recurrent urinary tract infections following intercourse?*

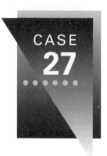

TUTORIAL

A 20-year-old woman with burning during urination

SCENARIO

Marie is a 20-year-old Caucasian female. She presents with complaints of frequency, urgency, and burning on urination. She has been in good health since her last physical exam 6 months ago. She lives with her boyfriend and works as a dancer in a local ballet company. She was fitted for a diaphragm and instructed in use of diaphragm and spermicide as a birth control method during her last exam. She chose a diaphragm and spermicide over other methods of birth control in order to avoid any hormonally induced weight gain from the other methods.

● TENTATIVE DIAGNOSES

Based on the information provided so far, what are the potential diagnoses?

DIAGNOSIS	RATIONALE
Urinary tract infection	Dysuria and frequent, urgent urination are classical symptoms of urinary tract infection.
Vulvovaginitis	It may be difficult for a patient to differentiate between dysuria and vulvar burning during urination (DeCherney and Pernoll, 1994).
Herpes infection	Urethritis and vulvitis owing to herpes infection both produce vulvar burning on urination (DeCherney and Pernoll, 1994).

● HISTORY

1. What are significant questions in the history for a woman with dysuria?

REQUESTED DATA	DATA ANSWER
Allergies	No food, drug, or insect allergies.
Current medication	Multivitamin daily and occasional NSAIDS.
Surgery	None.
Past medical history and hospitalizations	No adult illness; had chickenpox as child. All immunizations up to date. Minor auto accident 2 years ago, spent night for observation only. Last physical exam, normal, two years ago. Last GYN exam, normal, 1 month ago.
Social history	Works as a dancer in a local ballet company. Nonsmoker. Occasional social use of alcohol. No history of recreational drug use. Junior in college.
OB/GYN	LMP 2 weeks ago. G0P0A0. Last PAP smear WNL 1 month ago.
Sexuality	Heterosexual, has been with current boyfriend for 1 year, have been living together for 6 months, sexually active since 16 years old, 2 lifetime partners, uses condoms, no sexually transmitted infections. Denies sexual abuse.
Family history	Single but involved in a significant relationship. Both parents alive and well. Maternal Grandmother: 68 y/o, mild stroke 1990. Maternal Grandfather: 72 y/o, MI 1988. Paternal Grandfather: 75 y/o, prostate cancer. Paternal Grandmother: 74 y/o, HTN. Two siblings: Alive and well.

2. *What are the key points to cover on the review of systems?*

SYSTEM REVIEWED	DATA ANSWER
General	No fever, chills, or malaise. Generally feels good other than frequent urination that is beginning to interfere with activities.
Gastrointestinal	No nausea or vomiting. No weight gain or loss. Intermittent lower abdominal mild ache. No decrease in appetite.
Genital/urinary	C/o dysuria, frequency and urgency. No dyspareunia, discharge, blood in urine or odor. No history of urinary tract infections.
Genitalia	Recent gynecological exam, no complaints of vaginal discharge, odor, or itching.

● PHYSICAL ASSESSMENT

What are the significant portions of the physical examination that should be completed for Marie?

SYSTEM	FINDINGS
Vital signs	B/P: 106/58 P: 68 R: 16 T: 98.8
General appearance	Alert, oriented, well-developed, muscular 20-year-old Caucasian woman in no acute distress.
Abdomen	Flat, active bowel sounds in all four quadrants, generalized tympany to percussion, no organomegaly, mild suprapubic tenderness to palpation, no CVA tenderness. No masses or tenderness; active bowel sounds.
Genitalia	Deferred at present, recent GYN exam within normal limits.

● DIFFERENTIAL DIAGNOSES

What are the significant positive and negative data that support or refute your diagnoses for Marie?

DIAGNOSIS	POSITIVE DATA	NEGATIVE DATA
Lower urinary tract infection: urethritis or cystitis	Dysuria associated with frequency and urgency.	
Upper urinary tract infection: pyelonephritis	Dysuria.	No CVA tenderness, no chills, fever, or malaise (Stamm & Hooton, 1993).
Vulvovaginitis	Recent normal GYN Exam.	No change in sexual practice or partner. No complaints of vaginal discharge or itching.

● DIAGNOSTIC TESTS

Based on the history and physical assessment, what, if any, diagnostic tests would you obtain?

DIAGNOSTIC TEST	RATIONALE	RESULTS
Urine leukocyte esterase	Reflects the presence of white blood cells in the urine.	Positive.
Urine nitrite	Urinary nitrate is reduced in the presence of bacteria to nitrite.	Positive.
Urine protein		Negative.
Urine culture	The amount of bacteria and the species of the causative bacteria can be isolated. Especially useful for persistent infections.	*E. coli* 10^5 organisms/mL (not known at office visit; results returned 72 hours later).
Imaging	Uncomplicated UTIs that respond to treatment do not require imaging.	Not done.

● DIAGNOSES

What diagnoses are appropriate for Marie?

Lower urinary tract infection

Data Supporting the Diagnosis

1. Presents with the classical symptoms of dysuria, frequency, and urgency.
2. Recent history of use of diaphragm and spermicide.
3. Urine dipstick positive for leukocytes and nitrite.
4. Physical findings:
    Recent normal GYN exam
    Mild suprapubic tenderness.

● THERAPEUTIC PLAN

1. How can urinary tract infections be classified?

Urinary tract infections have been classified and categorized in many different fashions. One method of classification involves an anatomical categorization based on the urinary tract itself. This classification divides the urinary tract and subsequently urinary tract infections into two groups. The first group is lower urinary tract infections. This group consists of urethritis, cystitis, and prostatitis. The second group involves the kidneys and is therefore referred to as upper urinary tract infections. Examples of upper urinary tract infections are acute pyelonephritis and intrarenal or perinephric abscess (Stamm, 1994).

Although the anatomical classifications are obviously valid, another classification scheme was developed to help guide therapeutic decisions. In this classification there are three categories. They are acute uncomplicated urinary tract infections, acute uncomplicated bacterial pyelonephritis, and complicated urinary tract infections (Neu, 1992).

Acute uncomplicated urinary tract infections are infections that usually occur in women between the ages of 18–65 who present with the classic triad of symptoms (dysuria, frequency, and urgency). In order to be considered uncomplicated they must also have a temperature of less than 101°F and have no predisposing functional, metabolic, or anatomic factors (Williams, 1996).

Complicated urinary tract infections are infections that occur in patients (male and female) that may present with the classic symptoms but are also febrile (a temperature greater than 101°F) and may have other symptoms such as flank pain and tenderness of the costovertebral angle (CVA). Urinary tract infections are also considered complicated if they occur in association with metabolic factors such as an underlying disease such as diabetes, or functional and anatomic factors such as stones or obstruction (Williams, 1996).

Urinary tract infections in men are always considered complicated infections. These infections usually occur because of a partial obstruction from prostatic enlargement or as a result of genitourinary instrumentation. Another risk factor for men is being sexually active. Sexually active men may develop a urinary tract infection from anal sex or intercourse with an infected partner. These cases should have at least 7 days of treatment and the source of the infections should be considered when choosing the pharmacotherapy because they may involve pathogens other than the usual causative agent (Stamm & Hooton, 1993).

2. Why are these classifications important when developing a therapeutic plan?

An uncomplicated urinary tract infection is considered a superficial or mucosal infection. When developing a treatment plan for this type of infection, a high-dose, short-course treatment can be effective. In other words, a brief period with a high urinary concentrations should be sufficient to eradicate a superficial mucosal infection (Elder, 1992).

A complicated urinary tract infection involves a patient with a functionally, anatomically, or metabolically abnormal urinary tract. A complicated urinary tract infection can also be caused by a resistant organism. Patients who fall into this classification require longer treatment (7–10 days or more) and may require parenteral treatment (Stamm & Hooton, 1993).

3. What type of urinary tract infection does Marie have?

This is Marie's first urinary tract infection. She has no metabolic, functional, or anatomic abnormality. She is afebrile and does not appear acutely ill. Marie has an uncomplicated urinary tract infection (Hooton et al., 1996).

4. What criteria should be considered when developing a therapeutic plan for Marie?

An antibacterial agent should be chosen that fulfills specific criteria. These criteria include:

1. The causative organism must be sensitive to the antibacterial agent.
2. The agent must be capable of eradicating the organism from the vagina.
3. The agent must be capable of producing inhibitory drug concentrations in the urine.
4. The dosage should be convenient enough to enable compliance.
5. The cost of the agent should be taken into consideration (Wisinger, 1996).

5. *What pharmacotherapy choues whould you make for Marie?*

After considering these criteria, the agents of choice would be:

DRUG	DOSE	LENGTH OF TREATMENT
Trimethoprim-sulfamethoxazole (TMP-SMZ)	160/800 mg (1 double strength tablet) BID	3 days.
Nitrofurantoin macrocrystals (Macrodantin)	100 mg QID	3 days.
Nitrofurantoin macrocrystals (Macrobid)	100 mg BID	3 days.
Cefadroxil (Duricef)	500 mg BID	3 days.
Amoxicillin	500 mg TID	3 days.
Ciprofloxacin (Cipro)	250 mg BID	3 days.

Ewald & McKenzie, 1995.

Of these agents the TMP-SMZ was the most effective cost-efficient agent (approximately $0.40/day). The ciprofloxacin was also extremely effective but more expensive ($5.42/day), therefore it is usually reserved for patients that are allergic to or intolerant of the TMP-SMZ (Williams, 1996) (Grubbs et al., 1992).

6. *What is the rationale for a 3-day treatment plan?*

A 3-day treatment for uncomplicated lower urinary tract infections is effective due to the nature of the infection. In sexually active women who use diaphragms and spermacides, the vaginal environment is altered (changes vaginal pH and natural flora) in a manner that facilitates the growth of bacteria. Furthermore, the act of intercourse provides a mechanism for the migration of bacteria from the periurethral area to the bladder (Williams, 1996). The resulting infection is mucosal in nature.

The 3-day treatment with TMP-SMZ was shown to reduce *E. coli* carriage rates in the rectum, urethra, and vagina. If the symptoms persist for 2 weeks or a relapse occurs within 2 weeks, then Hooton (1995) recommends a 2-week treatment based on the results of the urine culture.

7. *What can Marie do to prevent future urinary tract infections?*

- Wipe from front to back: Although Denman and Murphy (1995) indicate that there is little evidence to support a specific wiping direction, it is known that *E. coli* is a normal fecal flora and the major causative organism of UTIs. The Mayo Clinic Health Letter (June, 1992) advocates wiping from front to back as a mechanism of keeping infectious bacteria from coming in contact with the urethra.
- Frequently empty bladder: Retaining urine after the urge to urinate may increase the risk of infection (Williams, 1996).
- Void after intercourse: Voiding after intercourse flushes bacteria that may have migrated up the urethra during intercourse. Failure of voiding soon after intercourse may facilitate the attachment of the bacteria to the urethral mucosa (Williams, 1996).
- Remove diaphragm: Remove diaphragm as soon as possible after intercourse (as soon as recommended by gynecologist in order to maintain birth control efficacy) and void after removal to enable efficient bladder emptying (Uphold & Graham, 1994).
- Drink plenty of liquids: Six to eight glasses of fluids a day can dilute your urine and help avoid urine stagnation (Mayo Clinic Health Letter, 1992).
- Drink cranberry juice: Cranberry and blueberry juice are frequently discussed as a prophylactic measure against urinary tract infections. They both have antibacterial properties and cranberry juice may acidify the urine. Theoretically the mechanisms of action are the antibacterial effect by which the urine is acidified and uropathogenic adhesion to the epithelial cells of the urinary tract is decreased (Hatton, Hughes, and Raymond, 1994). There has been a randomized, placebo-controlled trial documenting the effectiveness of cranberry juice. Although the results were not statistically significant, there was a trend in favor of a preventative effect (Hooton, 1995).

8. *What therapeutic options are available for young women with recurrent urinary tract infections following intercourse?*

Low-dose antibiotics for several months may be used for prophylaxis of UTI in young women with recurrent UTI's after sexual intercourse. This treatment is thought to reduce the bacterial attachment to the mucosal lining rather than inhibition of microbial growth (Hatton, Hughes, and Raymond, 1994).

Another option is postcoital prophylaxis. Studies have found postcoital treatment as effective as low-dose continuous treatment and, depending on sexual activity, may be less expensive (Hatton, Hughes, and Raymond, 1994). Cephalexin 250 mg, Cinoxacin 250 mg, Nitrofurantoin 50–100 mg, or TMP/SMX $\frac{1}{2}$–1 SS tablet are recommended for postcoital prophylaxis.

REFERENCES

Denman SJ. Murphy PA. Genitourinary infections, In Barker LR, Burton JR, Zieve PD (eds). *Principles of Ambulatory Medicine*. Baltimore: Williams & Wilkins; 1995; 319–324.

DeCherney AH, Pernoll ML (eds). *Current Obstetric & Gynecologic Diagnosis & Treatment*, 8th ed. Norwalk, CT: Appleton & Lange; 1994.

Elder NC. Acute urinary tract infection in women. *Postgrad Med* 1992; 92(6): 159–166.

Ewald GA, McKenzie CR (eds). *Manual of Medical Therapeutics*, 28th ed. Boston: Little, Brown; 1995.

Grubbs NC, Schultz HJ, Henry NK, Ilstrup DM, Muller SM, Wilson WR. Ciprofloxacin versus trimethoprim-sulfamethoxazole: Treatment of community-acquired urinary tract infections in a prospective, controlled, double-blind comparison. *Mayo Clin Proc* 1992; 67: 1163–1168.

Hatton J, Hughes M, Raymond CH. Management of bacterial urinary tract infections in adults. *Ann Pharmacother* 1994; 28: 1264–1272.

Hooton TM. A simplified approach to urinary tract infection. *Hosp Pract* 1995; 30(2): 23–30.

Hooton T, Scholes D, Hughes JP, Winter C, Roberts PL, Stapleton AE, et al. A prospective study of risk factors for symptomatic urinary tract infection in young women. *N Engl J Med* 1996; 335: 468–474.

Mayo clinic health letter. *Copy Ed* 1992; 10: 1–3.

Neu HC. Urinary tract infections. *Am J Med* 1992; 92: 4A-63S–4A-69S.

Stamm WE. Urinary tract infections and pyelonephritis, in Isselbacher KI, Braunwald E, Wilson J (eds). *Harrison's Principles of Internal Medicine*. New York: McGraw-Hill; 1994; 548–554.

Stamm WE, Hooton TM. Management of urinary tract infections in adults. *N Engl J Med* 1993; 329: 1328–1334.

Uphold CR, Graham MV. *Clinical Guidelines in Family Practice*, 2nd ed. Gainesville, FL: Barmarrae; 1994.

Williams DN. Urinary tract infection: Emerging insights into appropriate management. *Postgrad Med* 1996; 99(4): 189–201.

Wisinger D. Urinary tract infection: Current management strategies. *Postgrad Med* 1996; 100: 299–237.

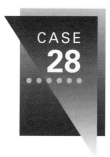

A 5 year-old-girl presents for a kindergarten physical

SCENARIO

Callie Johnson is a 5-year-old African-American female who presents to your office for a 5-year physical. She is 5 years, 2 months old. Her mother wants to determine if she is ready for kindergarten in the fall.

● TENTATIVE DIAGNOSES

Based on the information provided so far, what are potential diagnoses?

● HISTORY

1. *What are significant questions in Callie's history?*
2. *What are the key points on the review of systems?*
3. *What questions do you need to review with Callie's mother in terms of her development?*

● PHYSICAL ASSESSMENT

What are the significant portions of the physical examination that should be completed for Callie? What developmental assessment should be included in the exam?

● DIFFERENTIAL DIAGNOSES

What are the significant positive and negative data that support or refute your diagnoses for Callie?

● DIAGNOSTIC TESTS

Based on the history and physical assessment, what, if any, diagnostic tests would you obtain? Include your rationale for the tests.

● DIAGNOSIS

What diagnoses are being appropriate for Callie?

● THERAPEUTIC PLAN

1. *What immunizations does Callie need today?*
2. *What recommendations would you make for Callie's readiness for kinder-garten?*
3. *What anticipatory guidance issues would you discuss with Callie's mother?*
4. *What treatment options do you have for pinworms?*
5. *What recommendations will you share with Callie and her mother to pre-vent the occurrence of pinworms in the future?*
6. *How will the diagnosis of pinworms affect the rest of the family?*
7. *Does Callie need follow up for the pinworms?*
8. *When should Callie return for another well exam?*

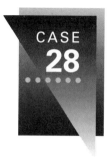

TUTORIAL

A 5-year-old girl presents for a kindergarten physical

SCENARIO:

Callie is a 5-year-old African-American female who presents to your office for a 5-year physical. She is 5 years, 2 months old. Her mother wants to determine if she is ready for kindergarten in the fall.

● TENTATIVE DIAGNOSES

Based on the information provided so far, what are the potential diagnoses?

DIAGNOSIS	RATIONALE
Not applicable at this time	Well visit. When reviewing this case, keep in mind that the school physical exam may be the only health maintenance visit for a school age child.

● HISTORY

1. What are significant questions in Callie's history?

REQUESTED DATA	DATA ANSWER
Allergies	NKA.
Current medications	None.

(continued)

REQUESTED DATA	*DATA ANSWER*
Birth history	Planned pregnancy. Had complete prenatal care, including amniocentesis. Born full-term, induced vaginal delivery. Mother had mildly elevated B/P shortly before delivery. $21\frac{1}{2}$ inches tall and 9 lbs. $5\frac{1}{2}$ oz. at birth. Content newborn, happy temperament.
Childhood illnesses	Chicken pox. Strep throat 2×/season.
Immunizations	Up to date: completed Hep B series, 4 DTP, 4 Hib, 3 OPV, 1 MMR.
Surgery	PE tubes inserted 5/92.
Past medical history and hospitalizations/fractures/injuries/accidents	Multiple otitis media episodes, with mild hearing loss noted. PE tubes inserted, no subsequent episodes.
Last complete PE	Last well child PE at age 4.
Appetite	Good. Mother notes she snacks very frequently.
Diet/24-Hour diet recall	No special diet. B: Dry cereal with water. L: Eats at day care, ex: pizza, applesauce, milk. D: Chili, salad, milk, fruit, dessert. S: Popsicle.
Sleeping	Sleeps approximately 12 hours per night, no naps.
Social history	Active child, inventive imagination.
Family history	Father: 40, arthritis, back problems, smokes $1\frac{1}{2}$ ppd. Mother: 42, HTN. PGF and MGF died at age 51 with MI. MGM, 63 HTN, PGM, 66, living and well.

2. *What are the key points on the review of systems?*

SYSTEM REVIEWED	*DATA ANSWER*
General	Mother feels Callie is doing well, no problems, no concerns.
HEENT	No problems. Callie has not lost any teeth yet. None appear to be loose. She brushes her teeth morning and before bed. Callie has gone to the dentist 2–3×, and uses fluoride toothpaste.

(continued)

SYSTEM REVIEWED DATA ANSWER

SYSTEM REVIEWED	DATA ANSWER
Respiratory	Able to do activities she wants, runs and plays with no difficulty. Denies SOB or cough.
Elimination	Had recent bout of fever with N/V, diarrhea. Resolved on its own. No problems with constipation, diarrhea, or dark stools. Complains of rectal itching in past week or so. Urination qs. No problems with bedwetting or incontinence.

3. *What questions do you need to review with Callie's mother in terms of her development?*

DEVELOPMENTAL AREA MOTHER'S REPORT

DEVELOPMENTAL AREA	MOTHER'S REPORT
Speech	No difficulties. No lisps. Very large vocabulary. Asks mother about what different words mean.
Emotional development	Callie seems very competent to manage daily routine. She picks out her clothes each day and seems to like the interaction of daycare.
Intellectual development	Enjoys learning; can count to 110, can even add some numbers. Enjoys puzzles, drawing, using markers. Sings songs, able to remember words to songs with little difficulty.
Work/home responsibilities	Has own responsibilities to take care of: feed fish, keep room clean, and set/clear table. Usually will do tasks with little argument. Gets along well with mother and father.
Social development	Has many friends. Plays with other girls in daycare. Has neighbor boy (7 y/o) with whom she plays occasionally. Seems to have difficulty agreeing on play activities with him.

● PHYSICAL ASSESSMENT

What are the significant portions of the physical examination that should be completed for Callie?

SYSTEM	RATIONALE	FINDINGS
Vital signs		B/P: 92/64 P: 92 R: 18 T: 97.8°F Ht. 48″ Wt. 43 lbs
General appearance/skin		Alert, interactive, playing. Body appears proportionate with appropriate muscle development. Good eye-to-eye contact. Participates in answering questions. Skin: no excessive bruises or burns. Has some bruises noted on anterior surface of legs.
HEENT		Equal tracking of eyes. WNL cover/uncover test. Ears: TMs with scarring, no erythema. Teeth in good repair. None missing. Throat with erythema. No exudate. Neck supple.
Lungs		CTA.
Heart		$S_1 S_2$ WNL, no murmurs.
Breasts		Appropriate for age. Extra nipple in MCL on Rt.
Abdomen		BS+, soft, no tenderness.
Genitalia		No erythema, irritation, discharge. Rectal area excoriated. No worms visualized.
Neurological/ musculoskeletal		Strength appropriate for age. Negative for scoliosis.

What developmental assessment should be included in the exam?

DEVELOPMENTAL AREA	FINDINGS
Coordination	Able to hop, skip, jump; able to walk on tiptoe. Can do duck walk; heel and toe walk. Able to balance on one foot × 5 sec.
Fine motor skills	Able to draw triangle, circle, square. Able to complete a stick figure drawing of man, including clothing.
Language development	Able to define nine words. Understands meanings of opposites. Able to identify words that rhyme. Able to recite alphabet.
Safety	Knows telephone number and address.

● DIFFERENTIAL DIAGNOSES

What are the significant positive and negative data that support or refute your diagnoses for Callie?

DIAGNOSIS	POSITIVE DATA	NEGATIVE DATA
Well-child exam	Appropriate growth and development. Attainment of developmental milestones.	None.
Pinworms	C/o rectal itching, excoriated rectal area, +daycare.	No pinworms vizualized.

● DIAGNOSTIC TESTS

Based on the history and physical examination, what, if any, diagnostic tests would you obtain?

DIAGNOSTIC TEST	RATIONALE	RESULTS
Visual acuity	Provides baseline to determine if further evaluation is needed.	OS 20/30 OD 20/30
Hearing screen	Provide indication if further workup is needed.	L/R 10dB: 500, 1000, 2000, 4000 Hz.
Tympanogram	Indicates functioning of TM and presence of middle ear effusion. Not invasive, relatively inexpensive test. Can be done in office.	Not done because hearing WNL, and no complaints of ear problems.
PPD	Required on admission to school.	0 mm reaction read 48 hours later.
Hemoglobin	Recommended once annually.	Hgb: 14.2.
U/A	Recommended once between 3–6 years.	U/A WNL.
Tape test	Test permits visualization of ova under microscope.	Ova visible.

● DIAGNOSES

What diagnoses are appropriate for Callie?

    Well 5-year-old exam
    Pinworms

● THERAPEUTIC PLAN

   1. What immunizations does Callie need today?

    DtaP (acellular is recommended)
    OPV
    MMR (recomended)

2. *What recommendations would you make for Callie's readiness for kinder-garten?*

Callie appears ready for school. She does not have any gross or fine motor dysfunction. Her language, speech, and behavior appear age appropriate (Shapiro, 1993).

Callie is currently attending day care, so she is able to spend time away from home. She interacts with adults other than her parents. She is able to accept behavior control expectations. In addition, she has sufficient self-esteem to carry on independent activity (Stephens, 1994).

3. *What anticipatory guidance issues would you discuss with Callie's mother?*

A. Injury prevention
   1. Discuss with mom the area of most likely injuries:
      a. Burns, falls, need to use car seatbelts, toxic substance ingestion, safety around mowers and tools (guns should be kept locked up). Supervision needed when playing around streets. Need to review stranger safety practices. Callie should know address, phone number, 911.
      b. Reminder about bike safety and wearing of bike helmet all the time.
B. Good parenting practices/discipline:
   1. Use of time out for behavior modification.
   2. Discourage use of corporal punishment.
   3. Ability of child to assume some responsiblities around home.
   4. Ability to begin simple money management with allowance.
   5. Encourage parents to interact, and act as role models for reading and decreased TV watching/set TV limits.
C. Sleep:
   1. Reinforce a regular bedtime for Callie.
   2. Napping is dependent on behavior.
D. Dental health:
   1. Encourage brushing at least two times a day. May begin using floss at this time.
   2. Encourage twice yearly preventive exams.

4. *What treatment options do you have for pinworms?*

The recommended treatment for pinworms is Mebendazole (Vermox) 100 mg, 1 chewable tablet, now and repeated in 2 weeks. Sitz baths may be helpful for rectal irritation. Desitin may be helpful for rectal excoriation (Dershewitz, 1993).

5. *What recommendations will you share with Callie and her mother to prevent the occurrence of pinworms in the future?*

   Callie should bathe daily. She should wash her hands after toileting and before eating. She should wear tight underpants during the treatment phase. She should change her underpants in the morning and at bedtime. She should have her bedding changed nightly. Reoccurrences are common (Boyton, Dunn, and Stephens, 1994).

6. *How will the diagnosis of pinworms affect the rest of the family?*

   The rest of the family may need to be treated simultaneously with Vermox. Handwashing will need to be emphasized since communicability is high. Towels, linens, and clothing will need to be washed in hot water.

7. *Does Callie need follow up for the pinworms?*

   Not generally indicated. If symptoms are not gone in 3 weeks, will need to call or return to the office.

8. *When should Callie return for another well exam?*

   Callie should return for a 6-year well visit.

REFERENCES

Boyton R, Dunn E, Stephens G. *Manual of Ambulatory Pediatrics*, 3rd ed. Philadelphia: Lippincott; 1994.

Dershewitz R. *Ambulatory Pediatric Care*, 2nd ed. Philadelphia: Lippincott; 1993.

Recommended childhood immunization schedule, US, July-December 1996, Advisory Committee on Immunization Practices, American Academy of Pediatrics, and American Academy of Family Practice Physicians.

Shapiro B. School readiness, in Dershewitz R (ed). *Ambulatory Pediatric Care*, 2nd ed. Philadelphia: Lippincott; 1993.

Stephens G. Well child care, in Boyton R, Dunn E, Stephens G (eds). *Manual of Ambulatory Pediatrics*, 3rd ed. Philadelphia: Lippincott; 1994.

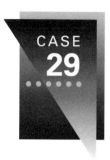

A 67-year-old man with a painful rash in the perineal area

SCENARIO

Gerald Fox is a 67-year-old African-American male complaining of a painful red rash in the perineal area. He states that he has had it for approximately 3 weeks. He has been applying hydrocortisone but has obtained little relief. He denies having intense itching and says it just hurts.

● TENTATIVE DIAGNOSES

Based on the information provided so far, what are potential diagnoses?

● HISTORY

What are significant questions in Gerald's history?

● PHYSICAL ASSESSMENT

What are the significant portions of the physical examination that should be completed for Gerald?

● DIFFERENTIAL DIAGNOSES

What are the significant positive and negative data that support or refute your diagnoses for Gerald?

● DIAGNOSTIC TESTS

Based on the history and physical assessment, what, if any, diagnostic tests would you obtain? Include your rationale for the tests.

● DIAGNOSIS

What diagnoses are appropriate for Gerald?

● THERAPEUTIC PLAN

1. *What treatment would you prescribe for Gerald?*
2. *What other instructions would you give Gerald?*
3. *How long can Gerald expect to have the itching and inflammation?*
4. *When should Gerald return for follow up?*

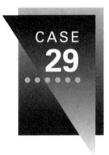

29

TUTORIAL

A 67-year-old man with a painful rash in the perineal area

SCENARIO

Gerald Fox is a 67-year-old African-American male complaining of a painful red raised rash in the perineal area. He states that he has had it for approximately 3 weeks. He has been applying hydrocortisone but has obtained little relief. He denies having intense itching and says it just hurts.

● TENTATIVE DIAGNOSES

Based on the information provided so far, what are the potential diagnoses?

DIAGNOSIS	RATIONALE
Contact dermatitis	Gerald c/o red rash.
Condylomata acuminata	Papules present in genitalia.
Psoriasis	Red raised rash in perineal area.
Scabies	Red raised rash in perineal area.
Herpes simplex	Painful rash in perineal area.

● HISTORY

1. What are significant questions in Gerald's history?

REQUESTED DATA	DATA ANSWER
Allergies	NKDA.
Current medications	Fosinopril (Monopril) 10 mg QD for HTN. Hydrocortisone for itching applied to genital area.
Surgery	Cholecystectomy 20 years ago, no transfusions.
Past medical history and hospitalizations/fractures/injuries/accidents	Healthy except for HTN (18 yrs).
Describe more detail about your rash: anyone else in family have a similar rash, relationship to anything else, new clothing, soap, medications, systemic symptoms.	Noticed red bumps in perineal area. Denies intense itching or discomfort initially. Noticed in gluteal fold first, then becoming increasingly red and painful. Denies any relationship to season, medications, or travel. No new clothes, soap, or medication. Denies any systemic symptoms such as fever, H/A, weakness, or weight loss. No one else in family has a rash. Just he and his wife are home, but frequently has grandchildren visit.
Sexuality	Monogamous relationship.
Social history	Tobacco: Smoked but quit 30 years ago. Alcohol: Social only, approx. 6 beers week. Drugs: Denies. Caffeine: Drinks about three cups coffee/day. Exercise: No regular.
Family history	Father: Died age 75, CHF. Mother: Died age 58, DM. Siblings: Two brothers, 72, 70, both have HTN. Wife: Age 60, healthy. Children: One daughter, 35, healthy. One son, 33, healthy.

2. *What are the key points on the review of systems?*

SYSTEM REVIEWED	DATA ANSWER
Skin	Rash only in perineal area—no rash noticed anywhere else.
Lungs	No problems with breathing.
Cardiac	Denies chest pain, pressure, numbness of arm.
GI/GU	Denies difficulty with urination or dysuria. C/o pain with BMs due to irritated buttocks. BM soft, brown QD.

● PHYSICAL ASSESSMENT

What are the significant portions of the physical examination that should be completed for Gerald?

SYSTEM	RATIONALE	FINDINGS
Vital signs	Provide baseline data.	B/P: 134/88 P: 88 R: 20 T: 99 Ht. 5'11" Wt. 178
General appearance	Provides overall indication of Gerald's status.	Sitting very still on table due to pain.
Lungs	Given his HTN history, should do a quick screen of chest.	CTA.
Heart	Given his HTN history, should do a quick screen of heart.	RRR. No MRG.
Perineal area	Need to evaluate the skin lesions.	Papular, vesicular rash of perineal area. Scattered, discrete multiple, crusted papules between gluteal fold with erythema/swelling. No burrows noted. Several papules noted on penis with crusting.

(continued)

SYSTEM	RATIONALE	FINDINGS
Skin	Whenever there is a dermatological problem, need to evaluate all skin surfaces, using a light source.	Rare papules found on stomach and Rt. upper arm. Hair and nails unaffected, mucous membranes intact, no lesions.

● DIFFERENTIAL DIAGNOSES

What are the significant positive and negative data that support or refute your diagnoses for Gerald?

DIAGNOSIS	POSITIVE DATA	NEGATIVE DATA
Contact dermatitis	Papular rash only involving perineal area.	Denies any change in routine— no new soaps, clothes, or medications.
Condylomata acuminata	Rash in genital area.	Painful rash, monogamous relationship, partner does not have them, no "raspberry"-like lesions.
Herpes simplex	Painful rash in genital area.	No painful ulcers in genital area, monogamous relationship, partner does not have lesions.
Psoriasis	Rash in perineal area.	No annular "salmon pink" rash. No plaques with sharply marginated borders/scales. No involvement of extensor surfaces.
Scabies	Papular/vesicular involvement of penis, perineal area.	Denies intense itching, no rash in partner, monogamous relationship, no burrows.

● DIAGNOSTIC TESTS

Based on the history and physical examination, what, if any, diagnostic tests would you obtain?

DIAGNOSTIC TEST	RATIONALE	RESULTS
Microscopic analysis	Provides diagnostic confirmation of scabies if burrow is found with resulting mites, eggs, or fecal pellets visible.	Scraping of papule revealed no confirmation of scabies.

● DIAGNOSES

What diagnoses are appropriate for Gerald?

Presumptive scabies

Data Supporting the Diagnosis

Papules and vesicles in perineal area. Papules and vesicles on penis are almost considered pathognomonic for diagnosis, once all others are ruled out (Fitzpatrick et al., 1997).

● THERAPEUTIC PLAN

1. *What treatment would you prescribe for Gerald?*

   Permethrin cream (Elimite) 5% applied to all areas of the body from the neck down to and including the soles of the feet. Particular attention should be paid to the fingernails. The cream should be left on for 8–12 hours and then showered off. One treatment is usually sufficient; however, the cream should be applied again in 1 week since scabicides are not ovicidal, so a repeat application is needed to kill newly hatched larvae (Boynton et al., 1994).

   Since Gerald is not complaining of intense itching, an antipruritic will not be ordered. Continued use of the hydrocortisone cream after treatment may help decrease the inflammatory response in the gluteal folds.

2. *What other instructions would you give Gerald?*

   Bedding and clothing should be decontaminated (machine washed or dried using heat or dry cleaned) or removed from body contact for at least 72 hours. Mites can remain alive for over 2 days on bedding and clothing, so direct skin-to-skin contact does not have to occur. Close or personal household contacts within the last month should be examined and treated (Fitzpatrick et al., 1997).

3. *How long can Gerald expect to have the itching and inflammation?*

Generalized itching may persist for a week or more after the treatment. This is caused by a hypersensitivity reaction to the remaining dead mites and mite products.

4. *When should Gerald return for follow up?*

No follow up is needed unless there is persistent pruritus after 2 weeks. Gerald should then return for a visit to repeat scraping of the lesion to determine the presence of mites.

REFERENCES

Boynton R, Dunn E, Stephens G. *Manual of Ambulatory Pediatrics*, 3rd ed. Philadelphia: Lippincott; 1994.

Fitzpatrick T, Johnson R, Wolff K, Polano M, Suurmond D. *Color Atlas and Synopsis of Clinical Dermatology*, 3rd ed. New York: McGraw-Hill; 1997.

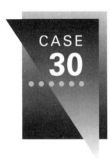

A 26-year-old woman with eye pain and tearing

SCENARIO

A 26-year-old African-American female, Jennifer, presents to the primary care clinic complaining of a foreign body sensation, increased lacrimation, mild photophobia, and pain to her right eye (OD) for 3–4 hours. She gives a history of a small fragment of a nutshell being propelled into her OD while cracking pecans at home with a hand-held nutcracker.

● TENTATIVE DIAGNOSES

Based on the information provided so far, what are the potential diagnoses?

● HISTORY

What are significant questions in the history of a person complaining of eye pain and lacrimation?

● PHYSICAL ASSESSMENT

What are the significant portions of the physical examination that should be completed for Jennifer?

● DIFFERENTIAL DIAGNOSES

What are the significant positive and negative data that support or refute your diagnoses for Jennifer?

● DIAGNOSTIC TESTS

Based on the history and physical assessment, what, if any, diagnostic tests would you obtain? Include your rationale for the tests.

● DIAGNOSIS

What diagnoses are appropriate for Jennifer?

● THERAPEUTIC PLAN

1. *What are elements of pain control for Jennifer related to the corneal abrasion?*

2. *How do you prevent a secondary infection for a patient with a corneal abrasion?*

3. *What is the current rationale for patching or not patching a person with a corneal abrasion?*

4. *What is a critical factor to know prior to patching a person's eye?*

5. *What is the current thinking regarding tetanus prophylaxis for corneal abrasions?*

6. *What are points that should be discussed in patient education and prevention?*

7. *When should Jennifer receive follow up for her corneal abrasion?*

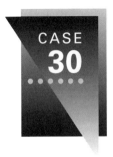

CASE
30

TUTORIAL

A 26-year-old woman with eye pain and tearing

SCENARIO

A 26-year-old African-American female, Jennifer, presents to the primary care clinic complaining of a foreign body sensation, increased lacrimation, mild photophobia, and pain to her right eye (OD) for 3–4 hours. She gives a history of a small fragment of a nutshell being propelled into her OD while cracking pecans at home with a hand-held nutcracker.

● TENTATIVE DIAGNOSES

Based on the information provided so far, what are the potential diagnoses?

DIAGNOSIS	RATIONALE
Traumatic corneal abrasion OD	Jennifer presents with eye pain, photophobia, and FB sensation after a traumatic injury to her OD. Corneal abrasions are commonly an outcome of a particulate FB to the eye (Kenyou & Wagoner, 1991).
Ocular FB OD	Jennifer c/o eye pain after a small particulate object was propelled into her OD. A small piece of the nutshell may be embedded in her cornea or trapped under the tarsal surfaces.
Acute traumatic iritis OD	Acute traumatic iritis may be seen after a blow to the eye. The patient presents with photophobia and eye pain.
Acute conjunctivitis OD	Jennifer presents with increased lacrimation.
Acute keratitis OD	Herpes simplex keratitis and herpes zoster keratitis can both present with pain and photophobia to the eye.

(continued)

DIAGNOSIS	*RATIONALE*
Penetrating injury to OD	Always consider a penetrating eye injury when any FB is projected into the eye (Kenyou & Wagoner, 1991).
Corneal abrasion to OD secondary to contact lens wear	Corneal abrasion secondary to contact lens wear can present with pain, photophobia, and FB sensation.

● HISTORY

1. *What are significant questions in the history of a person complaining of eye pain and lacrimation?*

REQUESTED DATA	*DATA ANSWER*
Exact mechanism of injury: A tangential blow from a human fingernail or from plant material usually causes a superficial corneal abrasion, but it has the potential for bacterial or fungal infection (Torok and Mader, 1996). Projectiles such as metal fragments and wood chips have the potential to cause penetrating wounds of the cornea, globe, and surrounding structures (Asbury and Sanitato, 1992).	Jennifer was cracking pecans with a simple hand-held spring type nutcracker and a small piece of a nutshell flew into her OD. The injury occurred approximately 3–4 hours ago.
Does the patient wear contact lens or any other type of corrective lens?	She does not wear contact lens or any other type of corrective lens.
Allergies	NKDA, no history of environmental allergies (to determine if symptoms are associated with an allergic conjunctivitis).
Current medications	Lo Ovral 28.
Immunizations (tetanus)	Last Td 3 1/2 years ago.
Past medical history and hospitalizations/fractures/injuries/accidents	Appendectomy at age 10.

(continued)

REQUESTED DATA	DATA ANSWER
Last eye exam	Approximately 4 years ago. No complaints of visual problems.
OB/GYN history	LNMP: 3 weeks ago. Contraception: Lo Ovral 28.
Family history	No family history of eye problems.

● PHYSICAL ASSESSMENT

What are the significant portions of the physical examination that should be completed for Jennifer?

SYSTEM	RATIONALE	FINDINGS
Vital signs	Provides baseline information, and screening of other problems.	B/P: 110/76 P: 72 R: 18 T: 98.2 Ht: 5' 7" Wt: 142 lbs
General appearance/skin	The general assessment gives a general idea about the status of the patient.	African-American female, in pain, holding hand over OD.
Visual acuity	Always check the VA first in assessing any ocular injury. If the patient wears corrective lens, but the lens are not available, check a pinhole VA. VA through a pinhole will assist in determining if VA changes are owing to trauma or a correctable astigmatism.	OD 20/25 OS 20/20 OU 20/20 without corrective lens.
External eye exam	After VA, the external structures should be thoroughly examined for evidence of trauma or FB.	Palpebral and bulbar conjunctiva mildly injected OD, + lacrimation, but no drainage noted from eyes. No hyphema, no subconjunctival hemorrhage. PERRLA, lids

(continued)

SYSTEM	RATIONALE	FINDINGS
		everted, no FB present below tarsal surfaces. Conjunctival cul-de-sac clear. No ciliary flush.
Cornea	The entire cornea and limbic structures need to be examined after any type of eye trauma to r/o abrasion, FB, or penetrating injury.	Fluorescein staining and examination with Woods lamp reveals a 1–2 mm superficial corneal abrasion at 7 o'clock on the periphery of the right cornea.

● DIFFERENTIAL DIAGNOSES

What are the significant positive and negative data that support or refute your diagnoses for Jennifer?

DIAGNOSIS	POSITIVE DATA	NEGATIVE DATA
Traumatic corneal abrasion OD	Eye pain OD, FB sensation, mild photophobia, + corneal abrasion with fluorescein stain. No FB present with exam. Normal VA, no ciliary flush.	Mild photophobia, FB sensation.
Ocular FB OD	+ FB sensation; mechanism of injury consistent with FB to cornea/eye; OD pain.	No FB seen with exam, lids everted and no FB trapped under tarsals.
Acute traumatic iritis OD	+OD pain; mechanism of injury mildly suggestive of traumatic iritis, +mild photophobia.	No VA changes, no ciliary flush present, + corneal abrasion with fluorescein stain.
Acute conjunctivitis OD	Injected palpebral and bulbar conjunctiva.	+Pain OD, mild photophobia, + corneal abrasion with stain, mild lacrimation, no mucosal or purulent d/c from OD.
Corneal abrasions to OD secondary to contact lens wear	None.	Jennifer does not wear contact lenses.
Penetrating injury to OD	Mechanism of injury might possible suggest penetrating ocular injury.	Mild eye pain, no visual changes, PERRLA, no FB present with exam or stain-

(continued)

DIAGNOSIS	POSITIVE DATA	NEGATIVE DATA
		ing, no change in iris or pupil noted.
Acute keratitis OD	None.	No evidence of herpes zoster or herpes simplex.

● DIAGNOSTIC TESTS

Based on the history and physical assessment, what, if any, diagnostic tests would you obtain?

DIAGNOSTIC TEST	RATIONALE	RESULTS
Slit lamp of external eye structures	If a slit lamp is available, it may be used for a more detailed exam of the external ocular structures. Unfortunately, this piece of equipment is not available in most primary care settings.	Not obtained; equipment not available.
Measurement of intra-ocular pressure (IOP) of OD	If acute iritis or acute glaucoma is suspected, the IOP should be measured. A Schiotz tonometer or a tonopen are commonly used to measure IOP in primary care settings.	Not obtained and not indicated.

● DIAGNOSES

What diagnoses are appropriate for Jennifer?

Corneal abrasion OD

Data Supporting the Diagnosis

FB sensation with pain and lacrimation are hallmark symptoms of a corneal abrasion. Exam reveals an injected conjunctiva, no FB, and a + corneal abrasion with fluorescein staining to OD (Poole, 1995).

● THERAPEUTIC PLAN

1. What are elements of pain control for Jennifer related to the corneal abrasion?

A. A local ophthalmic anesthetic such as ophthaine or ophthetic should only be used at the time of the exam to facilitate assessment of the eye. Never use topical anesthetics for prolonged control of eye pain since they may retard healing, mask pain, and aggravate keratitis (Torok and Mader, 1996).

B. Oral analgesics such as NSAIDS are usually effective for pain control of superficial corneal abrasions.

C. A short acting cycloplegic/mydriatic may be used to relieve pain caused by ciliary spasm that often occurs after corneal abrasion. Examples of short acting mydriatics/cycloplegics include Mydriacyl and Cyclogyl.

2. How do you prevent a secondary infection for a patient with a corneal abrasion?

Secondary infection can be prevented by installation of a topical ophthalmic antibiotic such as Erythromycin Ophthalmic, Sodium Sulamyd Ophthalmic, or Neosporin Ophthalmic ointments.

3. What is the current rationale for patching or not patching a person's eye with a corneal abrasion?

Recent studies have indicated that patching eyes after corneal abrasion does not affect pain (Patterson et al., 1996), shows no real increased healing rate (Hulbert, 1991; Kirkpatrick et al., 1993), and may decrease oxygen levels and increase corneal temperature that may lead to actual decreased corneal healing (Kirkpatrick et al., 1993).

Traditionally, eye patching for 24 hours with ophthalmic antibiotic ointment has been the treatment of choice for corneal abrasions not associated with contact lens wear. In light of recent findings, it is acceptable to treat small, noncentral corneal abrasions with topical antibiotics, cycloplegia, and no eye patch with follow up in 24 hours (Torok and Mader, 1996). Consider patching the eye with larger, central corneal defects.

4. What is a critical factor to know prior to patching a person's eye?

It is imperative to know whether a person wears contact lenses. Corneal abrasions that occur as a result of contact lens wear are susceptible to sight threatening *Pseudomonas* infections (Jampel, 1995). Therefore, a corneal injury associated with contact lens should be referred to an ophthalmologist for evaluation and management.

5. What is the current thinking regarding tetanus prophylaxis for corneal abrasions?

Tetanus prophylaxis is indicated following perforating eye injuries and eye injuries with signs of infection, devitalized tissue, and contaminants such as feces, soil, dirt, and saliva (Benson et al., 1993). Therefore, simple superficial corneal abrasions are not tetanus-prone wounds.

6. *What are points that should be discussed with Jennifer in terms of patient education and prevention?*

   A. If an eye is patched, caution the patient about alteration in depth perception. A patient with one eye patched should not drive, operate machinery, or work in an elevated setting.
   B. Inform patients that simple corneal abrasions usually heal within 24 hours, and it is expected to have some pain during this time. Take pain medication as directed and discuss potential side effects.
   C. Caution Jennifer to rest her eyes as much as possible. She should avoid eye straining activities such as computer work, reading, and so on. Even if the eye is patched, the affected eye will move in unison with the unaffected eye during any activities.
   D. Prevention is the best way to avoid eye injuries. Safety glasses with side shields should be worn while engaging in home and occupational activities in which FB may enter the eye.

7. *When should Jennifer receive follow up for her corneal abrasion?*

   Jennifer should seek follow up in 24 hours. All patients with a corneal abrasion should be rechecked in 24 hours. Most patients who are rechecked in 24 hours after a corneal abrasion will exhibit marked improvement or healed abrasions. If symptoms persist or are worse, Jennifer should be referred to an ophthalmologist for immediate evaluation.

REFERENCES

Asbury T, Sanitato J. Trauma, In Vaughn D, Asbury T, Riordan-Eva P (eds). *General Ophthalmology,* 13th ed. Norwalk, CT: Appleton and Lange; 1992; 363–370.

Benson W, Synder I, Granus V, Odom J, Macsai M. Tetanus prophylaxis following ocular injuries. *J Emerg Med* 1993; 11: 677–683.

Hulbert M. Efficacy of eye pad in corneal healing after corneal foreign body removal. *Lancet* 1991; 337: 643.

Jampel H. Patching for corneal abrasions. *JAMA* 1995; 274(19): 1504.

Kenyon K, Wagoner M. Conjunctival and corneal injuries, in Shingleton B, Hersch B, Kenyon K (eds). *Eye Trauma.* St. Louis: Mosby; 1991; 63–78.

Kirkpatrick J, Hoh H, Cook S. No eye pad for corneal abrasion. *Eye* 1993; 7: 468–471.

Patterson J, Fetzer D, Krall J, Wright E, Heller M. Eye patch treatment for the pain of corneal abrasion. *S Med J* 1996; 89(2): 227–229.

Poole S. Corneal abrasion in infants. *Pediatr Emerg Care* 1995; 11(1): 25–26.

Torok P, Mader T. Corneal abrasions: Diagnosis and management. *Am Fam Phys* 1996; 53(8): 2521–2529.

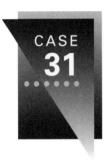

A 32-year-old woman
with a lump under her arm

SCENARIO

Grace Madison is a 32-year-old single Chinese-American female who presents with a nontender lump under her left arm. She detected this lump 2 weeks ago during a routine self breast exam. She also describes fatigue, scratchy throat, low-grade fever, and "occasional sweaty episodes that wake me up at night." She is interested in resuming the birth control pill. She has a 10-year history of oral contraceptives (OC), but discontinued the pill 1 year ago. "I thought I should give my body a rest." Her last gynecologic exam was 2 years ago. She had been sexually inactive for about 1 year until 4 weeks ago. She did not use a contraceptive but would like to resume OC.

Grace is employed by an international computer company with the majority of her travels in Singapore. Her latest trip was 4 weeks ago. She works approximately 14 hours a day.

● TENTATIVE DIAGNOSES

Based on Grace's presentation, what are your tentative differential diagnoses?

● HISTORY

What questions do you want to ask Grace to help develop a diagnosis?

● PHYSICAL ASSESSMENT

Based on subjective data, what parts of the physical exam should be performed and why?

● DIFFERENTIAL DIAGNOSES

Examine all the available data up to this point. Link the subjective and objective data to the appropriate differential diagnosis. Identify positive and negative data that support/refute the diagnosis.

DIAGNOSTIC TESTS

What additional data and/or diagnostic tests need to be performed to confirm the priority diagnosis?

DIAGNOSIS

After linking subjective, objective, and diagnostic data, what is your diagnosis?

● THERAPEUTIC PLAN

1. *How will you inform Grace of the diagnosis?*
2. *How can you develop a rapport with Grace and build a trusting relationship?*
3. *What is the current prognostic indicator for staging HIV?*
4. *When should Grace return for follow up?*
5. *What are the current therapies that should be considered for Grace?*
6. *What counseling and education will Grace need?*
7. *What issues will confront Grace and her family?*
8. *Identify information resources that might be helpful to Grace and her family.*
9. *What additional measures will you initiate to maintain health and prevent disease?*
10. *What gynecologic and family planning needs should you address with Grace?*

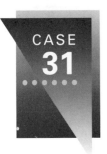

TUTORIAL

A 32-year-old woman with a lump under her arm

SCENARIO

Grace Madison is a 32-year-old single Chinese-American female who presents with a nontender lump under her left arm. She detected this lump 2 weeks ago during a routine self breast exam. She also describes fatigue, scratchy throat, low-grade fever, and "occasional sweaty episodes that wake me up at night." She is interested in resuming the birth control pill. She has a 10-year history of oral contraceptives (OC), but discontinued the pill 1 year ago. "I thought I should give my body a rest." Her last gynecologic exam was 2 years ago. She had been sexually inactive for about 1 year until 4 weeks ago. She did not use a contraceptive but would like to resume OC.

Grace is employed by an international computer company with the majority of her travels in Singapore. Her latest trip was 4 weeks ago. She works approximately 14 hours a day.

● TENTATIVE DIAGNOSES

Based on Grace's presentation, what are your tentative differential diagnoses?

Based on the brief presenting history, the nurse practitioner should have several different diagnoses in mind.

DIFFERENTIAL DIAGNOSIS	RATIONALE
Infectious mononucleosis	Grace complains of pharyngitis, fatigue, low-grade fever, and adenopathy. These symptoms may be related to exposure to Epstein-Barr virus, the viral agent responsible for infectious mononucleosis.

(continued)

DIFFERENTIAL DIAGNOSIS	*RATIONALE*
Tuberculosis (TB)	Night sweats, fatigue. Foreign travel may be seen with TB.
Breast cancer	Axillary node enlargement detected by BSE 2 weeks ago. 90% of breast masses are identified by the individual woman.
Hepatitis	Low grade fever, fatigue, foreign travel, and unprotected intercourse are all symptoms associated with hepatitis. Incubation period: 15–50 days: Hepatitis A virus (HAV) 45–160 days: Hepatitis B virus (HBV) 45–180 days: Hepatitis C virus (HCV)
Human immunodeficiency virus (HIV)	Unprotected intercourse, fatigue, night sweats, adenopathy, and travel to foreign regions with a high prevalence of HIV. Heterosexual transmission is the leading cause of HIV transmission to women worldwide.
Chronic fatigue syndrome	Night sweats, fatigue, adenopathy, pharyngitis are symptoms of chronic fatigue syndrome.

● HISTORY

What questions do you want to ask Grace to help develop a diagnosis?

REQUESTED DATA	*DATA ANSWER*
Allergies	Seasonal.
Medications	Over-the-counter allergy medications.
Childhood diseases	Chicken pox.
Immunizations	Last PPD was in 1994 = zero. All other immunizations up to date.
Surgery	None.
Transfusions	None.
Hospitalizations	None.
Fractures/injuries/accidents	None.
Adult illnesses	None.

(continued)

REQUESTED DATA | DATA ANSWER

REQUESTED DATA	DATA ANSWER
Medication history	Acyclovir; last used 1 year ago for genital herpes.
OB/GYN history	Menarche: Age 13. G 0 P 0 A 0. LNMP 1/15/97, menses every 32 days, duration 4–6 days. Last pap/pelvic December 1994, WNL.
Contraceptive history	Oral contraceptives used from 1985–1994. Discontinued 1 year ago. Condoms used occasionally.
Sexually transmitted infections	No prior history of gonorrhea, chlamydia, pelvic inflammatory disease, syphilis, or condylomata. Genital herpes diagnosed 1990. Outbreaks occurred one to two times yearly until 3 months ago. Presently every 4–6 weeks.
Sexual history	Heterosexual. "My last sexual partner was someone I met during a business trip. We did not use a condom or any contraception; I need to get back on the pill." No current partner.
Last complete PE	December 1994.
Weight changes	Stable.
24-Hour diet recall	Breakfast: Coffee, juice. Lunch: Salads, tuna, tea. Dinner: Chicken, baked potato, water/soda.
Sleeping pattern	Sleeps approximately 5–6 hours per night. Has awakened with night sweats two to three times in past month.
Family	Father: Age 54, hypertensive on medication. Mother: Age 52, healthy. Sister: Age 24, healthy.

Social habits
  Smoking:
  Alcohol:
  Other drugs:
  Caffeine:
  Exercise:
	
	No
	Wine: $\frac{1}{2}$ glass per night
	No
	10-12 cups per day
	No

Social groups	Recent relocation from Florida to Ohio. No established friendships yet.
Family relationships	Parents live in Florida. Phone three to four times per month. Sister in graduate school. Close family relationships.
Health care coverage	Full medical and dental coverage.
Home	Two-bedroom apartment close to work.

(continued)

REQUESTED DATA   DATA ANSWER

| Length of symptoms | "I've been tired for several weeks. I'm not sure if this is a result of my endless work demands and recent move, but this has gone on long enough." |
| What are the patient's primary concerns? | "There is no breast cancer in my family, but I am concerned about this lump under my arm. I need to get back on the pill and maybe vitamins will help my loss of energy. My doctor in Florida said my herpes outbreaks could increase under stress; I think he was right." |

● PHYSICAL ASSESSMENT

Based on subjective data, what parts of the physical exam should be performed and why?

SYSTEM	RATIONALE	FINDINGS
Vital signs	Baseline information.	HR: 68 RR: 18 B/P: 110/60 Temp. 98.4°F Ht: 5'6" Wt: 132 lbs
Skin color and character	Dermatologic changes may be important indicators of systemic disease.	Trunk: Erythematous, nonpruritic, maculopapular rash. No jaundice or bruises. Nail beds: within normal limits.
HEENT	Fundiscopic exam will determine changes related to cytomegalovirus associated with HIV. Oral cavity lesions of thrush, hairy leukoplakia, or aphthous ulcers are associated with HIV as is lymphadenopathy.	Fundoscopic exam: No AV nicking Disc well-marginated No plaques Tympanic membranes gray with light reflex present. Pharynx clear. Mucus membranes intact. Good dentition, no candida or mouth lesions. Frontal and maxillary sinuses—not tender.

(continued)

SYSTEM	RATIONALE	FINDINGS
		Bilateral posterior multiple cervical nodes enlarged, 1–2 cm. Thyroid within normal limits.
Thorax and lungs	Adventitious sounds and transmitted voice sounds may support diagnosis of TB or pneumocystitis pneumonia.	Inspection and percussion within normal limits. Clear to auscultation.
Heart sounds	Baseline data.	S_1 S_2 without murmur.
Breasts	Breast lump was chief complaint of Grace.	Left axillary node: 3 cm, discrete, nontender, mobile. Right axillae, infraclavicular, supraclavicular nodes: negative. Fibrocystic breast changes bilaterally. No nipple discharge, retraction, erosion, or erythema.
Abdomen	Hepatomegaly and splenomegaly are associated with both hepatitis and HIV.	Enlarged spleen 2 cm below left costal margin. Liver: No enlargement. Bowel sounds present and within normal limits. Inguinal node enlargement bilaterally, discrete, 2 cm.
Pelvic	Grace has not had a pelvic exam for 2 years. A gynecologic exam should be performed in association with resumption of OCs, and concern of possible STD.	Vulva: No lesions. Vagina: Mucus membranes within normal limits. Cervix: No cervical motion tenderness, no discharge. Uterus: Anteverted, mobile. Not tender, not enlarged. Adnexa: No masses or tenderness. Rectal: No masses noted.

● DIFFERENTIAL DIAGNOSES

Examine all the available data up to this point. Link the subjective and objective data to the appropriate differential diagnosis. Identify positive and negative data that support/refute the diagnosis.

DIAGNOSIS	POSITIVE DATA	NEGATIVE DATA
Infectious mononucleosis	"Scratchy throat," fatigue, night sweats.	Common in college age adults and children. Patient denies headache and CNS complications. No palatal rash. 95% of adults will have abnormal liver function.
Tuberculosis	Foreign travel, night sweats, fatigue, last PPD 2 years ago.	Stable weight, clear lungs, no cough.
Breast cancer	Early menarche, no prior pregnancies. 90% of patients with breast cancer have no familial breast cancer history. Presenting complaint for 70% of patients diagnosed with breast cancer is a breast lump.	First-degree relatives negative for breast cancer. No previous surgical breast biopsy procedure.
Hepatitis	History of unprotected intercourse, fatigue, night sweats.	No jaundice, dark urine, nausea. Stable weight, liver within normal limits.
HIV infection	History of unprotected intercourse, traveled to and lived in high endemic areas, fatigue, night sweats, adenopathy in greater than two noncontiguous areas, diffuse macular rash, increased frequency of genital herpes episodes, enlarged spleen, no prior HIV screen.	Negative drug history. Clear lungs and no history of pulmonary symptoms. Negative history of vaginal candidiasis and GI changes. Stable weight. Oral cavity exam is negative, i.e., no oral hairy leukoplakia or aphthous ulcers.
Chronic fatigue syndrome	Fatigue, night sweats, adenopathy.	No confusion.

● DIAGNOSTIC TESTS

What additional data and/or diagnostic tests need to be performed to confirm the priority diagnosis?

DIAGNOSTIC TEST	RATIONALE	FINDINGS
Monospot	90% of adults cases are iden-tified through monospot. If patient presents early in the disease course, monospot may be negative. Therefore, repeat the monospot in 7-10 days if still symptomatic. Consider collecting a throat culture for a rapid strepto-coccus test. If negative, collect a throat culture. 3–30% of mononucleosis cases will be positive for streptococcal infection.	Negative.
CBC with differential	In addition to hgb/hct, the leu-kocyte counts will provide important data about immu-nologic response to in-fection.	Hgb: 11.9 g/dL. Hct: 35.0%. WBC: 4,000/mm^3 Segs: 76%. Lymphs: 20%. Monos: 3%. Eosin: 2 %.
Chemistry panel	Baseline value for patients with questionable hepatitis, multisysytem complications, and potential future poly-pharmacy.	Lytes: WNL. AST: 30 U/L. ALT: 35 U/L.
Hepatitis profile	Serologic markers for acute hepatitis: IgM anti-HAV; HBSAG; IgM anti-HBc; Anti-HCV.	All tests negative.
PPD	Mantoux test to be read in 48 hours. Positive PPD is read according to induration not erythema. Criteria for Posi-tive Tuberculin Skin Test. ≥5 mm induration if patient is one of the following: is HIV$^+$;	0 mm.

(continued)

DIAGNOSTIC TEST　　RATIONALE　　　FINDINGS

| | has abnormal chest film; has S/S of TB; ≥10 mm; travels to high-prevalence countries; is foreign born, lives in long-term residential living, including prisons; intravenous drug user; has medical risk factors; employed in health care settings; ≥15 mm all other exposures.

If PPD is positive, sputum culture for mycobacterium tuberculosis is essential to confirm diagnosis; posterior–anterior chest film is needed to assess extent of bronchial involvement. | |

| ELISA/Western blot | Test results are reported as positive, negative, or indeterminant. A positive test requires both a positive ELISA as a screening test and a positive Western blot as confirmation. The most common cause of indeterminant results is a positive ELISA and a single band (usually p24) on a Western blot. This may reflect seroconversion in process, so the test should be repeated in 2–6 months. It is recommended that those who have positive results with no likely risk factors have repeated tests as well as those with negative results who continue to engage in risk behaviors. | Elisa: Positive.
Western blot: Indeterminate. |

| CD_4 CD_8 HIV RNA | Provides specific data related to HIV infection. | Elisa +, WB indeterminate.
CD 4 480/mm^3.
CD 8 750/mm^3.
HIV RNA >10^6/dL or 1,000,000/dL indicative of acute retroviral infection. Need to repeat in |

(continued)

DIAGNOSTIC TEST	RATIONALE	FINDINGS
		2–6 months. Would expect the below results at that time: Elisa +, WB +, CD 4 increased, HIV RNA decreased.
RPR or VDRL	Along with HIV screen, it is important to evaluate syphilis status. Grace presents with a rash that may represent second stage syphilis. Genital ulcer disease is highly correlated to the incidence of HIV.	RPR: Nonreactive.
Pap smear	Abnormal pap smears such as LSIL, HSIL, or cervical cacinoma are suggestive of HIV infection, particularly in young women at risk.	ASCUS: Abnormal cells of un-determined significance.
Gonorrhea and chlamy-dia cultures	Baseline information for sex-ually active unprotected women.	GC: Negative. Chlamydia: Negative.
Wet mount	If vaginal candidiasis is sus-pected, hyphae will be seen by microscopic exam. Candidiasis infections are common occurrences in HIV-infected women (Bardeguez & Johnson, 1994).	Negative.

● DIAGNOSIS

After linking subjective, objective, and diagnostic data, what is your diagnosis?

The correct diagnosis is acute retroviral HIV infection based on several laboratory tests. First, the Elisa is positive and Western blot indeterminate. This is a common laboratory response following acute HIV exposure. Second, positive HIV status is confirmed by a quantitative HIV RNA $>10^5/dL$ or 100,000/dL. This high value is indicative of acute viral replication and will sharply reduce as the patient moves into the seroconversion phase of HIV infection in 6–12 weeks after exposure. The quantitative viral load will begin to steadily increase with disease progression. Third, CD4 cell counts will demonstrate a transient drop during the acute viral syndrome phase, return to relatively normal values ($800–1050/mm^3$) and then decline markedly as disease continues. Early treatment with antiretrovirals and protease inhibitors can significantly alter these laboratory events. Clinical features of infectious mononu-cleosis-like illness with fever, adenopathy, hepatosplenomegaly, sore throat, myalgias, diffuse macular rash, mucocutaneous ulceration, diarrhea, leukope-nia with atypical lymphocytes are seen in 50–90% of patients during the acute viral syndrome phase. This patient is properly classified as Stage A2 HIV in-fection with a CD4 = 480 and HIV RNA >10^6/dL (Carpenter et al., 1996).

1993 Revised Classification System for HIV Infection and Expanded AIDS Surveillance Case Definition for Adolescents and Adults

CD4 + T-cell categories	CLINICAL CATEGORIES		
	(A) Asymptomatic, acute (primary) HIV, or PGL	(B) Symptomatic, not (A) or (C) condi-tions	(C) AIDS indicator conditions*
(1) > 500	A1	B1	C1
(2) 200–499	A2	B2	C2
<200 AIDS-indicator, T-cell count	A3	B3	C3

Shaded cells indicate AIDS; CDC, 1992.

AIDS Indicator Conditions

- HIV + persons with CD4 cell counts <200 or a CD4% <14%
- Candidiasis of bronchi, trachea, or lungs
- Candidiasis of esophageal
- Cervical cancer, invasive
- Coccidioidomycosis, disseminated or extrapulmonary
- Cryptococcosis, extrapulmonary
- Cryptosporidiosis, chronic intestinal (>1 month duration)
- Cytomegalovirus disease (other than liver, spleen, or nodes)
- Cytomegalovirus retinitis (with loss of vision)
- Encephalopathy, HIV-related
- Herpes simplex: chronic ulcer(s) (>1 month duration); or bronchitis, pneumonitis, or esophagitis
- Histoplasmosis, disseminated or extrapulmonary
- Isosporiasis, chronic intestinal (>1 month duration)
- Kaposi's sarcoma
- Burkitt's lymphoma (or equivalent term)
- Lymphoma, immunoblastic (or equivalent term)
- Lymphoma, primary, of brain

- *Mycobacterium avium* complex or *M. Kansasii* (disseminated or extrapulmonary)
- *Mycobacterium* tuberculosis, any site (pulmonary or extrapulmonary)
- *Mycobacterium,* other species or unidentified species, disseminated or extrapulmonary
- *Pneumocystis carinii* pneumonia
- Pneumonia, recurrent
- Progressive multifocal leukoencephalopathy
- Salmonella septicemia, recurrent
- Toxoplasmosis of brain
- Wasting syndrome owing to HIV

● THERAPEUTIC PLAN

1. *How will you inform Grace of the diagnosis?*

   The confirmation of HIV diagnosis is a traumatic experience for the patient. It is impossible to anticipate a patient's response, particularly if the patient does not suspect the possibility of this diagnosis. Until rapport is established between the patient and the nurse practitioner, it is not likely that patients will freely and honestly divulge their deep personal fears or ask revealing questions. Therefore, it is imperative that the nurse practitioner appreciate the intense impact on a patient who learns of a positive HIV diagnosis, possibly from a stranger with whom trust and rapport have yet to be established. When informing a patient of their positive status, very little information will be processed or integrated by the patient following confirmation of status. It is essential to have written information available that defines HIV infection, modes of transmission, and means of prevention. This should be short and succinct. Information that is essential for the present are names and phone numbers of health team members and a 24-hour emergency phone number. There can be a range of responses from depressive symptoms to suicide ideation or gestures. Not only do these feelings of overwhelming crisis occur with HIV diagnosis, but also may coincide with disease progression.

2. *How can you develop a rapport with Grace and build a trusting relationship?*

   We recognize that patients with long-term, life-threatening illnesses, as in HIV infection or AIDS, have unique needs in the patient/provider relationship. These needs include not only the diagnosis, medical, and psychological treatment of the patient, but extend ultimately to the lives of close family members, friends, and support systems. The establishment of a health care team is pivotal. This team not only works on behalf of the patient, but also for the individuals comprising the team. Health care team members have their own stressors associated with caring for the chronically ill and/or dying. This stress can be brought on by questions of competency, fear of exposure, emotional exhaustion derived from the deaths of previous patients, and ongoing confrontation with issues of morality and ethics. The practice of effective verbal and nonverbal communication among providers and between the patient and the provider are paramount in caring for the HIV-infected individual or family (Minkoff et al., 1995).

3. What is the current prognostic indicator for staging HIV?

Clinical guidelines for initiating antiretroviral therapy and maintaining therapy are changing rapidly. In light of recent publications, it is essential that the nurse practitioner work closely with a medical team well versed in recent advances in disease kinetics, more precise viral load assays, new FDA drugs, and the value of combination therapy versus monotherapy in all disease stages. The CD4, a subset of lymphocytes, has been the primary guide to staging HIV disease and thus the primary prognostic indicator. The CD4 value represents the immune response to increased viral production. Plasma HIV RNA determinations are rapidly becoming an important marker of disease progression. Additionally, HIV RNA copies per dL. are valuable under the following circumstances: 1) initiating antiretroviral therapy; 2) evaluating the effectiveness of therapy; or 3) determining treatment failure. CD4 and HIV RNA are independent predictors of clinical outcome; their combined use provides a more complete picture of the patient's status and response to treatment (Saag et al., 1996).

4. When should Grace return for follow up?

Grace will need an explanation of when medication will begin and on what basis that decision will be made. She needs reassurance of what is being monitored, why that information is needed, and the frequency of monitoring. The initiation of antiretroviral therapy will be a decision between the medical team and the patient. Grace will have scheduled visits every three to six months to include: CBC, CD4, HIV RNA, pelvic exam with pap smear, and appropriate immunizations. Scheduled visits will increase as indicated by decreasing CD4 and increasing HIV RNA copies per/dL. Opportunistic disease prevention will become increasingly important over time. There has been significant progress in the treatment and prophylaxis of *Pneumocystis carinii* pneumonia, toxoplasmosis, *Mycobacterium avium* complex, crytosporidiosis, cytomegalovirus, and fungal infections (Girard & Fineburg, 1994; CDC, 1995).

5. What are the current therapies that should be considered for Grace?

The following treatment guidelines for initiation of antiretroviral therapies must be thoughtfully selected in light of significant recent advances in drug development (Barlett, 1996). Therefore, these recommendations require periodic review and modification.

A. Indications to treat: CD4 count <500/mm; it is likely that future strategies will consider initiation of treatment with higher CD4 counts and viral burden of 20,000–75,000 copies/dL. as a possible independent indicator of treatment.

B. Monotherapy is generally not advocated although some considerations may justify exceptions.
   1. ddI (≥60 kg–200 mg tab bid; < 60 kg–125 mg tab bid)
   2. d4T (40 mg bid)
C. Combination therapy:
   1. Nucleoside analogs = AZT (200 mg tid) plus 3TC (150 mg bid)
   2. Protease inhibitor = Saquinavir (600 mg tid), or Indinavir (800 mg tid), or Ritonavir (600 mg bid), plus Nucleoside analog = AZT, or ddI, or ddC, or d4T, or 3TC
   3. Protease inhibitor plus 3TC (150 mg bid) + AZT (200 mg tid)
   4. AZT (200 mg tid) plus ddI (above dose) or ddC (0.75 mg tid)

6. *What counseling and education will Grace need?*

The following counseling and educational issues should be discussed with Grace as part of her treatment plan.

Services and use of clinical care:
- Differences between HIV and AIDS
- Natural history of HIV infection
- Role of CD4 and HIV RNA screening
- Transmission methods
- Pregnancy counseling and condom use
- Partner notification
- HIV treatments

7. *What issues will confront Grace and her family?*

Familial ties are challenged with chronic illnesses. There are several adaptive tasks that the patient and family will be faced with: 1) adjusting to diagnosis and disease development; 2) adjusting to daily living limitations and pain; 3) adjusting to hospital environments and medical procedures; 4) developing relationships with hospital and outpatient medical staffs; 5) learning how to maintain overall emotional balance; 6) preserving relationships; and 7) learning to live presently with the unsure future.

Responses to ill family members are a function of two factors: beliefs or values each family member holds specific to the patient diagnosis, and what families perceive to be acceptable and appropriate behavior in the presence of their ill family member. It is appropriate to consider psychological therapy for families facing HIV. The patient and their family need replenishing and nurturing so that the focus, the HIV infected family member, will not be lost in grief and fear. For Grace, she has described a family of close ties. This history of family support may enable her to move quickly to tell her family or to move cautiously to protect her family and to avoid the stigma associated with this disease. Grace may need assistance with role playing to prepare for family responses; she may need to tell her family in the presence of her medical team; she may decide not to tell her family for some time if at all. These and many other decisions will be fluid for Grace as she accepts the reality of the diagnosis. The health care team must accept vacillation and reordering of priorities (Minkoff et al., 1995).

8. *Identify information resources that might be helpful to Grace and her family.*

   Listed are many national resources; most larger cities have similar organizations that support persons and families with AIDS

   1. National AIDS Hotline 800 342-2437
      This number has everything a state hotline has, including trained counselors, and is open 24 hours a day. If you need referrals to local agencies or services, your state hotline number may have more up-to-date information.

   2. National AIDS Clearinghouse 800 458-5231
      This number gives you access to the full range of the CDC's published information. You can get referrals to AIDS service organizations and services, order publications, get information about AIDS in the workplace, find out about the latest clinical trials, or use automated service to get information by fax. You can also order a free catalog of HIV/AIDS education and prevention materials.

   3. National Institutes of Health . . . . 800 Trials
      AIDS Clinical Trails Information Service . . . . 800 Trials-A
      This number provides up-to-date information on clinical trials that evaluate experimental drugs and other therapies for adult and children at all stages of HIV infection.

   4. National Lesbian and Gay Health Association 202 939-7880

   5. National Minority AIDS Council 202 483-6622

   6. National Women's Health Network 202 347-1140

   7. National Hemophilia AIDS Foundation 800 424-2634

   8. Positively Aware
      Bimonthly publication
      1258 West Belmont Avenue
      Chicago, Illinois 60657-3292 . . . . 312 404-8726

   9. GMHC Treatment Issues
      The Gay Men's Health Crisis Newsletter of Experimental AIDS Therapies
      129 West 20th Street
      New York, N.Y. 10011
      (Excellent publication for not only gay men, but for all individuals infected with HIV).

9. *What additional measures will you initiate to maintain health and prevent disease?*

   Vaccination of HIV-infected adults is important because it helps prevent acquisition of other opportunistic infections. The following vaccination schedule should be adhered to:

Vaccination of HIV-Infected Adults

VACCINE	FREQUENCY	COMMENTS
Pneumococcal vaccine*	Once	HIV infection predisposes to pneumococcal infections.
Hepatitis B vaccine	Series of three vaccinations	Indicated if there is no prior hepatitis B exposure.
Influenza vaccine	Yearly	Prior to flu season (November) is the optimal time for maximizing protection.
Hemophilus influenza vaccine	Once	Should be considered. Efficacy is uncertain.
Measles	Once	Consider if patient was born after 1956. Safety and efficacy of the vaccine are unknown relative to HIV infection.
Diphtheria and tetanus	Every 10 years	Administer if a booster is indicated.

*Consider booster immunization every 5–7 years; CDC 1993

10. What gynecologic and family planning needs should you address with Grace?

It is the role of the nurse practitioner to initiate a discussion of sexuality, safe sex, contraception, and childbearing. These discussions evolve over time as the security and supportiveness of the relationship between the patient and nurse practitioner strengthens. Make no assumptions regarding their sexual preference, sexual history, and pregnancy plans. The nurse practitioner's role is to educate the patient about prevention of HIV transmission irrespective of the patient's sexual orientation or preferences. For heterosexual women, selection of a birth control method incorporates not only the specific needs and interests of the patient, but also the best selection in light of HIV status. Choosing the optimal method of contraception—barrier methods, spermicides, hormonal contraceptives (oral contraceptives, DMPA, Norplant), intrauterine devices, and sterilization—includes issues of method failure rate, dual efficacy of some methods in preventing pregnancy and sexually transmitted infections including HIV, the potential risk of increased HIV transmission owing to local genital irritation, potential contraception failure secondary to drug interaction with HIV-related therapies, potential drug toxicity secondary to interaction with HIV-related therapies, and the potential immunosuppressive effect of some agents (Bardeguez & Johnson, 1994).

Pregnancy in a seropositive woman carries a 15–35% risk of HIV infection; rates of HIV transmission increase for women with lower CD4 cell counts or high HIV RNA concentrations. Fetal transmission can be significantly reduced through the monotherapy, Zidovudine. Viral transmission may occur in utero, at delivery, or with breastfeeding (CDC, 1994).

There has been significant attention given to the question of gender-related differences in HIV-infected patients. There does not appear to be differences in the treatment of HIV disease or opportunistic infections between men and women except for gynecological care. Atypical Pap smears are common and require careful follow up quarterly or biannually, including colposcopy when abnormalities persist. Sexually transmitted infections, mucocutaneous candida infection, bacterial vaginosis, trichomonas, and human papilloma virus must be properly diagnosed and treated (Minkoff et al., 1995).

REFERENCES

Bardeguez A, Johnson MA. Women and HIV-1 infection. *AIDS* 1994; 8(Suppl 1): S261–S273.

Bartlett JG. *The Johns Hopkins Hospital Guide to Medical Care of Patients with HIV Infection.* Baltimore: Williams & Wilkins; 1996.

Carpenter CCJ, Fischl MA, Hammer SM., Hirsch MS, Jacobsen DM, Katzenstein DA, et al. Antiretroviral therapy for HIV infection. JAMA 1996; 276(2): 146–154.

Centers for Disease Control. 1993 revised classification system for HIV infection and expanded surveillance case definition for AIDS among adolescents and adults. *Morbid Mortal Wkly Rpt* 1992; 44(RR-17): 1–19.

Centers for Disease Control. Recommendations of the Advisory Committee on Immunization Practices (ACIP): Use of vaccines and immune globulins in persons with altered immunocompetence. *Morbid Mortal Wkly Rpt* 1993; 42(RR-4): 1–18.

Centers for Disease Control. Recommendation of the U.S. Public Health Service Task Force in the use of zidovudine to reduce perinatal transmission of human immunodeficiency virus. *Morbid Mortal Wkly Rpt* 1994; 43 (RR-11): 1–15.

Centers for Disease Control. USPHS/IDSA guidelines for the prevention of opportunistic infections in persons infected with human immundeficiency virus: A summary. *Morbid Mortal Wkly Rpt* 1995; 44(RR-8): 1–34.

Girard PM, Feinburg J. Progress and problems in AIDS-associated opportunistic infections. *AIDS* 1994; 8 (Suppl 1): S249–S259.

Minkoff H, DeHovitz JA, Duerr A. *HIV Infection in Women.* New York: Raven; 1995.

Saag MS, Holodniy M, Kuritzkes DR, O'Brien WA, Coombs R, Poscher M.E, et al. HIV viral load markers in clinical practice. *Nat Med* 1996; 2 (6): 625–629.

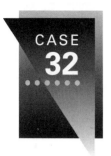

A 35-year-old man with LUQ abdominal pain with nausea and vomiting

SCENARIO

Ralph Turner is a 35-year-old Caucasian male who presents with severe sharp LUQ abdominal pain associated with nausea and vomiting. He states the pain started approximately 2 days ago after eating chili. The pain seems to come on as a spasm/cramping that is quite sharp then either goes away or turns into a burning sensation that goes to the chest. He states that over the past 7 years he has taken antacid for indigestion, and it does offer some relief.

● TENTATIVE DIAGNOSES

Based on the information provided so far, what are potential diagnoses?

● HISTORY

1. *What are significant questions in Ralph's history?*
2. *What are the key points on the review of systems?*

● PHYSICAL ASSESSMENT

What are the significant portions of the physical examination that should be completed for Ralph?

● DIFFERENTIAL DIAGNOSES

What are the significant positive and negative data that support or refute your diagnoses for Ralph?

● DIAGNOSTIC TESTS

Based on the history and physical assessment, what, if any, diagnostic tests would you obtain? Include your rationale for the tests.

● DIAGNOSIS

What diagnoses are appropriate for Ralph?

● THERAPEUTIC PLAN

1. *What factors contribute to gastric acidity?*
2. *What are issues to consider when deciding on treatment for PUD?*
3. *What are lifestyle changes that are recommended for PUD?*
4. *What are the pharmacological treatments for PUD?*
5. *What side effects of the regimen would you warn Ralph about?*
6. *What suggestions would you make for Ralph and his family in terms of dealing with family stresses?*
7. *Where can an NP obtain more information concerning PUD?*
8. *When should Ralph return for follow up?*

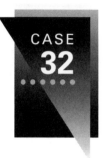

TUTORIAL

A 35-year-old man with LUQ abdominal pain with nausea and vomiting

SCENARIO

Ralph Turner is a 35-year-old Caucasian male who presents with severe sharp LUQ abdominal pain associated with nausea and vomiting. He states the pain started approximately 2 days ago after eating chili. The pain seems to come on as a spasm/cramping that is quite sharp then either goes away or turns into a burning sensation that goes to the chest. He states that over the past 7 years he has taken antacids for indigestion, and it does offer some relief.

● TENTATIVE DIAGNOSES

Based on the information provided so far, what are potential diagnoses?

DIAGNOSIS	RATIONALE
Gastric cancer	Ralph is presenting with abdominal pain, nausea, and vomiting. These may be presenting signs of gastric cancer.
Peptic ulcer disease (PUD)	Ralph describes abdominal pain that comes and goes, with a burning sensation in his chest. An antacid offers some relief. These are characteristic symptoms of PUD.
Angina	Angina can present as indigestion and burning in the chest.
Cholecystitis	Ralph presents with nausea, vomiting, and chest discomfort after eating spicy foods. These symptoms could be caused by cholecystitis.

(continued)

DIAGNOSIS	RATIONALE
Pancreatitis	Nausea and vomiting along with abdominal pain are symptoms of possible pancreatitis.
GERD	Indigestion and burning in the chest are common symptoms seen with GERD.

● HISTORY

1. What are significant questions in Ralph's history?

REQUESTED DATA	DATA ANSWER
Allergies	None known.
Current medications	Advil/Tylenol prn. Mylanta 1–2 tablespoons every 3–4 hours. Fluoxetine (Prozac) 20 mg QD. Laxative as needed.
Surgery/transfusions	Appendectomy at age 15.
Past medical history and hospitalizations/fractures/injuries/accidents	+ Depression, decreased ability to control anger. Gastritis. Measles. Chicken pox.
Immunizations	TB last year: Neg. Tetanus: 6 years ago.
Appetite/wt loss/gain	Spontaneous wt loss of 10 lbs in last 3 weeks.
24-Hour diet recall	B: Cold cereal or coffee. L: Sandwich, usually tuna, bologna, or peanut butter. Beer or glass of soda. D: Chili, cole slaw, soda, or beer.
Relationship of indigestion/abdominal pain to eating	Usually symptoms start right after eating. If I rest after eating the symptoms do not seem as bad.
Sleeping	No problems falling asleep. Sleeps 6 hours at night. Sometimes has indigestion at night too. Antacid helps.
Social history	Tobacco: $1\frac{1}{2}$ ppd. Alcohol: ~ a case of beer/day shared with friends. Caffeine: Seven to eight cups coffee or soda/day.

(continued)

REQUESTED DATA   DATA ANSWER

REQUESTED DATA	DATA ANSWER
	Drugs: None.
	Exercise: Rarely .
Family history	Father: Alive, 61, unsure of health, hx of alcohol abuse.
	Mother: 59, deceased, stroke.
	Siblings: Two sisters, one good health, one with psychiatric problems; one brother, healthy.
Relationship with family	Has girlfriend. She recently had a baby. He finds this very stressful since he is unemployed and has no income except for working on cars in the neighborhood. Lost his job about 3 months ago. Feels like all he and his girlfriend do now is shout at each other.
Home	Lives in one-bedroom apartment.
Last complete PE	2 years ago when he started a new job.
Income/insurance	Makes about $1,200/mo. Health insurance and unemployment will end in 3 months.
Depression history: How do you usually handle stress?	Strike out at those around me.
Have you ever thought of harming yourself?	No.
Describe how you feel now.	I feel sad, down in the dumps, and I want to get a job. In 3 months I won't be able to support myself.
CAGE questionnaire	States he sometimes feels guilty about how much beer he drinks, especially when he yells at his girlfriend. He gets angry when she suggests he should not drink as much now since he is a father. Usually does not drink in the morning. After a bad hangover he sometimes feels he should not drink since he feels so bad, but never seems to follow through.

2. *What are the key points on the review of systems?*

SYSTEM REVIEWED   DATA ANSWER

SYSTEM REVIEWED	DATA ANSWER
General	Overall, right now feels stressed and not healthy.
GI	Denies black, tarry, or bloody stools or emesis. Sometimes he has constipation.

(continued)

SYSTEM REVIEWED	DATA ANSWER
GU	Denies problems urinating, burning or frequency. No problem with emptying bladder.
Lungs	Denies SOB except when going up lots of steps or carrying the baby. Has a "typical" morning smoker's cough.
Cardiac	Denies sweating, radiation of pain into arm or neck. No SOB, or palpitations.

● PHYSICAL ASSESSMENT

What are the significant portions of the physical examination that should be completed for Ralph?

SYSTEM	RATIONALE	FINDINGS
Vital signs	Provides baseline data.	B/P: 110/70 HR: 96 R: 28 T: 97.8 Ht: 5'10" Wt: 175 lbs
General appearance/skin	Provides overall indication of status.	Neatly dressed, well developed, anxious. Hair thinning, dull, pale in color. Turgor fair, no jaundice.
Mouth	Gives indication of hydration status.	Lips dry, cracked, oral mucosa, pale pink. Tongue dry and tender to touch.
Lungs	Baseline data, checking for fluid or COPD, asthma signs.	CTA.
Heart	Need to evaluate because symptoms are similar to angina. Provides baseline data.	S_1S_2 WNL. No MRG.
Abdomen	Area where pain is occurring. Important to conduct complete, thorough exam of abdomen checking for pain, masses, organomegaly, and peritoneal symptoms (Schaik, 1993).	5 cm well-healed scar RLQ. No venous distention or striae. Symmetrical without obvious bulging. No visible peristaltic waves. High pitched, hyper active BS, no bruits or ve-

(continued)

SYSTEM	RATIONALE	FINDINGS
		nous hums. Liver percussed ~13 cm in MCL. C/O tenderness in epigastric area. Neg. Murphy's sign, psoas, and rebound.
Rectum	Important to evaluate because c/o of gastric problems, also to check stool for bleeding.	Small noninflamed external hemorrhoids. No rashes or irritation. No tenderness on palpation. Normal sphincter function. Prostate smooth. No masses. Hard brown stool, guaiac negative.

● DIFFERENTIAL DIAGNOSES

What are the significant positive and negative data that support or refute your diagnoses for Ralph?

DIAGNOSIS	POSITIVE DATA	NEGATIVE DATA
Gastric cancer	History of gastritis, male, age, diet, epigastric discomfort, vomiting.	No family history of cancer, no anorexia, abdominal mass, or ascites.
PUD	Age, male, gnawing, burning pain in epigastric area after meals, heartburn, diet high in irritating foods, history of NSAID use, food helps relieve pain, smoker.	No tarry, black or bloody stools, not awakened by pain at night.
Angina	Chest discomfort, increased stress, age, male, smokes.	Pain not relieved by rest, no FH, no radiation, diaphoresis.
Cholecystitis	Age, high fat diet, indigestion, nausea.	No peritonitis, no obesity, gender, no RUQ pain or shoulder pain, neg. Murphy's sign.
Pancreatitis	Alcohol consumption, diet, N/V, abdominal pain.	Severe abdominal pain that bores through to back, not accentuated by coughing or deep breathing, afebrile.

(continued)

DIAGNOSIS	POSITIVE DATA	NEGATIVE DATA
GERD	Indigestion relieved by antacids, alcohol intake, high fat intake.	No increase in indigestion with lying down after meals.

● DIAGNOSTIC TESTS

Based on the history and physical examination, what, if any, diagnostic testing would you obtain?

DIAGNOSTIC TEST	RATIONALE	RESULTS
CBC with differential	Able to see decrease in H/H with bleeding with hypochromic, microcytic anemia.	RBC: 4.21. WBC: 6.6. Hgb: 13.2. Hct: 39.1. MCV: 92.8.
Albumin	Helpful to determine nutritional status.	3.2 g/dL.
Electrolytes, liver function/renal	Baseline information of renal and liver functioning, especially important with alcohol intake (Schaik, 1993).	Na: 137. K+: 4.2. Cl: 97. CO2: 35. BUN: 8. Creat.: 0.7. AST: 51. ALT: 75. Alk. Phos.: 120.
H. pylori	Confirming presence of *H. pylori* is important because elimination of the bacteria is likely to cure PUD. Blood, breath, and stomach tissue tests may be performed to detect its presence. Tests highly accurate in detecting the bacteria (NIH, 1995).	Serum *H. pylori* +.

(continued)

DIAGNOSTIC TEST	*RATIONALE*	*RESULTS*
Abdominal X-ray	Good choice. Noninvasive study that provides considerable information about the GI system. Helps rule out perforation.	No evidence of bowel obstruction, no evidence of free intraperitoneal air.
Upper GI series	Used to diagnose esophageal lesions, gastric ulcers, and tumors, SBO, and small bowel lesions. Detects 90% of peptic ulcers.	No evidence of reflux or obstruction.
Endoscopy	Good choice if barium studies are negative. More expensive, but more sensitive and specific than barium. Becoming test of choice in many settings (Schaik, 1993).	Not done.

● DIAGNOSES

What diagnoses are appropriate for Ralph?

Peptic ulcer disease, duodenal
Alcohol abuse
Tobacco abuse
Depression/anxiety by history

Data Supporting the Diagnosis

Abdominal pain with indigestion, age, being male, alcohol intake, increased stress, and history of NSAID use. The National Digestive Disease group recognized three major causes of PUD (NIH, 1995):

- Infection with *H. pylori*
- Use of NSAIDS
- Pathologic hypersecretory states such as Zollinger-Ellison Syndrome

● THERAPEUTIC PLAN

1. *What factors contribute to gastric acidity?*

Psychogenic factors
Drug therapy
Trauma
Exposure to irritants
Genetic factors

Normal aging
Certain illnesses (pancreatitis, hepatic disease, Crohn's, etc)
Blood type (gastric, type A; duodenal, type O(Doughty, 1993)

2. *What are issues to consider when deciding on treatment for PUD?*

- pt ability to afford medication
- education of pt and significant other
- visits frequently enough to monitor compliance of regimen
- careful assessment of outcome radiology/endoscopy results

3. *What are lifestyle changes that are recommended for PUD?*

In the past, clinicians advised people with ulcers to avoid spicy, fatty, or acidic foods. However, a bland diet is now known to be ineffective for treating or avoiding ulcers. No particular diet is helpful for most ulcer patients. People who find certain foods irritating should avoid those foods. Smoking has been shown to delay ulcer healing and has been linked to ulcer recurrence; therefore, persons with ulcers should not smoke (Zakim, 1991).

4. *What are the pharmacological treatments for PUD?*

The most effective therapy, according to the NIH panel, is a 2-week, triple therapy. This regimen eradicates the bacteria and reduces the risk of ulcer recurrence in 90% of people with duodenal ulcers. People with stomach ulcers that are not associated with NSAIDS also benefit from bacteria eradication.

Inital treatment for 2 weeks with:

Tetracycline 500 mg qid
Bismuth subsalicylate 30 mL qid
Metronidazole 200–500 mg qid
Amoxicillin 250–500 mg qid may be tried as an alternative treatment.
Alternative to triple therapy:
Amoxicillin 250–500 mg two to four times a day, or clarithromycin tid
Omeprazole bid (NIH, 1995).

H2 receptor antagonists are used along with the triple therapy to provide acid suppression. These should be taken BID for 4–6 weeks.

Tagamet
Zantac
Pepcid

For patients in whom *H. pylori* has not been identified, but they have the typical PUD symptoms, a trial of H2 receptor antagonists is recommended for 4–6 weeks. If there is no improvement after 2 weeks, than further testing might need to be done (Heuman, Mills, and McGuire, 1997).

5. *What side effects of the regimen would you warn Ralph about?*

Inform the pt of the potential side effects of the regimen (superinfection, diarrhea, constipation).

6. *What suggestions would you make for Ralph and his family in terms of dealing with family stresses?*

   Appropriate interventions for Ralphs' family would be:

   - Education about PUD and the threapeutic management.
   - Family counseling; to learn ways to reduce stress and defuse potentially abusive situations.
   - Have emergency phone numbers close by: include number for NP/MD as crisis hotlines
   - Nutritional counseling for dietary/financial concerns (Doughty, 1993; Loeb, 1993).

7. *Where can an NP obtain more information concerning PUD?*

   - Local library should have a lot of information concering gastrointestinal diseases
   - National Digestive Diseases Information Clearinghouse (NDDIC)
     Bethesda, MD
     301 654-3810

8. *When should Ralph return for follow up?*

   Management is essentially symptomatic, emphazing drug therapy, physical rest, dietary changes, and stress reduction. The goal is to reduce gastric secretions, protect the mucosa from further damage, and relieve pain, providing emotional support and offering reassurance will optimize adherence to the treatment regimen. A small percentage of patients with duodenal ulcers require surgical intervention because of hemorrhage, obstruction, perforation, or intractibility.

   Follow up in 2–4 weeks to check on symptoms (response to medications, GI bleeding, adverse reaction to meds). For those with gastric ulcers document healing with UGI barium radiograph or endoscopy: 6 weeks for small ulcers; 12 weeks for large; imperative in gastric ulcers; unnecessary in uncomplicated duodenal ulcers (Salerno, 1994).

REFERENCES

Doughty D. *Gastrointestinal Disorders.* St. Louis: Mosby; 1993.

Heuman D, Mills A, McGuire H. *Gastroenterology.* Philadelphia: W.B. Saunders; 1997.

Loeb S. (ed). *Diseases: Causes and Complications: Assessment, findings, nursing diagnosis and interventions.* Springhouse, PA: Springhouse; 1993.

National Institutes of Health. *Stomach and Duodenal Ulcers* (NIH publication No. 95-38). Bethesda, MD: National Digestive Diseases Information Clearinghouse; 1995.

Salerno M. Gastrointestinal disorders. In Millonig VL (ed). *Adult Nurse Practitioner Certification Review Guide.* Potomac, MD: Health Leadership Associates; 1994; 240–250.

Schaik TV (ed). *Gastroenterology Nursing: A Core Curriculum.* St. Louis: Mosby; 1993.

Zakim DC. *Peptic Ulcer Disease and Other Acid Related Disorders.* Armonk, NY: Academic Research Associates; 1991.

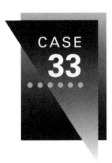

A 25-year-old man with a 3-day history of rhinorrhea, frontal headache, and maxillary tooth pain

SCENARIO

Randy is a 25-year-old Vietnamese male who works as a plumber. Two weeks ago he had a self-defined "cold" and used over-the-counter medications. Most of his symptoms resolved, but for the last three days he has still had rhinorrhea, a frontal headache that increases in intensity when he bends over, and a toothache that involves all his maxillary teeth.

● TENTATIVE DIAGNOSES

Based on the information provided so far, what are potential diagnoses?

● HISTORY

1. *What are significant questions in the medical history?*
2. *What questions should be reviewed regarding current problem?*
3. *What are key points that should be covered on the review of systems?*

● PHYSICAL ASSESSMENT

What are the significant portions of the physical examination that should be completed?

● DIFFERENTIAL DIAGNOSES

What are the significant positive and negative data that support or refute your diagnoses for Randy?

● DIAGNOSTIC TESTS

Based on the history and physical assessment, what, if any, diagnostic tests would you obtain. Include your rationale for the tests.

● DIAGNOSES

What diagnoses are appropriate for Randy?

● THERAPEUTIC PLAN

1. *What are the main goals in the treatment of sinusitis?*
2. *What pharmacological therapy is indicated in the treatment of sinusitis?*
3. *What common URI medication should be avoided in sinusitis? Why?*
4. *What are the most common causes of sinusitis?*
5. *What are the major organisms responsible for sinusitis?*
6. *What antibiotics provide appropriate coverage for the common causative organisms?*
7. *What nonpharmacologic treatments are helpful?*
8. *What major complications of sinusitis should the health care provider be aware of?*
9. *What instructions should the client be given?*

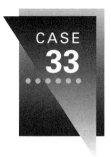

TUTORIAL

A 25-year-old man with a 3-day history of rhinorrhea, frontal headache, and maxillary tooth pain

SCENARIO

Randy is a 25-year-old Vietnamese male who works as a plumber. Two weeks ago he had a self-defined "cold" and used over-the-counter medications. Most of his symptoms resolved, but for the last three days he has still had rhinorrhea, a frontal headache that increases in intensity when he bends over, and a toothache that involves all his maxillary teeth.

● TENTATIVE DIAGNOSES

Based on the information provided so far, what are the potential diagnoses?

DIAGNOSIS	RATIONALE
Upper respiratory infection	Headache, rhinorrhea, and maxillary pain are complaints when involve the upper respiratory tract.
Allergic rhinitis	Rhinorrhea.
Vasomotor rhinitis	Rhinorrhea, recent URI symptoms.
Mechanical obstruction of nares?	Headache.
Viral influenza	URI symptoms.
Sinusitis	Recent URI, position-dependent headache, maxillary toothache, purulent nasal discharge (Williams et al., 1992).
Dental abscess	Maxillary toothache.

● HISTORY

1. What are significant questions in the past medical history?

REQUESTED DATA	DATA ANSWER
Allergies	No food, drug, or environmental allergies.
Current medication	OTC decongestant/antihistamine/analgesic combination.
Past history of upper respiratory illnesses or sinusitis	Average of two URI/year usually during weather changes or flu season. Has had sinusitis in past several times but not in the last 2 years.
Dental history	Exam every 6–9 months. Last exam included X-rays without any problems noted.
Childhood illnesses	Chicken pox.
Infectious disease exposure	No known exposure to active tuberculosis, no risk factors for HIV.
Immunizations	Childhood immunizations up to date.
Surgery	None.
Hospitalizations	None.
Injuries	Broke nose during high school football game. No problems with nose since that time.
Employment	Plumber.
Sexuality	Heterosexual, married, monogamous.
Substance use	No tobacco. Occasional social ETOH. No other substances.

2. What questions should be reviewed regarding current problem?

REQUESTED DATA	DATA ANSWER
Onset and duration of symptoms	URI 2 weeks ago. Three days with frontal headache and maxillary toothache
Fever, cough, and color of nasal discharge	No fever, occasional nonproductive cough, yellowish green nasal discharge.

(continued)

REQUESTED DATA   DATA ANSWER

Describe location of headache pain (include aggravating and relieving factors)	Above eyes and behind nose. Pain increases when bending over at work. Decreases after standing for a while without bending over, but is never totally relieved.
Past episodes of similar symptoms? Treatment of past episodes?	Years ago. Took some kind of antibiotic before it went away.

3. What are the key points on the review of systems?

SYSTEM REVIEWED   DATA ANSWER

HEENT	Recent upper respiratory infection. No visual changes. Intermittent patency of nares. Greenish yellow nasal discharge. No stiffness of neck.
Respiratory	Had some cough and shortness of breath with exercise during URI but much better now.
Cardiac	No history of chest pain, dizziness, or tachycardia with exercise.
Neurological	No history of head injury, no loss of consciousness, no syncope.
Skin	Concerned with acne on face, washes face with deodorant soap.

● PHYSICAL ASSESSMENT

What are the significant portions of the physical examination that should be completed for Randy?

SYSTEM   FINDINGS

Vital signs	B/P: 128/68 P: 80 R: 18 Temp: 99.4°F

(continued)

SYSTEM	FINDINGS
Height/weight	Ht: 78″ Wt: 175 lbs
HEENT	Sclera clear without injection. TMs intact bilaterally with bony landmarks visible and slight bulging on left. Posterior pharynx slightly erythematous without exudate. No lymphadenopathy. Maxillary and frontal sinuses tender to palpation. Toothache increases with percussion. Dull transillumination of rt maxillary sinus, left opaque. Frontal sinuses show dull transillumination. Nares erythematous and edematous bilaterally. Inferior and middle turbinates visualized easily after topical decongestant spray. Nares patient bilaterally after spray. Mucopurulent mucus visible bilaterally.
Chest	CTA.
Heart	RRR. No murmurs, gallops, or rubs.
Abdomen	No masses or tenderness, active bowel sounds, no organomegaly.
Neurological	Cranial nerves II-XII intact. Reflexes 2+.

● DIFFERENTIAL DIAGNOSES

What are the significant positive and negative data that support or refute your diagnosis for Randy?

DIAGNOSIS	POSITIVE DATA	NEGATIVE DATA
Upper respiratory infection	Headache, rhinorrhea, and maxillary pain are complaints which involve the upper respiratory tract.	None.
Allergic rhinitis	Rhinorrhea.	No history of allergies.
Vasomotor rhinitis	Rhinorrhea, recent URI symptoms.	None.
Mechanical obstruction of nares	Headache.	Patent nares with topical decongestants.

(continued)

DIAGNOSIS	POSITIVE DATA	NEGATIVE DATA
Chronic inflammatory rhinitis	Rhinorrhea.	Only infrequent history of symptoms.
Viral influenza	URI symptoms.	No fever or chills or muscle aches.
Acute sinusitis	Recent URI, position dependent headache, maxillary toothache, purulent nasal discharge, nonsmoker (Williams & Simel, 1993).	
Chronic sinusitis	None.	Only infrequent history of sinusitis type symptoms.
Rhinitis medicamentosa	Nasal congestion.	No use of topical decongestants, no substance abuse, no tobacco abuse.
Periodontal disease	Maxillary toothache.	Recent dental exam with X-rays WNL.

● DIAGNOSTIC TESTS

Based on the history and physical assessment, what, if any, diagnostic tests would you obtain?

Based on the classic symptoms presented, no diagnostic tests are needed. Tests would only be needed if symptoms do not resolve with treatment or if there is chronic sinusitis.

DIAGNOSTIC TEST	RATIONALE	RESULTS
Plain sinus radiographs	Indicated as primary imaging study. They provide a gross examination of the paranasal sinuses (Oppenheimer, 1992). Air fluid levels can be seen in acute sinusitis and mucosal thickening can be seen in chronic sinusitis	Not done.
Computed tomography (CT)	Most useful imaging study in sinusitis. Indicated when chronic sinusitis does not respond to treatment or	Not done.

(continued)

DIAGNOSTIC TEST	RATIONALE	RESULTS
	when recurrent episodes of acute sinusitis occurs. Much more specific than plain films. Demonstrates the type of disease. Good evaluation tool prior to surgery. Will show involvement of surrounding structures such as orbit or brain (Oppenheimer, 1992).	
Magnetic resonance imaging	More specific than CT scan, also more expensive, especially helpful in evaluating soft-tissue densities and therefore helpful indifferentiating benign for a malignant lesion (Oppenheimer, 1992).	Not done.
Endoscopic evaluation (rhinoscopy)	Provides direct visualization especially of mechanical obstruction. Polyps, foreign bodies, and anatomical anomalies can be directly visualized (Evans, 1994).	Not done.
CBC with differential	May help differentiate cause. Allergic: increased eosinophils. Bacterial: increased neutrophils.	Not done.
Allergy testing	Identifies allergen that may precipatate sinus infections.	Not done.

● DIAGNOSES

What diagnoses are appropriate for Randy?

1. Vasomotor rhinitis
2. Acute sinusitis

● THERAPEUTIC PLAN

1. *What are the main goals in the treatment of sinusitis?*

Control infection, reduce tissue edema, facilitate drainage, and maintain the patency of the sinus ostia (Oppenheimer, 1992).

2. *What pharmacological therapy is indicated in the treatment of sinusitis?*
   - analgesics as needed
   - mucolytics to promote drainage
   - systemic decongestants (promotes drainage through the ostia and effect deeper mucosal regions that topical agents cannot reach).
   - topical decongestants for no more than 3–5 days (promotes drainage through the ostia, but longer treatment may cause rebound edema).
   - consider topical and systemic corticosteroids for postacute phase of sinusitis caused by allergic rhinitis (Haugen and Ramlo, 1993).

3. *What common URI medication should be avoided in sinusitis? Why?*

   Avoid antihistamines because of drying effect (Haugen and Ramlo, 1993) and the tendency to slow the movement of mucus out of the sinuses (Uphold and Grahm, 1994). Antihistamines, however, may be considered for patients who have symptoms of allergy along with acute sinusitis during allergy season and to prevent recurrence in allergic patients after acute infection has cleared (Oppenheimer, 1992).

4. *What are the most common causes of sinusitis?*

   Allergies
   Complication of acute or chronic rhinitis
   Environmental irritants
   Nasal polyposis
   Viral infection (Godley, 1992)

5. *What are the major organisms responsible for sinusitis?*

   Streptococcus pneumoniae, Haemophilus influenzae, and *Moraxella catarrhalis* are the most common pathogens cultured in sinusitis (Godley, 1992); (Edelstein et al., 1993). Brook (1981) indicates that alpha-hemolytic *Streptococcus, Haemophilis influenzae,* and *Streptococcus pneumoniae* are normal flora of the nasal sinus area. Haugen and Ramlo (1993) describe an overgrowth of this normal flora damages the mucosa and cilia, resulting in the symptoms caused by pressure to the surrounding areas.

   Oppenheimer (1992) divided the causative organisms into two groups: anaerobic and aerobic. The causative pathogen depended on the environment of the sinus. If the ostial obstruction had been recent, then the causative organism was more likely to be aerobic which includes the previously mentioned pathogens and *Escherichia coli.* If the meatus has been obstructed consistently for a prolonged period then anaerobic bacteria such as *Propionibacterium* species, *Bacteroides,* and *Fusobacterium* can be found. To generalize aerobic bacteria usually are found in acute sinusitis and the anaerobic bacteria proliferate in chronic sinusitis.

6. *What antibiotics provide appropriate coverage for the common causative organisms?*

Acute sinusitis should be treated for 10–14 days (Haugen and Ramlo, 1993)

First-line therapy

Amoxicillin
Trimethoprim-sulfamethoxazol
Erythromycin

Second-line therapy (if little or no improvement in 5 days)

Cefaclor (Ceclor)
Cefuroxime (Ceftin)
Amoxicillin and clavulanic acid (Augmentin)
Cefixime (Suprax)
Loracarbef (Lorabid)
Azithromycin (Zithromax)
Clarithromycin (Biaxin)

Chronic sinusitis should be treated for 3 weeks with

Amoxicillin-clavulanate (Augmentin)
Clindamycin (Cleocin)
Metronidazole (Flagyl)

7. *What nonpharmacologic treatments are helpful?*

Moisture, saline nasal drops, sprays or irrigations
Heated mist, such as sauna, application of hot moist towels or showers
Increased fluid intake

8. *What major complications of acute sinusitis should the health care provider be aware of?*

- Chronic sinusitis
- Orbital and central nervous system complications owing to direct extension of infection to contiguous structures or seeding of bacteria via venous drainage (Haugen and Ramlo, 1993).
- Mucoceles: Chronic cystic lesions that expand slowly and cause symptoms through pressure, erosion, and extension beyond the sinus (Haugen and Ramlo, 1993).
- Intracranial complications: Subdural empyema, frontal lobe abscess, superior sagittal sinus thrombosis, and osteomyelitis are some of the possible intracranial complications (Haugen and Ramlo, 1993).

9. *What instructions should the client be given?*

Return for evaluation if symptoms not improved within 48 hours.
Return if there is swelling in periorbital area.
Humidify the air and increase fluid intake.

Avoid allergens.

Avoid swimming during acute phase.

Avoid antihistamines unless otherwise directed by heath care provider.

Avoid smoking (Uphold & Graham, 1994).

REFERENCES

Brook I. Aerobic and anaerobic bacterial flora of normal maxillary sinuses. *Laryngoscope;* 1981; 91: 372–376.

Edelstein DR, Avner SE, Chow JM, Duerksen RL, Johnson J, Ronis M, et al. Once-a-day therapy for sinusitis: A comparison study of cefixime and amoxicillin. *Laryngoscope;* 1993; 103: 33–41.

Evans KL. Diagnosis and management of sinusitis. *Brit Med J* 1994 309: 1415–1422.

Godley FA. Chronic sinusitis: An update. *Am Fam Phys* 1992; 45; 2190–2199.

Haugen JR, Ramlo JH. Serious complication of acute sinusitis. *Postgrad Med* 1993; 93(1): 115–125.

Oppenheimer RW. Sinusitis: How to recognize and treat it. *Postgrad Med* 1992; 91(5): 281–290.

Uphold CR, Graham MV. *Clinical Guidelines in Family Practice.* Gainesville, FL: Barmarrae; 1994.

Williams JW, Simel DL. Does this patient have sinusitis? Diagnosing acute sinusitis by history and physical examination. *JAMA* 1993; 270: 1242–1246.

Williams JW, Simel DL, Roberts L, Samsa GP. Clinical evaluation for sinusitis: Making the diagnosis by history and physical examination. *Ann Int Med* 1992; 117: 705–709.

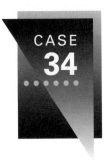

A 31-year-old woman with fatigue

SCENARIO

Rose Hall, a 31-year-old Hispanic female, presents to the health center with a history of tiring easily over the past 2 months. She is married and has two children. She works full time as a secretary.

● TENTATIVE DIAGNOSES

Based on the information provided so far, what are potential differential diagnoses?

● HISTORY

1. *What are significant questions in Rose's history?*
2. *What are the key points to cover on the review of systems?*

● PHYSICAL ASSESSMENT

What are the significant portions of the physical examination that should be completed for Rose?

● DIFFERENTIAL DIAGNOSES

What are the significant positive and negative data that support or refute your diagnoses for Rose?

● DIAGNOSTIC TESTS

Based on the history and physical assessment, what, if any, diagnostic tests would you obtain? Include your rationale for the tests.

● DIAGNOSIS

What diagnoses are appropriate for Rose?

● THERAPEUTIC PLAN

1. *How is hepatitis classified?*
2. *What influence does the classification of hepatitis have on the therapeutic treatment plan?*
3. *What will the management of Rose's hepatitis B consist of?*
4. *When should Rose be referred to a specialist and to whom?*
5. *What patient education should you provide for Rose?*
6. *What impact does this illness have in terms of being contagious to Rose's family, friends, and coworkers?*
7. *What suggestions can you make to Rose for her fatiguability?*
8. *When should Rose return for follow up?*
9. *What community resources are available to the NP and Rose?*

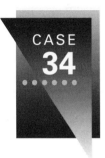

TUTORIAL

A 31-year-old woman with fatigue

SCENARIO:

Rose Hall, a 31-year-old Hispanic female, presents to the health center with a history of tiring easily over the past 2 months. She is married and has two children. She works full time as a secretary.

● TENTATIVE DIAGNOSES

Based on the information provided so far, what are the potential diagnoses?

DIAGNOSIS	RATIONALE
Anemia	Rose presents with a recent history of easy fatiguability. Her employment is physically undemanding. There are no indications of blood loss.
Viral infection	The vague presentation of symptoms and the incubation period are appropriate for a viral-induced infection. Viral induced etiologies include: Hepatitis. HIV. Cytomegalovirus. Epstein-Barr virus.
Chronic fatigue syndrome	More prevalent in women, especially those under age 45. Etiology unknown. Major criteria: fatigue unresolved with bed rest, affects daily activity, and persists for at least 6 months (Norris, 1993).
Acquired hypothyroidism	A possibility, because acquired hypothyroidism begins with an insidious onset of fatigue. Other symptoms include dry skin, weight gain, cold intolerance, constipation, and heavy menses.

(continued)

DIAGNOSIS *RATIONALE*

. . . .

Depression	Diagnosis of elimination that presents with depressed mood, loss of interest in activities, weight loss/gain as well as fatigue.

● HISTORY

1. What are significant questions in Rose's history?

REQUESTED DATA *DATA ANSWER*

. . . .

Allergies	NKA.
Current medications	OCs. OTC meds for occasional H/A, minor aches/pains.
Surgery/transfusions	C-section × 2, no transfusions.
Past medical history and hospitalizations/fractures/injuries/accidents	Chicken pox, mumps, and measles as child. Sutures on forehead from MVA—no sequelae.
Adult illness	Past history of duodenal ulcer 4 years ago.
OB/GYN history	LNMP: 2 weeks ago, normal flow and duration. Last pelvic: Approx. 9 months ago. Mammogram: None. SBE: Regularly for past year. G2P2A0.
Appetite/weight change	No changes in appetite, no weight changes since last pregnancy. Has weighed the same for past 9 years.
Social history	Tobacco: Never. Alcohol: None. Caffeine: Two to three cups coffee/day. Two to three colas/day. Drugs: None. Exercise: Occasional walks approximately 1 mile.
Family history	Father: age 54, good health. Mother: 52, good health. Brother: 33, good health. Sisters: Two, ages 29 and 28, good health. Spouse: 33, good health. Children: Son, 11; daughter, 9; good health.

(continued)

REQUESTED DATA	*DATA ANSWER*
Social organizations	First Baptist Church, children-oriented activities at church/school.
Relationship with husband	Both are monogamous. Married 12 years. They have sex about 3×/week and both enjoy the act. Husband works at a blue-collar job near home on first shift.
Relationship with children	Both she and her husband value their time with the children in evenings. She makes children's outfits for school plays and Halloween costumes. The couple purposefully explore activities the family can do together.
Income/insurance/home	She and her husband make decent wages. Both jobs are secure. Medical and dental insurance through husband's job. They own their own home.
Length of symptoms	Easy fatiguability for the past 2 months. No memory of any acute infection prior to fatiguability. Fatigue occurs every day. Makes it through work shift ok, but then has to nap for approx. 1 hour. Has been sleeping approximately 10 hours/night.
How has this affected your ADLs?	Fatigue alters energy level. Has not been able to do things with the children. Comes home and naps daily. Decreased libido related to fatigue. Only has enough energy to maintain work responsibilities. Husband has been helping with daily household chores, as have the children.
How do you manage stress?	Enjoys walking. Enjoys activities at church and school. Occasional leisurely walks with children. Does some creative sewing at times.
Any evidence of blood loss (stool, heavy menses, hemoptysis, urine, etc)?	No changes in stool or urine elimination. Menstrual cycles fine. No hemoptysis or hematemesis.
Have you traveled recently?	No recent travel history. Last trip was with the family 1 year ago to Walt Disney World in Florida.
Have you had any recent tattoos or body piercing procedures?	No exposure to procedures involving needles.
Has anyone else in the family been sick?	No.
Have you noticed any change in skin color?	No.

● PHYSICAL ASSESSMENT

What are the significant portions of the physical examination that should be completed for Rose?

SYSTEM	RATIONALE	FINDINGS
Vital signs	Baseline data.	B/P: 128/82 Rt arm: HR 80 R: 20 T: 98.8 Ht: 5'6" Wt: 175 lbs
General appearance/skin	Gives general indication of patient's overall status.	Alert, NAD. Skin warm and dry, No spider angiomata. Color natural. No pallor or jaundice.
HEENT	Should be included because one possible diagnosis is mononucleosis. Important to check for lymphadenopathy or any oral lesions that might indicate HIV.	Normocephalic, no sinus tenderness, Tms gray and WNL, Nose pink and moist with septum midline, oral mucosa moist and pink. Uvula midline. No pharyngeal erythema or oral lesions noted. No LA, supple neck. Thyroid nonpalpable, no masses.
Lungs	Can be done as a quick screening to r/o pulmonary problems.	CTA.
Heart	Should be done as a quick screening even though no indications of problems.	S_1S_2 WNL, no MRG.
Abdomen	Important to do as screening because one possible diagnosis is hepatitis.	BS +, soft, no splenomegaly. Liver palpable just below rt. costal margin, mild liver tenderness on deep palpation. No ascites. No lymph adenopathy.
Neurological	Important to do as basic screening. Some of the possible diseases may show changes in neuro tests, such as hypothyroid.	Alert and oriented, gait normal. Strength/sensation intact. DTRs 2+. No liver flap.

(continued)

SYSTEM	RATIONALE	FINDINGS
Rectum	Need to obtain stool for occult bleeding.	Normal rectal exam. Small amount brown stool.
Extremities	Basic screen.	Pulses 2+. No edema noted.

● DIFFERENTIAL DIAGNOSES

What are the significant positive and negative findings that support or refute your diagnoses for Rose?

DIAGNOSIS	POSITIVE DATA	NEGATIVE DATA
Anemia	Fatigue, past history of duodenal ulcer.	No active blood loss subjectively or objectively. No pallor.
Viral induced: hepatitis	Incubation period appropriate. Even though no known exposure, certain percentage are unknown etiologies. Mild hepatic tenderness on deep palpation. Liver palpable below costal margin.	No known exposure, not in high risk population or occupation. No splenomegaly. No jaundice. No spider angiomata.
Viral induced: HIV	Fatigue.	No known exposure, not in high-risk population. No weight loss, cough, or dyspnea. No yeast infections. Afebrile.
Viral induced: cytomegalovirus	Vague presentation of symptoms. Mild tenderness of liver with deep palpation.	Afebrile, no dyspnea, no jaundice, no spider angiomata.
Viral induced: Epstein Barr/infectious mononucleosis	Incubation period appropriate, hepatomegaly, fatigue.	Afebrile, no sore throat or palatal petechial rash. No lymphadenopathy, no splenomegaly.
Chronic fatigue syndrome	Fatigue.	Diagnosis of elimination. Although her fatigue is affecting ADLs, it is resolved with bed rest. Decreased libido, < 6 months duration, no change in concentration.

(continued)

DIAGNOSIS	POSITIVE DATA	NEGATIVE DATA
Acquired hypothyroidism	Insidious, vague onset of symptoms, fatigue.	No thyroid enlargement. No skin dryness, no recent change in weight, normal Bms. Normal menses.
Depression	Fatigue, deceased libido.	No sleep disturbances, no crises, no previous history of depression, has interest in daily activities, no sadness, crying.

● DIAGNOSTIC TESTS

Based on the history and physical assessment, what, if any, diagnostic tests would you obtain?

DIAGNOSTIC TEST	RATIONALE	RESULTS
Endoscopy	Not first-line test—would not obtain unless evidence of blood loss (microcytic anemia).	Not done.
CBC with diff	Provides information regarding H/H for anemia, as well as WBC for info about possible infection. H/H will be low if bleeding from GI tract. Lymphocytosis with > 10% atypical cells is characteristic for Epstein-Barr. Leukopenia is common with Hep A.	Hgb: 15.6. Hct: 43.1. WBC: 7.4.
Mono spot	R/O mononucleosis. Mono test is inexpensive and results quickly obtained.	Negative.
CXR	Cytomegalovirus may demonstrate bilateral, diffuse white infiltrates. CXR can wait until you have serology tests back, depending on how strongly you feel the H&P leans toward CMV.	Normal CXR.

(continued)

DIAGNOSTIC TEST	*RATIONALE*	*RESULTS*
Thyroid screen	TSH will be elevated with hypothyroidism. Free T4 will be low in hypothyroidism.	TSH: 4.6. T4: 7.8 U/l.
Electrolytes, renal panel, LFT	Basic screening lab work. Important to do LFT owing to enlargement of liver. AST is maximally elevated in acute phase of hepatitis (>1000) then tapers off. AST and ALT levels do not always correlate with degree of liver damage. Total and direct bili will be elevated with hepatitis. Jaundice usually detectable with total bili levels >2 mg/dL. Jaundice does not reflect disease severity (Norris, 1993).	AST: 60. ALT: 121. Alk Phos: WNL. Total bili: 2.0
HIV	R/O HIV infection.	Negative.
HbsAG	Hepatitis B surface antigen confirms diagnosis of Hep B (Groer & Shekleton, 1979). Anti HBs is detectable later in the convalescence and generally indicates termination of infection.	+HBsAG. Anti HBs neg.
IgM anti Hbc	Hepatitis B core antibodies confirms acute Hep B infection. Occurs early, except in young infants.	Positive.
Liver biopsy	Determines extent of the disease. Not usually performed until the disease is believed to be chronic as defined by clinical history of unresolved symptoms with AST and ALT elevations of 6 months or longer. Does not provide useful prognostic value in acute hepatitis.	Deferred until blood work returns.

● DIAGNOSES

What diagnoses are appropriate for Rose?

Hepatitis B: resolving acute vs chronic
Fatigue

Data Supporting the Diagnosis

Fatigue
Hepatomegaly
Tenderness of liver
Elevated LFTs,
+ Hep B surface
Core antibodies

● THERAPEUTIC PLAN

1. How is hepatitis classified?

	HEPATITIS A	HEPATITIS B	HEPATITIS C	HEPATITIS D	HEPATITIS E
Causative agent	RNA virus	DNA virus with surface and core components	RNA virus	RNA with HBsAG coat	RNA virus
Transmission	Fecal–oral	Parenteral sexual	Parenteral	Parenteral	Fecal–oral contaminated water supply
Incubation	15–50 days	45–180 days	60–180 days	28–180 days	45–60 days
Period of infectivity	Late incubation to early clinical phase	When HBsAG positive	Unknown	When anti-HDV seropositive	Unknown
Chronic state	No	Common	Common	Common	No

Adapted from Shulman S, 1992.

2. What influence does the classification of hepatitis have on the therapeutic treatment plan?

The classification of hepatitis will determine what level of treatment and follow up is needed for Rose.

3. *What will the management of Rose's hepatitis B consist of?*

The main therapeutic plan managing Rose's hepatitis will be to follow her liver enzyme levels and closely observe her symptoms.

The possible treatments for hepatitis consist of:

- Observation: Only with monitoring of the disease process can the decision be made to use interferon. Observation allows the body time to heal itself while eliminating addition side effects or metabolic labor for the liver (i.e., d/c all meds if possible).
- Interferon: The interferon is used to eradicate viral replication and end the chronic hepatitis infection. Common side effects of interferon are flu-like symptoms, especially at initiation of treatment which tend to decrease with continued therapy. The flu-like symptoms can be minimized by being well-hydrated and administering the dose at bedtime. Acetaminophen 30 min before the interferon also may help (Zeldis & Friedman, 1997).

4. *When should Rose be referred to a specialist and to whom?*

If Rose's liver function tests remain elevated or progressively elevate, Rose should be referred to a gastroenterologist for a possible liver biopsy to assess the extent of hepatic damage. If the enzymes continue to be elevated, a liver biopsy will be performed and interferon might be used in an attempt to eradicate viral replication and end the chronic hepatitis infection.

5. *What patient education should you provide for Rose?*

Talk to Rose about the fact that many cases of hepatitis where the etiology is never determined (Shulman, 1992). The liver performs many tasks for the body, such as metabolism and excretion of products for the body (Groer & Shekleton, 1979). It is important not to take any medications unless she checks first with the health care provider. Hepatitis can be transmitted sexually, so condom protection should be used for intercourse. The OCs should be discontinued. Rose should know that the liver is able to withstand and repair damage remarkably. Complete regeneration can occur even when 70% of the liver is destroyed. For this reason it is important to monitor the progression/regression of the disease process so that hepatic fibrosis does not impact on the hepatic architecture and eventually hepatic function.

6. *What impact does this illness have in terms of being contagious to Rose's family, friends, and coworkers?*

The family impact of any infectious disease is worrisome and guilt-provoking if the disease is inadvertently passed on to loved ones. A highly effective HBV vaccine is available. Rose's husband was tested and demonstrated immunity (HBsAG positive). The two children were tested and do not demonstrate immunity. They will be given a course of Hep B immunization injections to attenuate/prevent infection. The United States initiated neonatal hepatitis B immunizations in 1994. Prompt use of hepatitis B hyperimmune globulin (HBIG) and HBV is effective in providing treatment and immunization to unimmunized individuals with needle sticks or sexual exposure, and to neonates with vertical transmission (Zeldis & Friedman, 1997).

7. *What suggestions can you make to Rose for her fatiguability?*

Fatigue is a common symptom of hepatitis; it difficult to manage since there is no specific therapy that can be prescribed. Fatigue will be managed by increasing Rose's knowledge of its etiology and behavioral management, giving her permission and control over it as the primary symptom of hepatitis. Assist Rose in assessing her home/work situation to identify where she can conserve energy. Give her encouragement to ask for help and set up a schedule to get the needed assistance. Since the whole family knows there is a reason for the fatigue, it will be easier to enlist family support for various household tasks.

8. *When should Rose return for follow up?*

Rose will be followed on a monthly basis to assess her symptoms. Obviously, if she presents with an increased severity of symptoms, she will be assessed more frequently. Blood work will be done every 2 months or if the symptoms become worse.

9. *What community resources are available to the NP and Rose?*

> American Liver Foundation
> Hepatitis/Liver Disease Hotline
> 800 223-0179
> (Provides printed material and reference to the nearest support group)
> Local health department

REFERENCES

Groer M, Shekleton M. Disorders of digestions, absorption, excretion, and metabolism, in Groer M, Shekleton M (eds). *Basic Pathophysiology: A Conceptual Approach.* St. Louis: Mosby; 1979; 344–376.

Norris J. Infection, in McMahon E, Ambrose M, Deutsch D (eds). *Diseases.* Springhouse, PA: Springhouse; 1992; 209–211.

Norris, J. Gastrointestinal disorders, in Norris J, et al. (eds). *Diseases.* Springhouse, PA: Springhouse; 1993.

Shulman S. Viral hepatitis, in Shulman S, Phair J, Sommers H (eds). *The Biologic and Clinical Basis of Infectious Diseases.* Philadelphia: W.B. Saunders; 1992; 312–326.

Uphold C, Graham M. *Clinical Guidelines in Family Practice,* 2nd ed. Gainesville, FL: Barmarrae; 1994.

Zeldis J, Friedman, L. Acute and chronic viral hepatitis, in Rakel R (ed). *Conn's Current Therapy.* Philadelphia: Saunders; 1997; 488–495.

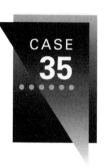

A 68-year-old woman with severe dizziness

SCENARIO

Grace Brown is a 68-year-old, slender Hispanic female who presents with complaints of severe dizziness, nausea, and vomiting. She states she has had bouts of dizziness over a 3-day period, and the nausea had increased to the point that she has had four violent vomiting episodes since awakening early this AM. She complains of weakness.

● TENTATIVE DIAGNOSES

Based on Grace's presentation, what are the tentative differential diagnoses?

● HISTORY

What questions do you want to ask Grace to assist you in developing a diagnosis?

● PHYSICAL ASSESSMENT

1. *What parts of the physical examination are needed?*
2. *Are there any special maneuvers that need to be included in the exam?*

● DIFFERENTIAL DIAGNOSES

What are the significant positive or negative data that support or refute the differential diagnoses for Grace?

● DIAGNOSTIC TESTS

What additional data or diagnostics are needed to confirm the priority diagnosis? Include your rationale for the tests.

● DIAGNOSIS

After combining subjective and objective data with test findings, what is the diagnosis? Identify data that support this diagnosis.

● THERAPEUTIC PLAN

1. *What is the basic teaching you will offer Grace about BPPV?*
2. *What self-care measures would be helpful for Grace in terms of exercise, diet, and monitoring?*
3. *What referrals would be appropriate for Grace?*
4. *What medications might be appropriate for Grace based on the severity of her symptoms?*
5. *What follow up should be planned for Grace?*
6. *What impact might BPPV have on her family? Identify needed education for the family.*
7. *What resources are available to Grace and her family?*

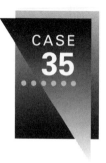

TUTORIAL

A 68-year-old woman with severe dizziness

SCENARIO

Grace Brown is a 68-year-old, slender Hispanic female who presents with complaints of severe dizziness, nausea, and vomiting. She states she has had bouts of dizziness over a 3-day period, and the nausea had increased to the point that she has had four violent vomiting episodes since awakening early this AM. She complains of weakness.

● TENTATIVE DIAGNOSES

Based on Grace's presentation, what are the tentative differential diagnoses?

DIFFERENTIAL DIAGNOSIS   RATIONALE

DIFFERENTIAL DIAGNOSIS	RATIONALE
I. Peripheral vertigo	Peripheral vestibular disorder, trauma, or age-related changes of the inner ear can cause the sensation of spinning or motion.
a. Benign paroxysmal positional vertigo	Accumulation of organic debris in post-semicircular canal. Grace complains of a spinning sensation with position change. All of these symptoms are associated with BPPV.
b. Peripheral vestibulopathy	A spinning sensation of dizziness with nausea is an indicator of vestibulopathy. A primary cause of vestibulopathy is labrynthitis caused by tertiary syphilis.
c. Meniere's disease	Grace complains of dizziness: a symptom of Meniere's disease.

(continued)

DIFFERENTIAL DIAGNOSIS   RATIONALE

d. Post traumatic vertigo	Dizziness can be caused by trauma. Until recent trauma is ruled out, this diagnosis needs to be considered.
e. Ototoxic drugs	Various drugs can cause the adverse effect of dizziness and nausea. Drugs such as aspirin, aminoglycosides should be considered potential causes of dizziness.
II. Central vertigo	Neoplastic and vascular disorder of the lower brain stem and cerebellum can cause unsteadiness, imbalance, and a feeling that a fall is imminent.
a. Acoustic neurinoma	Grace complains of vertigo. One symptom of acoustic neurinoma is dizziness.
b. Vertibrobasilar arterial disease	Hearing loss and vertigo are symptoms of inadequate bloodflow to the brain.
III. Syncope/near syncope	These conditions are caused by cardiovascular, cerebrovascular or psychogenesis with feelings of lightheadedness, fainting, or impending loss of consciousness.
a. Hypotension, from vasodilating drugs and decreased blood volume.	Dizziness and nausea are indicators of hypotension. Until blood loss from recent trauma is ruled out, it must be considered a potential diagnosis.
b. Cardiac disease, such as aortic stenosis, arrhythmia, carotid sinus hypersensitivity, and diminished vascular reflexes of the elderly.	Grace's complaint of dizziness supports the possible diagnosis of cardiac disease. In addition, given her age, cardiac causes need to be considered a possibility of etiology.
c. Metabolic conditions, such as hypo- or hyperglycemia, hypothyroidism, and anemia.	Dizziness is a possible symptom for increased glucose, or decreased glucose or thyroid function. Elderly women are at risk for developing hyperglycemia and hypothyroidism. In addition, anemia with its resultant lowered hemoglobin could cause dizziness and must be considered.
d. Intracranial conditions, such as seizure disorder, migraine, and increased intracranial pressure.	Grace's complaints of dizziness and nausea can be the primary symptoms noted for an intercranial lesion.
e. Psychiatric disorders, such as anxiety, depression, psychosis.	Because you do not know Grace's living situation, coping abilities, or social situation, dizziness and nausea should be considered symptoms of psychiatric disorders. A vague history along with stress can indicate psychogenic disorders (McGee, 1995).

● HISTORY

What questions do you want to ask Grace to assist you in developing a diagnosis?

QUESTION	ANSWER
Allergies?	No known allergies.
Current medications?	Prescribed: Atenolol (Tenormin) 50 mg po qd × 3 years Hydrochlorothiazide 25 mg po qd × 3 years OTC: Tylenol Extra Strength prn for pain (approximately two × month)
When did the symptoms start?	About 3 days ago.
How long does the dizziness last?	Not long—a few seconds, then it stops. Then I feel sick to my stomach.
Do you have a sensation of spinning or the room moving around you?	Mostly spinning, like the room is moving. Then I feel a little off-balance.
Does any certain movement precipitate the dizziness?	It seems to start first thing in the morning when I roll over to get out of bed. And then, when I try to lay down on the couch because I'm sick at my stomach, the dizziness starts over again.
Do you have any changes in vision with the dizziness?	No.
Elimination	Denies problems with urinating. Denies dark, tarry, or bloody stools.
Have you had any other illness in the past 3 months?	No.
Do you have any pain with the dizziness?	No.
Do you have any loss of balance with the dizziness or any loss of consciousness (Ruchenstein, 1995)?	No.
Have you noticed any hearing loss or ringing in your ears?	My daughter says I'm getting hard of hearing, but I haven't noticed it getting worse. No ringing of the ears.
Difficulty walking or weakness?	I feel weak today because I can't keep anything down. I've thrown up four times today. It is difficult to walk when you are so dizzy and sick.

(continued)

QUESTION	ANSWER
Any history of seizures or convulsions?	No.
Have you hit your head lately or been in any kind of accident where you might have hit your head?	No.
Do you feel like you're going to pass out or faint?	No.
Any history of heart disease for you or your family?	No.
Have you ever had this type of dizziness before?	No.
Describe your diet for the past 24 hours.	Breakfast: One piece toast, cup of hot tea. Lunch: Sliced tomato and tuna with crackers, glass of milk. Dinner: Chicken and rice frozen dinner, tea.
Have you been able to maintain your normal activities since you have been sick?	Can't do my volunteer job at the library. I've had to call in sick the last 3 days. When I bend over to clean up at the bathroom sink, I feel like the dizziness is going to start again, and I just can't get any of my housework or yard-work done. My neighbor and I take a walk every night after dinner, and I haven't felt like doing that.
Do you live alone?	Yes, my husband passed on 8 years ago. I stay busy with my friends and children, and I do volunteer at the local library a few hours in the mornings. I love books and I love to read. I'm usually able to drive, but today felt too sick to drive.
Have you had a recent weight gain or loss?	No.
Do you have any problems sleeping?	I usually get 7–8 hours a night. Haven't had any problems with sleeping, but in the last couple of days, I have this dizziness in bed sometimes, especially when I roll over to look at the clock. It makes getting to sleep hard.

Social habits
  Tobacco:
  ETOH:
	
	No.
	Occasionally have a cocktail when out to dinner with friends one to two × month.

● PHYSICAL ASSESSMENT

What parts of the physical examination are needed?

EXAMINATION	RATIONALE	FINDINGS
Vital signs	Baseline information. Orthostatics indicated for hypovolemia.	Supine BP RA: 136/88 LA 138/88, HR 76 Standing BP RA: 134/86 LA: 136/86 Standing BP RA: 134/86 HR: 78 Resp: 20 Temp: 97.4°F oral
Skin and mucous membranes	Check for hydration status.	Pale, dry, turgor fair. Mucus membranes and nailbeds pink. No jaundice, bruising, spider angiomas noted.
Eye	Indicated to check for visual changes as well as spontaneous nystagmus in both peripheral and central vestibular dysfunction. Also important to evaluate secondary to HTN (Williams et al., 1994).	No AV nicking. No exudate, hemorrhage noted. Disk well marginated. EOMs intact, peripheral vision intact. Visual acuity OD 20/40, OS 20/30 corrected with glasses.
Ear	Indicated for evaluation of hearing loss, a symptom of Meniere's syndrome.	Denies tenderness of external ear. TM's gray, light reflex present. Rinne/Weber WNL hearing handicap inventory for the elderly—score of 6—A score of 8 shows probable. Screening version hearing loss.
Neck	Indicated to check for bruit, which may be a manifestation of blockage of vessels, and a cause of dizziness.	Thyroid nonpalpable. No venous hum over neck vessels, no carotid bruits heard.
Chest	Baseline data.	Clear to auscultation.
Heart	Baseline data. Allows for evaluation of irregular heart rhythm that may have impact on dizziness, as well as CHF resulting from HTN.	S_1 and S_2 within normal limits. No murmur or extra heart sounds auscultated.

(continued)

EXAMINATION	*RATIONALE*	*FINDINGS*
Abdomen	Important to evaluate because of nausea and vomiting.	Soft, nontender BS + in all quads. No hepato or splenomegaly. No bruits.
Neurological	Important data related to chief complaint.	Alert and oriented x 3. CN I-VII, IX-XII intact. VIII diminished bilaterally to whisper test. No spontaneous nystagmus. Motor function/muscle strength gait normal. Romberg test negative. DTRs 2+ Heel/toe walking normal, slow on turn. Extremities equal in strength. Sensory function: intact pain discrimination in all extremities.

Are there any special manuevers that need to be included in the exam?

SPECIAL MANUEVER	*RESULTS*	*RATIONALE*
Barany maneuver (Hallpike Dix)	Barany maneuver. Nystagmus elicited in 10 seconds with head turned 45 degrees to the right. Nystagmus movement: upward fashion toward the right ear.	Allows for observation of nystagmus, dizziness, and vertigo when head is rotated into a horizontal position with the affected posterior semicircular canal 30–45 degrees below the horizontal plane. Direction of nystagmus helps to distinguish BPPV from other types of positional vertigo. Nystagmus goes counterclockwise when the Rt. ear canal is abnormal and clockwise when the Lt. ear is abnormal (Ojaln & Palo, 1991).

● DIFFERENTIAL DIAGNOSES

What are the significant positive or negative data that support or refute the differential diagnoses for Grace?

DIFFERENTIAL DIAGNOSES	POSITIVE DATA	NEGATIVE DATA
Benign positional vertigo	Positive: Spinning sensation of dizziness with positional change. Nausea. Positive nystagmus elicited with Barany maneuver.	Hearing deficit.
Peripheral vestibulopathy	Spinning sensation of dizziness with nausea.	TM's gray, with light reflex present. No erythema or exudate of oropharynx. Nasal passages normal. Breath sounds clear. Abdomen soft, nontender. No hearing deficit. No spontaneous nystagmus.
Meniere's disease	Vertigo.	Tinnitus, ear discomfort, tandem gait normal. No hearing deficit.
Post traumatic vertigo		No history of recent trauma to head, fall or whiplash type injury. No Battle's sign.
Ototoxic drugs	Atenolol and HTCZ both have the possible adverse effects of dizziness and N/V.	No history of taking aminoglycosides, salicylates, ethacrynic acid, or furosemide. Tinnitus, Rinne and Weber tests normal.
Acoustic neuroma	Vertigo.	No unsteadiness or loss of balance when upright, no unilateral hearing loss, tinnitus, V and VII cranial nerves intact.
Vertibrobasilar arterial disease	Weakness, vertigo, nausea, and vomiting.	No visual changes, perioral numbness, clumsiness, ataxia, unilateral hearing loss.

(continued)

DIFFERENTIAL DIAGNOSES	POSITIVE DATA	NEGATIVE DATA
Volume depletion/anemia	Nutritional intake history, vertigo, weakness, nausea and vomiting. Diuretic: hydrochlorothiazide.	Fair skin turgor; B/P and P within normal range; no significant orthostasis; mucus membranes and nailbeds pink.
Cardiac disease, hypotension, arrhythmia, syncope		Vital signs stable, no significant orthostasis, HR regular, S_1S_2 without murmur, denies fainting feeling or LOC.
Cerebellar disease	Vertigo, N/V.	No truncal ataxia.
Hypothryoidism	Vertigo, weakness.	No weight gain, hoarseness, depression, bradycardia, thickened skin, hypersomnia.
Psychiatric illness	At-risk because living alone, loss of spouse, advanced age.	No history of recent stress, no vague history, denies depressed mood, weight gain or loss, sleep disturbances, impaired concentration, or substance abuse.

● DIAGNOSTIC TESTS

What additional data or diagnostics are needed to confirm the priority diagnosis? Include your rationale for the tests.

DIAGNOSTIC TEST	RATIONALE	RESULTS
Vestibulo-ocular reflex evaluation (VOR)	Blurring occurs as well as image movement with head movement. With loss of VOR function, visual acuity decreases by more than one line on the Snellen chart during passive horizontal and vertical head oscillations. VOR deficits are owing	Not done.

(continued)

DIAGNOSTIC TEST	RATIONALE	RESULTS
	to bilateral labrynthine damage, usually the result of ototoxic drugs.	
Caloric test	Normal response with use of WARM water is nystagmus toward warm irrigation. Normal response with use of COLD water is nystagmus away from cold irrigation. This test causes profound discomfort and nausea.	Not done.
TSH	Vertigo and decreased hearing may be symptoms of hypothyroidism. If elevated, suspect hypothyroidism.	1.3 mU/L.
HGB/HCT	To check for anemia as possible cause of vertigo. Further testing with CBC is warranted if any abnormalities are found.	12.5/38.
Fasting blood sugar	Initial screening for diabetes mellitus.	92 mg/dL.
Electronystagmography	Useful in Meniere's disease and persistent BPPV to determine the degree and progression of vestibular deficit, side affected, and surgical intervention if called for. Done by audiologist on referral. Also provides objective data for cases with client with psychogenic vertigo who need reassurance that no organic diseases are present.	Not done.
MRI	Very expensive. Indicated if diagnosis of central vertigo is suspected. Small lesions can cause significant symptoms. Bone structures can cause artifact with CT scans, and enhanced resolution makes MRI preferable to CT (Weinstein & Devons, 1995).	Not done.

(continued)

DIAGNOSTIC TEST	RATIONALE	RESULTS
FTA-ABS	Inflammatory labyrinthitis may be caused by syphilis, and nontreponemal tests may be negative in tertiary syphilis. Patients with symptoms of peripheral vertigo should be screened for syphilis.	Negative.
Audiometry with speech discrimination	Provides screening for acoustic neuroma hearing loss of Meniere's disease.	Not done.
ECG/Holter monitor	Allows for identification of cardiac arrhythmias.	Not done.

● DIAGNOSIS

After combining subjective and objective data with test findings, what is the diagnosis? Identify data that support this diagnosis.

DIAGNOSES	RATIONALE
Benign paroxysmal positional vertigo (BPPV)	Hallpike-Dix /Barany maneuver is positive for latent nystagmus elicited with upward movement, and torsionally counterclockwise toward the right ear. Episodes of dizziness do not last more than 1 minute individually, though the episodes have occurred in clusters in the past 3 days. No neurological signs found, indicating more serious illness (Neatherlin et al., 1994).

● THERAPEUTIC PLAN

1. What is the basic teaching you will offer Grace about BPPV?

A. Most cases of BPPV are self-limiting in weeks to months.

B. Some people with BPPV have a course of remissions and reoccurrence for months to years.

C. Some have permanent symptoms, and they may be candidates for surgery (Clark, 1994).

   D. Follow-up visits may be necessary if present symptoms do not subside, and will be extremely important if other accompanying symptoms should occur. Atypical results of follow-up assessment may indicate need for referral.
   E. Periods of dizziness and associated nausea from BPPV usually are very brief and intense, and use of sedating medications can cause impaired mental alertness and clarity, with a resulting change in lifestyle for this active woman.

2. *What self-care measures would be helpful for Grace in terms of:*

   A. Exercise: Positional exercises (Brandt's exercises) should be taught to the patient, and prescribed to be done every 3 hours or 3 times a day until symptom-free for 2 consecutive days. Exercises that can be performed by an otolaryngologist or a neurologist are the Liberatory Maneuver of Siment and/or the Canolith Repositioning Procedure. These exercises are done in an effort to move free-floating deposits out of the semicircular canal (Brandt & Darof, 1980).
   B. Diet: A diet low in Na^+ and MSG may benefit Grace. Both of these lead to fluid retention and increase the production and retention of endolymph, which deflates the cupula of the semicircular canal.
   C. Monitoring: Teach Grace to keep a log of activities and symptoms, so that she learns which movements should be adjusted.

3. *What referrals would be appropriate for Grace?*

   Refer to audiologist for hearing loss determination.

4. *What medications might be appropriate for Grace based on the severity of her symptoms?*

   Treatment with an antivertigo medication may provide relief of symptoms, although it remains controversial owing to the side effects, especially in the elderly.

   First- and second-line choices:

   Meclazine (Antivert) 25–100 mg/day in divided doses
   Antihistamine, antiemetic
   Dimenhydrinate (Dramamine) 50–100 mg po, antiemetic
   Diphenidol (Vontrol) 25–50 mg po, antiemetic
   Diazepam (Valium) CNS depressant
   Scopolamine, anticholinergic

   These medications have adverse effects of dizziness, drowsiness, ataxia, sedation, and scopolamine may cause depressed respirations.

5. *What follow up should be planned for Grace?*

   Test results of TSH, HCT, blood glucose, FTA-ABS per phone call if normal as soon as results are available. Follow up in 2–4 weeks after prescribing at-home Brandt's exercises and diet changes for re-evaluation, looking for evidence of other causes of vertigo.

Serial follow-up visits to reevaluate, looking for evidence of other possible causes of dizziness. If at-home exercises and diet changes have not alleviated the symptoms, may refer to audiologist, otolaryngologist, or neurologist for further testing/treatment. Surgical follow-up for clients whose dizziness and accompanying symptoms are chronic may include posterior semicircular canal occlusion, and laser partitioning of the labyrinth to create semicircular occlusion.

6. *What impact might BPPV have on her family? Identify needed education for the family.*

   - Teach family about the nature of BPPV, and exercises that may relieve the vertigo.
   - Follow up should occur earlier than the 2–4 wk appointment if symptoms worsen or continue for a prolonged period, or if other symptoms appear.
   - If medication is prescribed, family should be educated on possible side effects, especially of sedation and possible respiratory depression. Family may need to stay with Grace when medicated to monitor ambulation, as she would be at high risk for falls.
   - Family/friends may be needed to do grocery shopping, essential errands until episodes have been abolished. For safety reasons, she should not drive at this time, nor while taking antivertigo medication.
   - Teach about prognosis and alternatives to care.
   - Teach family to be supportive of Grace's continuing her present active independent lifestyle as much as possible (Barker et al., 1995).

7. *What resources are available to Grace and her family?*

   Vestibular Disorders Association
   PO Box 4467
   Portland, OR 97208-4467
   (503) 229-7705
   Call or write for further educational materials for client and family.

REFERENCES

Barker L, Burton J, Zieve P. *Principles of Ambulatory Medicine,* 4th ed. Baltimore: Williams & Wilkins; 1995; 1198–1207.

Brandt T, Darof R. Physical therapy for benign paroxysmal positional vertigo. *Arch Otolaryngol* 1980; 106: 484–485.

Clark M. Chronic dizziness: An integrated approach. *Hosp Pract* 1994; 29: 57–64.

McGee S. Dizzy patients: Diagnosis and treatment. *W J Med* 1995; 162: 37–42.

Neatherlin J, Egan J. Benign paroxysmal positional vertigo. *J Neurosci Nurs,* 1994; 26: 330–335.

Ojaln M, Palo J. The aetiology of dizziness and how to examine a dizzy patient. *Ann Med,* 1991; 23: 22–230.

Ruchenstein M. A practical approach to dizziness. Questions to bring vertigo and other causes into focus. *Postgrad Med,* 1995; 97: 70–81.

Weinstein B, Devons C. The dizzy patient: stepwise workup of a common complaint. *Geriatrics* 1995; 50: 42–50.

Williams J, Schneiderman H, Algranati P. *Physical Diagnoses: Bedside Evaluation of Diagnosis and function.* Baltimore: Williams & Wilkins; 1994; 156, 158.

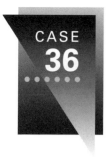

A 36-year-old woman with lower back pain

SCENARIO

Joan Beckett, a 36-year-old Caucasian female, presents with the chief complaint of lower back pain. She called this morning saying she needed to be seen because she was in so much pain that she could not work and she needed a work excuse.

● TENTATIVE DIAGNOSES

What are the potential diagnoses you have identified based on Joan's brief history?

● HISTORY

1. *What additional information do you need before making a diagnosis?*
2. *What information do you need regarding Joan's employment?*
3. *What are Joan's risk factors associated with lower back pain?*
4. *Does Joan have any "red flags" for potentially serious conditions related to lower back pain in her history?*

● PHYSICAL ASSESSMENT

1. *Is a complete physical exam necessary?*
2. *What parts of the exam would you include and why?*
3. *What are specific tests for malingering?*
4. *Does Joan have any "red flags" for potentially serious conditions related to lower back pain in her physical exam?*

● DIFFERENTIAL DIAGNOSES

List and prioritize your most probable differential diagnoses. With each diagnosis, list the positive and negative data that validate or refute the diagnoses.

● DIAGNOSTIC TESTS

What, if any, additional data should be obtained? Would any diagnostic tests be appropriate in this case? Include your rationale for the tests.

● DIAGNOSIS

What is your conclusive diagnosis? What positive and negative data assisted you in arriving at your decision?

● THERAPEUTIC PLAN

1. *What group of pharmacologic agents would you use for Joan, if any?*
2. *What is your rationale for choosing these particular agents?*
3. *What are some alternatives to this treatment? Include nonpharmacological alternatives.*
4. *What ergonomic issues need to be examined in Joan's job? How might they be addressed?*
5. *What patient education does Joan need?*
6. *What follow-up care will Joan need?*

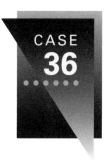

TUTORIAL

A 36-year-old woman with lower back pain

SCENARIO

Joan Beckett, a 36-year-old Caucasian female, presents with the chief complaint of lower back pain. She called this morning saying she needed to be seen because she was in so much pain that she could not work and she needed a work excuse.

● TENTATIVE DIAGNOSES

What are the potential diagnoses you have identified based on Joan's brief history?

DIFFERENTIAL DIAGNOSES   RATIONALE

DIFFERENTIAL DIAGNOSES	RATIONALE
Lumbosacral strain	Most common cause of back pain. Joan c/o lower back pain.
Herniated lumbar disc	A common cause of back pain. Joan c/o lower back pain.
Sciatica	Lower back pain could be due to sciatica.
Possible vertebral fracture	Back pain could be caused by fracture. Need to determine if Joan had recent trauma to back.
Possible tumor or infection	One of serious conditions that need to be r/o as a possible cause of back pain.
Possible cauda equina syndrome	A serious neurological condition that needs to be r/o with every case of back pain.
Abdominal aortic aneurysm	Back pain could be related to AAA, although it is unlikely in some one of her age. Needs to be r/o.

(continued)

DIFFERENTIAL DIAGNOSES   *RATIONALE*

Malingering	Back pain is a frequent excuse for people not to go to work or to seek narcotics or muscle relaxants.
Substance abuse	Back pain is a frequent excuse for people not to go to work or to seek drugs.

● HISTORY

1. *What additional information do you need before making a diagnosis?*
2. *What information do you need regarding Joan's employment?*
3. *What are Joan's risk factors associated with lower back pain?*
4. *Does Joan have any "red flags" for potentially serious conditions related to lower back pain in her history?*

REQUESTED DATA   *DATA ANSWER*

Allergies	NKDA.
Medication	None.
Recent changes in health	None.
Chief complaint/present illness Onset, location, quality, aggravating/alleviating factors	Joan described noticing a minor pain in her back the evening before while at work. She went to sleep as usual; however, when she awakened she was in a lot of pain and was very stiff. The pain was described as a "bad aching" but was worse in the Rt lumbosacral area. The pain radiated to her Rt buttock. It hurt her to stand up or find a comfortable position. Pain worsens after bending or lifting. The ache is present even at rest, but worsens with movement.
Associated manifestations	No history of UTI symptoms. No vaginal discharge or dyspareunia. No change in bowel or bladder habits. Denies weight loss or fever.
History of previous back pain/ injury/trauma	None.
Risk factors for back pain	Works at local garment factory where she stands most of the day and lifts bundles of fabrics. No previous history of back injury.
Past medical history	Normally healthy. No hospitalizations or surgeries. G1P1.

(continued)

REQUESTED DATA	DATA ANSWER
History of back injuries/problems in family members	Her older brother injured his back while stocking grocery shelves. He recovered without any difficulty and returned to work.
Ability to pay for care	In debt "way over her head." No health insurance benefits.
"Red flags" for potentially serious back problems	Denies muscle weakness, paresthesia, loss of sensations, no severe or progressive neurological deficit in lower extremity. No history of cancer, or risk factors for spinal infection (no IV drug abuse, UTI, immune suppression).
Family system	Single mom. Ex-husband not involved financially or physically in care of child. Parents live 100 miles away. One brother in town. Joan only has a few close friends. She has no church involvement.
Support systems	Few friends, not close; sees brother seldom.
Satisfaction with job	Sees job only as a means of providing income for her and her daughter.
Coping abilities	Considers herself a strong and independent woman.

● PHYSICAL ASSESSMENT

1. *Is a complete physical exam necessary?*
2. *What parts of the exam would you include and why?*
3. *What are specific tests for malingering?*
4. *Does Joan have any "red flags" for potentially serious conditions related to lower back pain in her physical exam?*

SYSTEM	FINDINGS	RATIONALE
Skin	Skin is pink and supple, no lesions noted.	Overall quick assessment of visible skin should be performed. Particular attention should be given to the face.
Heart sounds	S_1S_2 normal, without murmur.	Provides baseline information.
Breath sounds	Clear to auscultation.	Allows the NP to determine if there has been respiratory involvement.

(continued)

SYSTEM	FINDINGS	RATIONALE
Vital Signs	T: (oral) 98^8 HR: 86 RR: 20 BP: 134/84 Wt: 175 Ht: 63"	Gives an indication of possible infection.
Gait/posture	Flexed forward at 15 degrees, walked slowly with a wide-based stance, and grimaced with movement. Heel and toe walking intact.	Important to evaluate gait/posture because back pain is chief complaint.
Spinal column	No kyphosis, scoliosis, or lordosis; unable to extend or rotate. Lateral movement: bilaterally to 20 degrees. All attempts at ROM produced pain. Rt. Paravertebral muscle spasm noted in lumbar area.	Important to evaluate spinal column because back pain is chief complaint.
Neurological	DTRs: patellar, Achilles 2+; strength of lower extremities equal bilaterally, vibratory and proprioceptive sensation intact bilaterally. Full ROM of hip and knee. Normal plantar flexion.	Information allows the NP to r/o disc or other joint involvement as factors causing symptoms.
Traction maneuvers	SLR negative, Patrick test negative, crossed SLR negative.	Allows the NP to determine the probability of disc involvement as a cause of symptoms.
Malingering tests	No overreaction, negative axial loading, distracted SLR negative, Magnuson's test reproducible, no unusual motor or sensory findings. No "giving way" of any muscles.	Provides information to help determine if Joan is faking symptoms for possible secondary gain.
"Red flags"	No laxity of anal sphincter, no sensory or perineal sensory loss. No noted major motor weakness: knee extension, ankle plantar flexors, evertors, and dorsiflexors.	Helps r/o potentially serious conditions, such as cauda equina syndrome or nerve compression.

● DIFFERENTIAL DIAGNOSES

List and prioritize your most probable differential diagnoses. With each diagnosis, list the positive and negative data that validate or refute the diagnosis.

DIAGNOSIS	POSITIVE DATA	NEGATIVE DATA
Acute lumbosacral strain	Minimal discomfort initially followed by increased pain and stiffness 12–36 hours later, SLR, crossed SLR, heel and toe walking were intact. All malingering tests were negative. No muscular weakness or loss of sensation. DTRs were equal and not depressed. Babinski negative. Spasms noted in paravertebral muscles.	Pain in buttocks.
Herniated lumbar disc	Pain in buttocks.	SLR and crossed SLR, no muscular weakness or loss of sensation. DTRs equal and WNL.
Sciatica	Pain in back/buttocks.	No lower limb symptoms suggesting lumbosacral nerve root compromise.
Possible vertebral fracture	Low back pain.	No history of major trauma, minor trauma.
Possible tumor or infection	Low back pain.	Age not over 50, no history of cancer, no recent fever, chills, or unexplained weight loss. No risk factors for spinal infection (UTI, IVDA, immune suppression). Pain does not increase when supine.
Possible cauda equina syndrome	Low back pain.	No loss of bowel or bladder function. No saddle anesthesia loss of sensation. No progressive loss of neurological function in lower extremity. No laxity of anal sphincter or other indications of major motor weakness.

(continued)

DIAGNOSIS	POSITIVE DATA	NEGATIVE DATA
Abdominal aortic aneurysm	None.	No increase in abdominal aorta width. No lateral pulsations.
Malingering	None.	No overreaction, negative axial loading, distracted SLR negative, Magnuson's test reproducible, no unusual motor or sensory findings. No "giving way" of any muscles.
Substance abuse	None.	Denies substance abuse. No history of prior substance abuse. No indications of malingering.

● DIAGNOSTIC TESTS

What if any, additional data should be obtained? Would any diagnostic tests be appropriate in this case? Include your rationale for the tests.

DIAGNOSTIC TEST	RATIONALE	RESULTS
None needed	Because of the diagnosis of acute lumbosacral strain without radicular pain, no radiographic tests were necessary. Magnetic resonance imaging (MRI) is able to detect anatomical lesions in the lumbar spine with greater sensitivity than other radiographic techniques (Barker, Burton, and Zieve, 1995), but because of expense, a decision for utilization of this technique should be held in reserve for those persons exhibiting signs of nerve root irritation. Also, as there were no acute constitutional symptoms, there is no need for labora-	No tests done.

(continued)

DIAGNOSTIC TEST	RATIONALE	RESULTS
	tory tests. Had there been any of the above, consultation or referral to a physician would have been necessary.	

● DIAGNOSIS

What is your conclusive diagnosis? What positive and negative data assisted you in arriving at your decision?

DIAGNOSIS	RATIONALE
Acute lumbosacral strain	Minimal discomfort initially followed by increased pain and stiffness 12–36 hours later, -SLR, -crossed SLR, heel and toe walking were intact. All malingering tests were negative. No muscular weakness or loss of sensation. DTRs were equal and not depressed. Babinski negative. Spasms noted in paravertebral muscles.

● THERAPEUTIC PLAN

1. What group of pharmacologic agents would you use for Joan, if any?

Joan is probably most interested in relief of pain. Nonprescription drugs such as acetaminophen, aspirin, and ibuprofen will provide relief for most persons. If these analgesics are not effective, other nonsteroidals (NSAIDS) with a rapid onset of action are appropriate (Barker, Burton, and Zieve, 1994; Gorroll, May, and Mulley, 1995; Tierney, McPhee, and Papadakis, 1996). Muscle relaxants appear to be no more effective than NSAIDS (Bigos et al., 1994) and should be reserved for those whom NSAIDS do not help (Gorroll, May, and Mulley, 1995). When muscle relaxants are used they should be limited to courses of 1–2 weeks, and they should be avoided in older patients who are at risk of falling (Gorroll, May, and Mulley, 1995). Opiates usually are not necessary in the management of lumbosacral strain. If opiates are used, they should be taken for only a short period of time. Poor patient tolerance, risk of drowsiness, decreased reaction time, clouded judgment, and potential misuse/dependence have been reported in up to 35% of patients (Bigos et al., 1994).

2. What is your rationale for choosing these particular agents?

NSAIDs usually are effective for low back patients that are able to take them. They are appropriate for use with back strain because they are anti-inflammatories and will help decrease inflammation through the inhibition of prostaglandins.

3. What are some alternatives to this treatment? Include nonpharmacological alternatives.

Up to 90% of persons with a diagnosis of lumbosacral strain respond to a course of conservative therapy (Barker, Burton, and Zieve, 1994), and recover completely by 4 weeks (Gillette, 1996a). Most patients will not require bed rest. Recent studies demonstrate that no bed rest and continuation of daily activities as tolerated is preferred. Bed rest is reserved for those persons with more severe leg pain (Bigos et al., 1994; Gillette, 1996b; Tierney, McPhee, and Papadakis, 1996).

Until Ms. Beckett returns to her usual activities, aerobic (endurance) conditioning exercises such as walking, swimming, stationery biking, or even light jogging may be recommended to avoid debilitation. The level of activity prescription will depend on her level of activity prior to low back pain (i.e., Ms. Beckett was sedentary, so walking was recommended).

Aerobic exercises may be started in the first 2 weeks, with a goal of 20–30 minutes daily. Ms. Beckett understands that even though her symptoms may increase initially, she should work through the pain unless it is intolerable (Bigos et al., 1994).

Ms. Beckett said she had a back belt worn earlier by her brother and asked if it would help. The NP explained that back corsets and belts are not beneficial; their only benefit is in reminding the person wearing them to use proper body mechanics. Other therapies that are of no benefit include shoe lifts (unless the legs are of differing lengths), biofeedback, and TENS units. Hand-held electrical stimulators appear to cause the release of endorphins, which may decrease the need for medication.

Other therapies provide some relief, if used for 3 weeks or less and are utilized as an adjunct to prescribed therapy; these adjunct therapies include ultrasound and massage. Manipulation, if desired, has been found to be safe and effective in the first month (Bigos et al., 1994). Local application of ice may help initially in decreasing both edema and pain; after 2–3 days, either heat or ice may be applied (Gillette, 1996b).

4. What ergonomic issues need to be examined in Joan's job? How might they be addressed?

Ms. Beckett, because of her job, would increase stress on her back by bending, twisting, and lifting; therefore, she may need 3–7 days off work, or she may be able to perform other duties until her symptoms abate. Once Ms. Beckett returns to her usual work routine, the NP recommends that she rest one foot at a time on a low stool and to change feet every 15–20 minutes to relieve stress on her back. Guidelines for sitting and unassisted lifting should be followed in planning care. If sitting, chairs with straight backs or lumbar supports are preferred. Knees should be higher than hips. While driving to work, Ms. Beckett is encouraged to position her seat so that she is not stretching to grasp the steering wheel.

5. *What patient education does Joan need?*

The management plan and its discussion is the time to go over the expected outcomes for the complaint. The discussion should include the expected course of the problem, when the patient may return to work, and what are the likely scenarios if the recovery does not go as expected. This is also an excellent time to discuss any compliance issues that may have arisen with prior treatment(s) and if compliance was a problem discuss the reason(s). A *brief* assessment of family, support systems, difficulty taking or getting medications or treatments, financial, and transportation resources can also be performed at this time.

Sleeping may be facilitated by lying on either side with knees flexed. Pillows under the head or between the knees do not interfere. Ms. Beckett said she slept on her back so the NP recommended that she put pillows under her knees and a small pillow under her lower back.

One of the most important aspects of care provided by the NP involves prevention. NPs should teach proper body mechanics involved in lifting; stress weight loss if necessary, and encourage overall muscular conditioning.

Available community resources may include physical therapists, exercise programs, swimming pools, and walking trails. Some resources are too difficult to access or expensive for persons to incorporate in their care, so education is invaluable in assisting the person to assume responsibility for his or her own care.

6. *What follow-up care will Joan need?*

Acute lumbosacral strain usually resolves rapidly and the person is able to return to his or her usual activities (Deen, 1996), but some may perceive it as catastrophic and disabling, and this perception may have a negative impact on efforts to get better (Gillette, 1996a). Effective management of persons who exhibit chronic pain behavior test the provider's patience and skill. Attempting to build a trusting relationship and encouraging the person to take on responsibility for self-care minimize the chance of dependence. Those persons whose symptoms do not improve and progress to chronic disorder represent only one-tenth of the total number of persons with low back pain, but represent a health care and social problem of alarming dimensions (Gillette, 1996a).

The NP should inquire about the person's job satisfaction, as this is the single most important predictive factor in returning to work (Weinstock and Neids, 1996). Other stressors also affect progress: prior personal and family responses to illness, support systems, access to resources, financial well-being, locus of control, and coping methods. The NP, by assessing the person holistically and emphasizing self-care and education, is an ideal provider to guide the person with low back pain to more positive ways of thinking.

The NP schedules Ms. Beckett to return in 2 weeks, but she also tells her that if she has questions or feels she is not improving to call for an earlier appointment.

REFERENCES

Barker LR, Burton JR, Zieve PD (eds). *Principles of Ambulatory Medicine.* Baltimore: Williams & Wilkins; 1995.

Bigos BS, Bowyer RO, Braen G, Brown KC, Deyo RA, Haldeman S, et al. Acute low back problems in adults. *Clinical Practice Guideline, Quick Reference Guide, Number 14,* Rockville, MD: U.S. Department of Health and Human Services, Public Health Service, Agency for Health Care Policy and Research, AHCPR Pub. No. 95-0643; 1994.

Deen HG. Concise review for primary care physicians. *Mayo Clin Proc* 1996; 71: 283–287.

Gillette RD. Behavioral factors in the management of back pain. *Am Fam Phys* 1996a; 53: 1313–1318.

Gillette RD. A practical approach to the patient with back pain. *Am Fam Phys* 1996b; 53: 670–676.

Gorroll AH, May LA, Mulley AG (eds). *Primary Care Management.* Washington: American Psychological Association; 1995.

Tierney LM, McPhee SJ, Papadakis MA (eds). Current Medical Diagnosis and Treatment. Norwalk, CT: Appleton & Lange; 1996.

Weinstock MB, Neides DM (eds). The Resident's Guide to Ambulatory Care. Columbus, OH: Anadem Publishing; 1996.

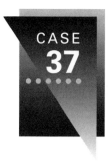

A 65-year-old man with elevated blood pressure

SCENARIO

Denzel Armstrong is an obese 65-year-old African-American male who is new to the clinic. His previous physician retired 1 year ago and he is now seeking care for his hypertension. He also has complaints of urinary frequency and nocturia three to four times/night for 2 weeks. He denies dysuria or fever, but admits to urgency and mildly decreased force of stream. Denzel reports 8–12 bathroom visits per day. He denies previous problems with urination and states that his only medical problem is high blood pressure, for which he takes hydrochlorothiazide 25 mg/day.

● TENTATIVE DIAGNOSES

Based on Denzel's presentation, what are your tentative differential diagnoses?

● HISTORY

What questions do you want to ask Denzel to assist you in developing a diagnosis?

● PHYSICAL ASSESSMENT

Based on the subjective data you have obtained, what parts of the physical examination should be performed and why?

● DIFFERENTIAL DIAGNOSES

Examine all the data up to this point. Link the subjective and objective data to the appropriate differential diagnosis. Identify both positive and negative data that support or refute the diagnoses.

● DIAGNOSTIC TESTS

What additional data and/or diagnostic tests need to be performed to confirm the diagnosis and assist in the development of the plan of care?

● DIAGNOSIS

What is your conclusive diagnosis? What was your rationale to support the diagnosis?

● THERAPEUTIC PLAN

1. *What are issues that need to be considered when deciding on treatment?*
2. *What is the goal B/P to strive for?*
3. *What choices are available relative to pharmacologic therapy? What is the rationale behind choosing the antihypertensive agent?*
4. *What counseling should be done relative to dietary changes that need to be made?*
5. *What recommendations would you give prior to Denzel beginning an exercise regimen?*
6. *What other preventive medications would you have Denzel begin?*
7. *What is the influence of his COPD, BPH, and NIDDM relative to his HTN? Discuss each diagnosis and indicate your plan of care for each.*
8. *What alternative treatments might be appropriate to assist Denzel in the overall treatment plan?*
9. *When should Denzel come back for follow up?*
10. *On a return visit 1 week later, Denzel's B/P is 146/90 sitting and standing. His fasting blood sugar is 142. What changes would you make to the plan of care based on this information?*
11. *What would a long-term therapeutic plan look like for Denzel?*
12. *What impact might the diagnoses of HTN and NIDDM have on Denzel's family?*
13. *What resources are available for Mr. Armstrong related to his HTN and DM?*
14. *What other health care professionals might be consulted to develop a holistic treatment plan for Denzel?*

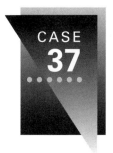

TUTORIAL

A 65-year-old man with elevated blood pressure

SCENARIO

Denzel Armstrong is an obese 65-year-old African-American male who is new to the clinic. His previous physician retired 1 year ago and he is now seeking care for his hypertension. He also has complaints of urinary frequency and nocturia three to four times/night for 2 weeks. He denies dysuria or fever, but admits to urgency and mildly decreased force of stream. Denzel reports 8–12 bathroom visits per day. He denies previous problems with urination and states that his only medical problem is high blood pressure, for which he takes hydrochlorothiazide 25 mg/day.

● TENTATIVE DIAGNOSES

Based on Denzel's presentation, what are your tentative differential diagnoses?

DIFFERENTIAL DIAGNOSES	RATIONALE
Hypertension (HTN)	Denzel states he has had high blood pressure for a while. He is not sure when it was diagnosed. He currently takes medications for HTN.
Benign prostatic hyper-plasia (BPH)	Mr. Armstrong is complaining of polyuria, nocturia, and a decrease in his urinary stream. He may have BPH because he is a male over the age of 50.
Diabetes mellitus—non-insulin dependent (NIDDM)	NIDDM needs to be considered for Denzel because he is complaining of polyuria and nocturia. He is also obese, which is a sign of NIDDM.
Obesity	Denzel appears overweight. No information is available yet concerning his lifestyle or diet.

(continued)

DIFFERENTIAL DIAGNOSES	*RATIONALE*
Urinary tract infection (UTI)	Denzel complains of urinary frequency and urgency with a recent onset, all symptoms of a UTI.

● HISTORY

What questions do you want to ask Denzel to assist you in developing a diagnosis?

REQUESTED DATA	*DATA ANSWER*
Allergies	None.
Medications	HCTZ 25 mg QD. Albuterol MDI 2 puffs QID prn. Denies OTC medications.
Childhood diseases	Measles, chicken pox.
Immunizations	Yearly influenza vaccine. Cannot remember last tetanus shot. Had negative TB test at age 20 (military). No Pneumovax.
Surgery	None.
Transfusions/hospitalizations	None.
Fractures/injuries	None.
Adult illness	Bronchitis every winter.
Last PE	One year ago with retired MD. B/P was okay using medicine. No rectal exam.
Dental exam	2 years ago.
Vision exam	2 years ago. Denies blurring, wears reading glasses.
Weight	Denies change in weight.
Appetite	Hungry all the time, has a sweet tooth.
Thirst	Complains of dry mouth, drinks pop, lemonade, and sweetened ice tea all day long (10–15 glasses).
Urination	C/o frequency, urgency, and decreased force of stream. Denies dysuria, hematuria, foul odor, or cloudy urine. States this has occurred over the past year and

(continued)

REQUESTED DATA   DATA ANSWER

REQUESTED DATA	DATA ANSWER
	worsened in the past 2 wks. Denies prior UTI or STD, no history of prostate exam or problems. Worried that he has sugar diabetes because of all the urination.
Past history of HTN	Diagnosed with HTN 12 yrs ago, on HCTZ for past 4 years. Has B/P checked at senior center two to three times each year, and it has been good. One B/P was 160/96.
24-Hour diet recall	B: Two eggs, bacon, three toast with jelly, oatmeal with sugar, juice. L: Cheese sandwich, cookies, grapes, juice, lemonade. S: Chocolate candies (whole bag), chips, sodas (four to six) sweetened ice tea (three to four). D: Pork chops (three), rice, gravy, corn, bread, ice tea, banana. S: Cake and ice cream before bed. Eats what he wants—no diet followed.
Describe breathing problems you have had	SOB increases with exertion, able to walk four to five blocks before SOB. No paroxysmal nocturnal dyspnea. AM cough with production four to five × per year when sick; no hospitalization, no children with asthma. Denies occupational exposure to asbestos, chemicals, dust, or second-hand smoke. Smoked one pack/day for 25 years; quit smoking 20 years ago.
Family history	Father: Died at 59 of heart problems. Mother: Died at 68 of stroke and sugar. Never took insulin. Siblings: Brother, age 57 with HTN; sister, age 59, sugar and breast CA; sister, age 63, living and well. Cousin with IDDM. Children: Four, all living and well.
Social history	Married × 43 years. Wife does all cooking and shopping. Wife is good, supportive, and monogamous, in good health. He is retired truck driver. Four children and 10 grandchildren. Close family with grandchildren visiting frequently. Has lots of candy around for the children. Social activity is full with family. Feels his life is happy.
Lifestyle	No exercise: walks dog 1×/day. No alcohol except special occasions. Smoked 25 pack years/quit 20 years ago.
Sleep	Sleeps about 6 hours/night; only interrupted to urinate. Occasional naps in front of TV.
Religion/spirituality	"Churchgoing" Christian.
Income/insurance	Retired on fixed income < $25,000; owns home. Medicare A and B.

(continued)

REQUESTED DATA	*DATA ANSWER*
Preventive measures	Wears seat belt, smoke detector in home and changes battery each Christmas. No guns in house, railings on steps, no scatter rugs. House in good repair.
Review of systems	Denies numbness/tingling/swelling in hands/feet. Denies chest pain (Lowther et al., 1991).

● PHYSICAL ASSESSMENT

Based on the subjective data you have obtained, what parts of the physical exam should be performed and why?

SYSTEM	*RATIONALE*	*FINDINGS*
Vital signs	Baseline information	B/P: 160/100 RA: sitting and standing, large cuff. 164/92 LA sitting. P: 72 R: 18. Height: 5'10". Weight: 221 lbs. Temp: 97.8°F.
Skin	Important to look for any lesions with his hyperglycemia symptoms.	Warm, dry, without lesions, scars.
HEENT	Important to evaluate eyes in terms of fundus for hemorrhage, AV nicking because of longstanding history of HTN	Normocephalic, PERRLA, EOMs intact, fundoscopic: Red reflex present, no nicking or hemorrhage. TM intact bilaterally. Pharynx: swallows without difficulty, no erythema; Neck: thyroid nonpalpable, no carotid bruits.
Lungs	Recent addition of MDI for medication. Need to evaluate chest for problems.	AP/Lateral diameter WNL, slight wheeze on forced expiration, clear to auscultation, no prolonged expiration, resonance to percussion.

(continued)

SYSTEM	RATIONALE	FINDINGS
Cardiovascular	Important to evaluate heart size, rate, rhythm because of HTN.	Regular rate and rhythm, no murmurs or gallops; peripheral pulses 2+, no peripheral edema.
Abdomen	With history of HTN, important to evaluate for bruits and organomegaly.	BS present, obese, no organomegaly or masses, no abdominal bruits.
Rectum	Need to evaluate because he is c/o frequency and nocturia.	Prostate firm, slightly enlarged without nodule; no masses. Negative for occult blood.
Neurologic	Important to evaluate because he may have NIDDM.	Alert and oriented, gait coordinated; perceives light touch and pain in extremities bilaterally; vibratory sense intact; no apparent neurological deficits. Brachial and patellar DTRs 2+.
Feet	Important area to evaluate since he may have NIDDM.	No open areas, no excessive callus formation. Nails in good repair.

● DIFFERENTIAL DIAGNOSES

Examine all the data up to this point. Link the subjective and objective data to the appropriate differential diagnosis. Identify both positive and negative data that support or refute the diagnoses.

DIAGNOSIS	POSITIVE DATA	NEGATIVE DATA
HTN	Previous diagnosis. B/P reading 164/90.	No target organ damage.
DM	Polyuria, polydipsia, polyphagia, obese, elderly African-American, + family history, inactivity, diet high in sugar.	No peripheral neuropathy, no visual changes, no weight loss.
BPH	Enlarged prostate, nocturia, frequency, decreased force of stream, elderly male.	No history of prostate problems or prior UTI, no family history of prostate CA, no incontinence.

(continued)

DIAGNOSIS	POSITIVE DATA	NEGATIVE DATA
UTI	C/o urinary frequency, urgency, enlarged prostate.	No dysuria, fever, hematuria, cloudy or smelly urine.
COPD	History of smoking 25 years, expiratory wheeze, frequent bronchitis, + response to bronchodilator.	Normal AP/lateral diameter. No prolonged expiration, no hyperresonance on percussion.
Obesity	Ht: 5'10". Wt: 221. High-calorie diet, inactivity.	

● DIAGNOSTIC TESTS

What additional data and/or diagnostic tests need to be performed to confirm the diagnosis and assist in the development of the plan of care?

DIAGNOSTIC TEST	RATIONALE	RESULTS
CBC	May identify anemia or polycythemia as a cause of SOB. Baseline data for future changes.	HGB: 14. HCT: 45. WBC: 6.2. RBC: 4.5. Platelets: 323.
Glycosylated hemoglobin	Gives a picture of the range of blood sugars during the past 3 months.	HgbA1C: 9.8.
Renal panel, including FBS, BUN, creatinine	Fasting glucose >140 strong indicator of DM. BUN and creatinine may be elevated with nephropathy and end organ damage from HTN; sodium and potassium may be abnormal with diuretic use and dehydration.	Glucose: 175. Sodium: 143. Potassium: 3.8. Chloride: 101. Co2: 23. BUN: 11. Creatinine: 0.8.
Calcium/magnesium	Calcium deficiency is associated with increased prevalence of HTN. Magnesium deficiency may also be associated with HTN.	Calcium: 9.0. Magnesium: 2.1.
Uric acid	Increased level may indicate impaired renal function.	Uric acid: 5.3.

(continued)

DIAGNOSTIC TEST	RATIONALE	RESULTS
Thyroid function (T$_4$ and TSH)	Hyperthyroidism causes increased cardiac output that tends to increase systolic pressures.	WNL.
Lipids	Fasting cholesterol, HDL, Triglycerides and LDL are indicators of cardiovascular risk. Increased risk is present in someone with HTN, DM, inactivity and high-fat caloric diet.	Cholesterol: 209. Triglycerides: 244. HDL: 36. LDL: 167.
Prostate specific antigen (PSA)	May be elevated in prostate cancer.	PSA: 2.0.
Urinalysis	Leukocytes, nitrites, RBCs are indicators of infection. Glucose may be present in DM and protein in renal dysfunction.	Hazy appearance, pH 5.5, protein negative, glucose 500 mg/dL, ketone negative, bilirubin negative, blood negative, no leukocytes, no nitrites; urobilinogen 0.2 mg/dL, specific gravity: 1.010.
Liver function tests	Baseline before initiating any hepatotoxic drugs like lipid lowering agents or weight loss medication.	WNL.
EKG	Good indicator of left ventricular hypertrophy, ischemic changes or arrhythmias.	NSR, minimal voltage criteria for LVH.
CXR	Shows any cardiac enlargement as well as pulmonary changes.	No evidence of cardiomegaly, early changes associated with COPD.

● DIAGNOSIS

What is your conclusive diagnosis? What was your rationale to support the diagnoses?

   A. Hypertension
      1. BP elevated on two occasions on HCTZ
      2. EKG: minimal voltage criteria for LVH, NSR
      3. CXR: no evidence of cardiomegaly
      4. U/A: negative protein, neg. blood

     5. Renal: WNL for sodium, potassium, chloride, BUN, creatinine

     6. Calcium, magnesium, uric acid WNL

     7. CBC: WNL

     8. No evidence of target organ involvement of kidneys, eyes, or brain

     9. Obesity

   10. High sodium diet and inactivity (SHEP, 1991)

 B. Diabetes mellitus

     1. Fasting blood glucose and U/A glucose elevated

     2. Obesity

     3. Subjectively, polyuria, polydipsia, polyphagia; inactivity

     4. High sugar/calorie diet; family history of diabetes

 C. Obesity

     1. Weight greater than 20-30% of ideal body weight (IBW) is considered obese

     2. Lipid profile: cholesterol minimally elevated

     3. Admits to high-calorie, high-fat, hig-sodium diet and inactivity

 D. COPD

     1. CXR: early changes associated with emphysema

     2. Wheezing on forced expiration

     3. Subjectively, history of 25 pack years tobacco smoking, DOE, response to bronchodilators

 E. BPH

     1. PSA 2.0

     2. Prostate slightly enlarged on rectal exam

     3. Subjectively, decreased force of stream (FOS) and frequency of urination; nocturia

     4. Elderly male

● THERAPEUTIC PLAN

1. What are issues that need to be considered when deciding on treatment?

   1. Knowledge deficit: Denzel needs to be assessed for interest in education and understanding of chronic illnesses, dietary restrictions, and lifestyle modifications and taught based on assessment.

   2. Family support: Family also needs to be assessed and educated to offer support and encouragement. If Mrs. A. does most of the grocery shopping and meal planning, then her assistance is crucial to this patient's compliance with any dietary restrictions.

   3. Motivation: Patient's motivation level needs to be assessed and his willingness to try lifestyle changes and medication options.

2. What is the goal B/P to strive for?

Hypertension: Denzel needs to have his BP 130/85 or less (BP goal is lowered because of concomitant condition of diabetes) (National HBP Education Working Group, 1994).

3. *What choices are available relative to pharmacologic therapy? What is the rationale behind choosing the antihypertensive agent?*

The B/P goal is not being accomplished with the HCTZ 25 mg QD, and the diuretic may be aggravating the urinary frequency and may worsen glucose tolerance, increase insulin resistance, and raise fasting blood sugar. Reduction in sodium intake and loss of weight may be sufficient to control blood pressure in some patients. It may be helpful to discontinue the HCTZ and start an angiotension converting enzyme (ACE) inhibitor. ACE inhibitors have been found to reduce proteinuria and renal damage and slow the loss of renal function in diabetic hypertensive patients. Beta-blockers should be avoided in patients with COPD as bronchial constriction may be worsened, and in patients with DM, hypoglycemic symptoms may be masked and glucose tolerance decreased (Joint National Committee, 1993).

Stop HCTZ and start Lisinopril 5 mg QD. Monitor renal function and serum potassium closely while on ACE inhibitor.

4. *What counseling should be done relative to dietary changes that need to be made?*

Dietary counseling to reduce weight, sodium, fat; no salt shaker, limit fast foods and prepared foods; use frozen or fresh vegetables and fruits rather than canned; skim and trim fat from foods; limit fried foods; read labels for calories, fat, and sodium content. Consider a dietitian/nutritional counseling referral.

Limit ETOH to 1 oz ethanol (2 oz of whiskey, 8 oz wine, or 24 oz beer) per day should he decide to drink ETOH socially.

5. *What recommendations would you give prior to Denzel beginning an exercise regimen?*

Plan to begin exercise slowly with increasing aerobic activity as tolerated. Walking 15 minutes per day is a good starting plan.

6. *What other preventive medications would you have Denzel begin?*

ASA 325 mg QD. ASA recommended as prevention for MI and CVA.

7. *What is the influence of his COPD, BPH, and NIDDM relative to his HTN? Discuss each diagnosis and indicate your plan of care for each.*

A. Diabetes: Denzel needs to have his HgbA1C (glycosylated hemoglobin) within normal range of 4-8. As patient has not been previously diagnosed, nonpharmacological interventions of diet, exercise, and weight control are recommended initially. Help the patient to understand the chronic nature of diabetes with long-term commitment to lifestyle change to maximize health. Reinforcement with educational literature and motivation needs to be done at each visit.

1. Start on sugar/calorie restricted diet; eliminate simple sugars such as soda, candy, pastry, ETOH, and encourage complex carbohydrates, protein, and fresh fruit and vegetables. Artificial sweeteners can be used in moderation.
2. No hypoglycemics will be started for Mr. A. until trial of diet and exercise for several months.
3. Refer for annual eye exam to rule out diabetic retinopathy.
4. Foot and skin examination at each visit and encourage patient to do checks daily. Diabetics have delayed wound healing and are more likely to be unaware of injuries because of peripheral neuropathy.

B. Obesity: Denzel needs to reduce weight to decrease hypertension, and lower blood sugar and lipids. Weight loss is potentially the most important intervention for diabetics to reduce morbidity and mortality. The combination of diet modification and exercise program is critical to successful weight loss.
1. Referral to a dietitian is often needed. Continued support of the patient by professional and family is needed for this difficult lifestyle change. Support groups such as Overeaters Anonymous, Weight Watchers, and walking groups are helpful.

C. COPD: Denzel needs to be aware of chronic nature of COPD, the need to try to prevent pulmonary infection and to report change in color, amount, and consistency of sputum or need for increased use of inhaler.
1. Influenza vaccination yearly and pneumococcal vaccination once.
2. Exercise to increase tolerance of activity and reduction of O_2 consumption.
3. Avoid environmental pollutants, such as tobacco smoke.
4. Continue use of Albuterol inhaler qid, prn.
5. If symptoms worsen, PFT's may be a helpful diagnostic test.

D. BPH: Denzel needs to be aware of signs and symptoms of obstruction if condition worsens, such as UTI, retention, decreased flow, and post-voiding fullness.
1. Yearly rectal exam and PSA.
2. May consider use of Hytrin, a long-acting Alpha-1 blocker beginning with 0.5 mg at bedtime as the initial dose (caution: first dose hypotension) and may increase to 2–10 mg at hs. This category of drug may relieve some of the symptoms of BPH and in the case of Mr. A, may also further reduce blood pressure.

8. *What alternative treatments might be appropriate to assist Denzel in the overall treatment plan?*
   • Relaxation techniques, such as therapeutic touch, biofeedback, visualization, prayer, meditation, Tai Chi, music, Yoga may promote health through stress reduction.

- Health food supplements: Although research does not support the efficacy of herbal substances for the treatment of hypertension, diabetes, or obesity, encourage patients to discuss anecdotal information about the use of herbs and their health effects.

9. *When should Denzel come back for follow up?*

   Denzel was treated with Lisinopril 5 mg QD and educated about lifestyle modifications of diet and exercise and health maintenance activities for risk factor reduction. He was given pneumovax and tetanus booster and will receive a flu vaccine in the Fall. He is to continue Albuterol inhaler, prn. He will return to the clinic in 1 week for fasting blood sugar, renal panel, and blood pressure check (Uphold & Graham, 1994).

10. *On a return visit 1 week later, Denzel's B/P is 146/90 sitting and standing. His fasting blood sugar is 142. What changes would you make to the plan of care based on this information?*

    - On the return visit, Mr. A's weight is unchanged although he claimed to be following diet and exercise plan. BP: 146/90 sitting and standing; potassium: 4.1; creatinine: 0.8, and BUN: 12; FBS is 142.
    - Increase Lisinopril to 10 mg QD.
    - Nutrition consult and encourage patient to bring his wife.
    - Offer encouragement and reinforce need to persevere with plan for health.
    - RTC in 4 weeks for BP check, weight, fasting finger stick for glucose.
    - Explore how he feels about change in lifestyle, health belief, and locus of control; discuss risk factors.
    - Encourage patient to bring wife and family to clinic visits (WHO/ISH, 1993).

11. *What would a long-term therapeutic plan look like for Denzel?*

    - Long-term follow up will depend on progress toward control of blood pressure and blood sugar, reduction of weight, and adequacy of exercise. ACE inhibitor dosage may need to be increased or a second drug such as calcium channel blocker may be needed. May consider adding Hytrin as described earlier. Oral hypoglycemic agent may be needed if blood sugar does not normalize with nonpharmacological intervention. Since major lifestyle change is required, allow ample time for patient and family to adjust (Kaplan, 1994).

12. *What impact might the diagnoses of HTN and NIDDM have for Denzel's family?*

    - Mr. A. has indicated that his wife and family are supportive of him. Because Mrs. A. does the shopping and preparation of food it is important to have her present for clinic and dietitian meetings. She will need to be well informed and supportive of Denzel's lifestyle changes, but should expect him to be responsible for his health behaviors. Feelings about the future health and well being of the family given his diagnosis should be explored. Each family member should be informed not only about Denzel's condition and needs, but also about each of their needs for health care maintenance and disease prevention. Discussion of clinic and community support services should be discussed with the family (Sadowski & Redeker, 1996).

13. *What resources are available for Mr. Armstrong related to his HTN and DM?*

   • Information about health concerns of Denzel can be obtained from community organizations such as The American Diabetes Association, American Heart Association, American Lung Association, American Dietetic Association, National Institutes of Health, Heart, Blood and Lung Institute, and exercise support groups.

14. *What other health care professionals might be consulted to develop a holistic treatment plan for Denzel?*

   • Interdisciplinary collaboration may include nurse, physican, health educator, dietitian, pharmacist, podiatrist, ophthalmologist, exercise physiologist, psychologist, social worker, and urologist. There are numerous professionals at hospital and community organizations to provide supportive health care to Denzel and his family.

REFERENCES

Joint National Committee. *The fifth report of the joint national committee on detection, evaluation, and treatment of high blood pressure.* Bethesda, MD: National Institutes of Health, 1993.

Kaplan NM. *Clinical Hypertension,* 6th ed. Baltimore, MD: Williams & Wilkins, 1994.

Lowther N, Carter V, Herrmann J. Hypertension, in Baas L. (ed). *Essentials of Cardiovascular Nursing.* Gaithersburg, MD: Aspen; 1991.

National High Blood Pressure Education Program Working Group. National high blood pressure education program working group report on hypertension in diabetes. *Hypertension* 1994; 23:145.

Sadowski A, Redeker N. The hypertensive elder: A review for the primary care provider. *Nurse Pract* 1996; 21:99.

Systolic Hypertension in the Elderly Program (SHEP) Cooperative Research Group. Prevention of stroke by antihypertensive drug treatment in older persons with isolated systolic hypertension. *JAMA* 1991; 265:3255.

Uphold C, Graham M. *Clinical Guidelines in Adult Health.* Gainesville, FL: Barmarrae Books; 1994.

WHO/ISH. Guidelines for the management of mild hypertension. Memorandum from a world health organization/international society of hypertension meetings. *J Hypertens* 1993; 11:95.

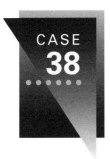

A 2-year-old boy presents for a well-child visit

Max Ingram is a 24-month-old Caucasian male. He has been brought to clinic for his "checkup and shots." His family is new to the area and this is his first time to be seen in this facility. His mother did not bring any prior medical records along other than his immunization booklet.

● TENTATIVE DIAGNOSES

Based on the information provided so far, what are potential differential diagnoses?

● HISTORY

1. *What are significant questions in Max's history?*
2. *What are the key points to cover on the review of systems?*

● PHYSICAL ASSESSMENT

What are the significant portions of the physical examination that should be completed for Max?

● DIFFERENTIAL DIAGNOSES

What are the significant positive and negative data that support or refute your diagnoses for Max?

● DIAGNOSTIC TESTS

Based on the history and physical assessment, what, if any, diagnostic tests would you obtain? Include your rationale for the tests.

● DIAGNOSIS

What diagnoses are appropriate for Max?

● THERAPEUTIC PLAN

1. *What anticipatory guidance will you review with Max's mother?*
2. *What anticipatory guidance would you review with Max's mother based on their recent move?*
3. *When should Max return for follow up?*

TUTORIAL

A 2-year-old boy presents for a well-child visit

SCENARIO

Max Ingram is a 24-month-old Caucasian male. He has been brought to clinic for his "checkup and shots." His family is new to the area and this is his first time to be seen in this facility. His mother did not bring any prior medical records along other than his immunization booklet.

● TENTATIVE DIAGNOSES

Based on the information provided so far, what are potential differential diagnoses?

DIAGNOSIS	*RATIONALE*
Potential diagnoses are not applicable at this point	Inadequate database. Unless there are ill visits this may be the only opportunity to see Max. A complete health assessment identifies immediate problems and establishes a baseline against which future changes are evaluated. There is no reference point at this time.

● HISTORY

1. What are significant questions in Max's history?

REQUESTED DATA	RESPONSE
Reason for contact	"Checkup and shots."
Past health history	Seen by family practice physician for all routine and episodic health care at clinic where family resided prior to this—never been to ED.
Childhood illnesses	Denies having chicken pox or other xanthemous diseases.
PMH	About three episodes of fever with vomiting and diarrhea when began daycare. Per advice of clinic, did not need to be seen by physician (did not last beyond 24 hrs). Treated with diet and Kaopectate. Recent cold (3 mos. ago)—took to physician, was prescribed "pink" antibiotics—claims completed until finished. Does not know name of medicine.
Birth history	Prenatal: Planned pregnancy, P2G2. Prenatal care initiated in first trimester—no complications. Prenatal vitamins. Denies use of alcohol, drugs, and tobacco. L&D: Full-term, 18 hr. labor, vaginal delivery with epidural. Weight: 8 lbs. 11 oz. Length: 20.5 in. APGAR unknown but states infant cried vigorously at birth. Postnatal: Some jaundice, did not require phototherapy. Formula-fed, tolerated well. Went home with mother after 24 hours.
Newborn history	Newborn: Denies problems with feeding, sleeping, behavior. "Easy baby, ate well, and gained weight."
Current health	Other that episodes of ear infections and recent cold—"healthy."
Allergies	Denies food, drug, or environmental allergies.
Medications	Denies use of vitamins. Gives one full dropper of Tylenol for comfort and fever only with ear infections—not with teething.
Immunizations	2 mos. HBV, DPT, Hib, OPV. 4 mos. HBV, DPT, Hib, OPV. 6 mos. DTP, OPV. 12 mos. Hib. 15 mos. HBV, DTP, MMR, TB Tine.

(continued)

REQUESTED DATA   RESPONSE

Developmental history	Growth: 24 lbs., 30 in. at 1 year.
Milestones	**Gross Motor:** Rolled over at 4 mos., sat alone at 6 mos., crawled at 10 mos., walked at 13–14 mos., runs and kicks. **Fine Motor:** Feeding self at 1 yr., uses spoon and fingers to eat, scribbles. **Language:** Saying words at 1 yr., three to four word sentences at present, "understands everything." **Personal-Social:** Responsive smile at 2 mos. Plays interactively with brother and parents—ball, tag, hides. Imitates parent activity, tries to help.
Habits	Pacifier much of waking time—especially if tired/irritable. If pacifier not available, does not appear to substitute thumb.
Sleep	Sleeps about 9 PM to 7 AM, seldom awakens. Usually naps 1–4 PM. Moved from crib to twin bed about 1 mo. ago—was starting to climb out of crib. Never sleeps with parents, has own bedroom. Has bedtime routine of bath, snack, brushing teeth, story. Has night light and security blanket that he sleeps with.
Temperament	Generally in a happy mood. Fussy if tired, and has begun to refuse to cooperate on occassions. Has never been disciplined.
Diet history	Formula during first year. Initiated baby foods at 4 mos. Off bottle completely by 15 mos. Feeds self with some assistance. Table foods at present—prefers grains and fruits, eats vegetables. Mother knows food pyramid and tries to offer variety, though meat, bread, and potatoes are staple. Family eats meals out 1–2 days per week, usually fastfood. One to two cups 2% milk, and two to three cups juice daily—sometimes substitutes Kool-Aid. Eats sweets though seldom offered. Appetite not as good as usual, getting "picky."
24-Hour intake	B: 1/2 cup cereal + 1/2 cup milk, 1/2 cup orange juice S: 1/2 bananna + 1/2 cup milk L: 1/2 hot dog (refused bun), 1/2 banana, 1 cup "Juicy Juice" S: 2 peanut butter cookies, 1/2 cup "Juicy Juice" D: 1/4 bologna sandwich, 1/2 cup applesauce, 1/2 cup milk B: 1/2 cup milk, 1/2 cup "Juicy Juice" States as a "pretty good day" for child. Dinner atypical owing to recent move, usually has hot meal.

(continued)

REQUESTED DATA	*RESPONSE*
Family health history	PGF: Deceased at 65 yrs. from stroke—had hypertension. Was heavy smoker. PGM: Mid 60's, mild hypertension, and smokes. Otherwise good health. MGF: Deceased at 65 yrs. from liver cancer. Also had heart attack 2–3 yrs. prior. Smoked entire adult life. Notable family history for lung cancer and eczema. MGM: 62 yrs., severe arthitis, hypertension—family history of mental illness—mood disorders. Father: 30 yrs., good health. Mother: 29 yrs., good health. Brother: 5 yrs., good health.
Social history	Both parents high-school educated. Father works assembly equipment, mother is a secretary.
Relationship with sibling	Relationship with older brother is good—play and interact well. Has been in daycare since 6 mos. Will continue to attend same facility, which is near mother's work.
Relationship with family	Relationships with extended family are good—is one reason for moving closer. Grandmothers and parents' siblings regularly help with children. Family socializes frequently.
Environmental history	Family rented an old farmhouse about 50 miles away but moved because of buying a newer home, to be in safer community and closer to families, and reduce commute to jobs. Has taken precautions in past to store cleaning and other supplies away from children. Has not yet in new home—still in process of moving everything, is "hectic." New home built in 1950s, is on corner lot, street is moderately busy. Yard is fenced with gate that can be locked, and is in good condition. Previous owners left sandbox, swing set.

2. *What are the key points on the review of systems?*

SYSTEM REVIEWED	*DATA ANSWER*
General	Denies any physical concerns at this time—is aware of potential hearing loss associated with ear infections but feels this is not a concern.

(continued)

SYSTEM REVIEWED   *DATA ANSWER*

SYSTEM REVIEWED	DATA ANSWER
HEENT	Denies problems with clumsiness or falling or visual difficulties.
Ears	Seems to hear OK—cleans ears daily with cotton swabs. Otitis media ×4.
Mouth	Stuffiness/discharge with cold. Teething uneventful—scrubs teeth for child once daily. Unsure whether water is fluoridated.
Cardiorespiratory	Denies SOB, wheezing, change in color, or difficulty with exertion. No known heart murmur or anemia.
Gastrointestinal	Generally good appetite, no colic as infant. Denies food intolerances. Minor bouts with vomiting and diarrhea (see Past Health History). Two bowel movements daily—soft and formed, does not strain. Beginning to notify adults when diaper soiled.
Genitourinary	Circumcised at birth. Denies difficulty with urination—color pale and nonmalodorous. Beginning to remain dry for longer periods though seldom dry in the morning.
Neuromusculoskeletal	Denies problems with gait, balance, coordination, or weakness. Executes gross and fine motor activities with ease expected for age. Unable to identify hand preference. Denies joint problems.
Skin and endocrine	Denies unusual skin discoloration or pigmentation. Only rash occured in buttocks region with diarrhea. Denies dry, itchy, or scaling skin. Bathed with hair washed daily to every other day. Denies temperature intolerances, though describes as a "hot" child. Is very warm at night and sweats mildly—damp in morning.

● PHYSICAL ASSESSMENT

What are the significant portions of the physical examination that should be completed for Max?

SYSTEM	RATIONALE	FINDINGS
Vital signs	Provides baseline data.	B/P: unable to obtain due to child's protests T: 99.8°F P: 128 R: 30
Growth	Provides baseline data.	Weight: 31 lbs. (<90th percentile) Length: 36 in. (>75th percentile) Head circumference = 51 cm. (90th percentile).
General appearance	Provides overall view of patient's status.	Well-developed white male. Is clean, appropriately attired, color pink, and appears well-nourished. Skin is warm, dry, and supple, no diaphoresis or lesions noted. Behavior and appearance consistent with stated age of 24 mos.—content to be seated in mother's lap, curious, and mildly wary of examiner.
HEENT	Because this is a well check-up, it is important to conduct athorough exam to make sure all systems are intact.	Normocephalic. Hair light brown, evenly colored and distributed, clean, and soft. No scalp lesions or pediculosis. Facial symmetry at rest and with movement. Trachea ML, shoddy tonsilar nodes, remaining nonpalpable. Full AROM. Perpherial eye structures unremarkable. Conjuntivae pink, sclerae white. Reflex blink intact, corneal light reflexes correspond, EOMs ×6. Red reflex present bilaterally. Small ears, normal alignment. No external le- *(continued)*

SYSTEM	*RATIONALE*	*FINDINGS*
		sions, swelling, or erythema. Canals clean, no redness. TMs intact, pearly gray, and mobile. Light reflects normally bilaterally. Turns to voice. Nares symmetrical, patent, no drainage. Tongue ML, pink, with normal rugae. 16 deciduous teeth, aligned, clean, no caries noted. No posterior molar eruption. Gums, oral mucosa, and pharynx pink and unremarkable. Tonsils +1–2. Uvula ML and gag reflex intact.
Lungs	Provide baseline info about breathing.	Breathing easy and regular, no retracting. Thorax symmetrical, 1:1 AP:lateral ratio. Resonant to percussion and clear to auscultation throughout.
Heart	Provide baseline information about cardiovascular status.	Sinus arrythymia with inspiratory S2 split. No murmurs noted.
Abdomen	Allows for exam of abdominal organs, looking for masses or organomegaly.	Protuberant, umbilicus ML, inverted, no herniation. No vascular patterns noted. Active bowel sounds, pitch moderate. No masses or enlargement, liver at RCM.
Genitalia	Provides information about care of genitalia, particularly in light of circumcision. Also indicates whether testes have descended.	Unremarkable male anatomy. Circumcised, testicles decended bilaterally, moderate scrotal rugae.
Neurologic	Neurological screen indicates how well system has matured and developed.	CN II, III, IV, VI, VIII, X, XII intact CN V, VII, XI—symmetry observed CN I and IX not assessed. Alert, oriented to name and place—is "at doctor's." Displays characteristic behaviors for age. Tandem, coordinated gait. Jumps in place, kicks ball. In supine,

(continued)

SYSTEM	*RATIONALE*	*FINDINGS*
		curls at ML to sit then stand. Sensory deferred. DTRs 2+. Babinski negative.
Extremities	Combined neurological and cardiovascular screen for arms and legs.	Gross AROM is symmetrical and without obvious weakness or discomfort. Flexes elbows and supinates hands without difficulty or complaint of discomfort. Slightly wide-based gait with medial weight-bearing and mild pronation. No visible or palpable joint swelling or anomolies. Spine straight, negative Trendelenburg. Capillary refill less than 3 seconds ×4. Pulses 2+.
Developmental		DDST II normal.

● DIFFERENTIAL DIAGNOSES

What are the significant positive and negative findings that support or refute your diagnoses for Max?

DIAGNOSIS	*POSITIVE DATA*	*NEGATIVE DATA*
Well 2-year-old exam	Max has completed all immunizations and developmental milestones appropriate for his age.	

● DIAGNOSTIC TESTS

Based on the history and physical assessment, what, if any, diagnostic tests would you do? Include your rationale for the tests.

DIAGNOSTIC TEST	RATIONALE	RESULTS
Lead level	Annual lead screening is advised for children 9 mos. to 6 yrs. who are at risk for lead toxicity. This family lived in an old farmhouse before their move, and have moved into one built in the 1950s. Prior to 1950 paint contained lead, and 70% of houses built prior to 1960 are estimated to have lead paint (Center for Disease Control, 1991).	3 µg/dL.
Hematocrit or hemoglobin	Iron deficiency anemia occurs most commonly between 9 and 24 mos. Max's milk intake is not excessive. (Greater than 1 quart/day is a common cause.) However, he is not receiving vitamin supplements, and his eating patterns have changed. Routine screening is recommended during early childhood or preschool visits (American Academy of Pediatrics Committe on Practice and Ambulatory Medicine, 1991).	Hct: 38%. Hgb: 12 g/dL.
Screening audiogram	Follow up to infection and evaluation of hearing loss is routine. Max's history of language and speech development is well within normal limits, as was the physical exam. Thus screening rather than diagnostic testing is suggested.	Normal.

● DIAGNOSIS

What diagnoses are appropriate for Max?

Well child exam: 2 years

● THERAPEUTIC PLAN

1. What anticipatory guidance will you discuss with Max's mother?

AREA — ANTICIPATORY GUIDANCE

AREA	ANTICIPATORY GUIDANCE
Development	Behavior changes that accompany a child's transition into toddlerhood need to be discussed and/or reinforced. The tendency to react to situations with intensity and negativity should be explored with Mrs. Ingram. Her expectations and her understanding of normal changes and temperament associated with toddlerhood, as well as her approach to discipline should likewise be assessed (Dixon & Stein, 1992).
Safety	Poisoning, burns, drowning, and motor vehicle accidents comprise the major safety risks for this age group. Choking is less of a concern but warrants consideration. Toddlers are seeking to become more autonomous. Thus, they tend to become adventuresome and yet are too immature to recognize the inherent dangers in most situations.
	Mrs. Ingram should be encouraged to take the necessary precautions to prevent Max from accessing cleaning supplies, medications, and other solvents and/or chemicals (e.g., that might be located in the garage and basement). The local poison control number should be provided to her.
	Turning the hot water heater down to 140 degrees helps to prevent burns from tub faucets. Taking precautions to keep hot pots and pans from the edge of the stove can help prevent Max from pulling hot contents down onto himself.
	Toddlers need to be constantly supervised around pools and in the bath. Due to their low center of gravity, it is also possible for toddlers to topple into toilets and large, deep water pails and become trapped and drown.
	Max should be closely supervised outdoors especially given the corner location the new home and report of moderate traffic. The history did not indicate the Ingram's utilization of car seats. The need to be consistent with the use of car seats should be stressed. Guidelines for appropriate safety seat selection and placement should be provided to Mrs. Ingram.
	Max's toys and environment still needs to be monitored for small objects that he might place in his mouth. Buttons, small toys, and toy parts, balloons, and such are common considerations. Food risks continue to be hot dog chunks, peanuts, and the like. Counsel Mrs. Ingram accordingly and provide her with information regarding CPR and choking rescue techniques (Boynton, 1994).

(continued)

AREA	ANTICIPATORY GUIDANCE

Behavior and discipline

Confronting testing behaviors with consistent responses, and timeout for repeated unacceptable social behavior is recommended for children at this age. If the family employs corporal discipline, it is only recommended to deter persistent behavior that threatens the child's physical safety (such as teasing a dog).

When toddlers are able to successfully partake in daily rituals, especially those associated with routines accompanying meals and bedtime, it helps them to achieve and maintain a sense of autonomy and control. Reinforce Mrs. Ingram's ongoing use of rituals with Max. In addition, she can further facilitate Max's autonomy by encouraging him partake in simple daily activities such as getting out eating utensils at mealtime. Although he is too young to independently assume responsibility for daily chores, he should be coaxed to start helping with simple tasks such as placing his dirty clothes in the hamper following baths (Burns et al., 1996).

Toilet training

Review Mrs. Ingram's knowledge of readiness for toilet training, and her anticipated approach. In light of the family's recent move, any thoughts Mrs. Ingram may have about initiating training might be postponed for a few months. Physical and psychological readiness is usually present by the end of the second year. Max displays some signs of readiness—intact necessary gross motor skills of walking and sitting, regular bowel movements, increasing periods of dryness, and notifying adults of having defecated. As he begins to remain dry for longer periods and more consistently on waking, demonstrates curiosity regarding his brother's and/or parent's toileting, and begins to become intolerant of being wet and/or soiled, training will be more successful (Hoekelman et al., 1997).

Nutrition

Near the second year, there is a deceleration in physical growth and resultant decrease in nutritional needs. The resultant picky, fussy, and mercurial appetite is normal. Mrs. Ingram should be encouraged to continue to offer Max a balanced variety—the same that is prepared for and consumed by the other family members. A tablespoon of solid food per year of age constitutes an adequate serving size during the early childhood years. Special foods and efforts to coax/force Max to eat are not recommended (Pipes & Trahms, 1993).

Milk continues to be an essential source of calcium and phosphorous. Max should be receiving about 3 cups of milk daily. A minimum of 2% milkfat is still needed for growth and energy needs. Milk should not be replaced with fruit juices (or Kool-Aid). The daily fluid requirement for a toddler is 115 mL/kg (approximately 54 oz. for Max). Milk and juices should be limited to this so that they do not interfere with the consumption of other foods.

Other

The sandbox in the yard left behind by the prior owners could harbor dangerous objects (e.g., broken toys, glass), or harmful matter (e.g., animal feces, parasites). Mrs. Ingram may wish to consider discarding the existing sand, and cleansing the box before refilling it and allowing the children to play in it. The swingset likewise needs to be assessed for its safety, and be anchored firmly in the ground.

2. *What anticipatory guidance would you review with Max's mother based on their recent move?*

Max's mother should closely monitor the environmental and social elements of the family. Accidents are more likely to happen in a chaotic environment, as might occur during or after a recent move. Resources for coping may not be available for a newly relocated family, although their extended families are here and should provide a source of support.

3. *When should Max return for follow up?*

Max should return in 1 year for a 3-year well-child visit.

REFERENCES

American Academy of Pediatrics Committee on Practice and Ambulatory Medicine. Recommendations for preventative pediatric health care. *AAP News* 1991; 19.

Boynton RW, Dunn ES, Stephens GR. *Manual of Ambulatory Pediatrics,* 3rd ed. Philadelphia: J.B. Lippincott; 1994.

Burns C, Barber N, Brady M, Dunn, A. *Pediatric Primary Care: A Handbook for Nurse Practitioners.* Philadelphia: W.B. Saunders; 1996.

Center for Disease Control. *Preventing Lead Poisoning in Young Children.* Washington, DC: U.S. Department of Health and Human Services/Public Health Services; 1991.

Dixon S, Stein M. *Encounters with Children: Pediatric Behavior and Development,* 2nd ed. St. Louis: C.V. Mosby; 1992.

Hoekelman R, Friedman S, Nelson N, Seidel H, Weitzman M. *Primary Pediatric Care,* 3rd ed. St. Louis: C.V. Mosby; 1997.

Pipes P, Trahms C. *Nutrition in Infancy and Childhood,* 5th ed. St. Louis: C.V. Mosby; 1993.

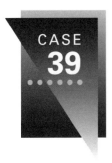

A 55-year-old woman with a rash on her arm

SCENARIO

Nancy is a 55-year-old Russian female complaining of a rash on her arm for the past 3 weeks. She states it is red, with little itching, but sometimes it has an open area.

● TENTATIVE DIAGNOSES

Based on the information provided so far, what are potential diagnoses?

● HISTORY

1. *What are significant questions in Nancy's history?*
2. *What are the key points on the review of systems?*

● PHYSICAL ASSESSMENT

What are the significant portions of the physical examination that should be completed for Nancy?

● DIFFERENTIAL DIAGNOSES

What are the significant positive and negative data that support or refute your diagnoses for Nancy?

● DIAGNOSTIC TESTS

Based on the history and physical assessment, what, if any, diagnostic tests would you obtain? Include your rationale for the tests.

● DIAGNOSES

What diagnoses are appropriate for Nancy?

● THERAPEUTIC PLAN

1. *What is the acute management for contact dermatitis?*
2. *What medications are commonly prescribed for contact dermatitis?*
3. *What follow up is needed for Nancy?*

TUTORIAL

A 55-year-old woman with a rash on her arm

SCENARIO:

Nancy is a 55-year-old Russian female complaining of a rash on her arm for the past 3 weeks. She states it is red, with little itching, but sometimes it has an open area.

● TENTATIVE DIAGNOSES

Based on the information provided so far, what are the potential diagnoses?

DIAGNOSIS	RATIONALE
Lichen simplex chronicus	A localized chronic disorder caused by repeated scratching and rubbing.
Contact dermatitis	Rash located in exposed or contact areas.
Scabies	Common rash seen on arms.
Nummular dermatitis	Eczematous plaques most commonly located on dorsa of hands and forearms.
Tinea corporis	Scales located on hands or forearms may be manifestations of tinea.
Carcinoma, squamous cell	Nodule located on hand or forearm may be cancerous.
Atopic dermatitis	Inflammation of dermis and epidermis.

● HISTORY

1. What are significant questions in the history for Nancy?

REQUESTED DATA	DATA ANSWER
Allergies	PCN: rash. Local anesthetics: bradycardia?
Current medications	Indapamide (Lozol) 2.5 mg QD Verapamil (Verlan) SR 120 mg QD ASA 365 mg QD Conjugated estrogen (Premarin) .625 QD Alprazolam (Xanax) 1 mg TID prn for anxiety Retin A applied at HS to face.
Surgery	Hysterectomy/Marshall Marchetti 8 years ago for cystocele. Blepharaplasty 4 years ago.
Past medical history and hospitalizations/fractures/injuries/accidents	HTN × 15 years. Thrombophlebitis/DVT 1 year ago; on Heparin IV and then Coumadin 2.5 QOD × 3 months. Multiple rib fractures 6 years ago/fell off chair. Solar keratosis on face, small basal cell carcinoma removed from forehead.
Chief complaint	Noticed red rash on left wrist about 1 month ago.
Present illness	Denies anything new in past month. Denies intense itching or lesions anywhere else. She does have dry skin and uses lotions all the time, increased in winter. No other associated symptoms. Works as a cafeteria cook part time. No new exposures at work. No changes in routine, washing, lotions. Has new watch, but got it 2 months ago, has worn without difficulty. Never has reaction to jewelry. Usually not allergic to anything. Does seem to have a reaction to cutting green peppers, gets red, burning hands. Works outside a lot in summer mowing grass. Wears sunscreen on face, not sure about hands. Has tried lotion with little relief. No one else in family has rash.
OB/GYN history	LNMP: Hysterectomy. Last pelvic/pap: 3 years ago. Last mammogram: 1 year ago, WNL. G3P3A0
Social history	Tobacco: Smoked 30 years, from 2 1/2 ppd to 4 1/2 ppd. stopped 8 years ago. Alcohol: None. Drugs: Denies. Caffeinated beverages: Tea four to five glasses/day. Exercise: Walks, but sporadic.

(continued)

REQUESTED DATA	DATA ANSWER
Family history	Father: Died at 80, CVA, prostate CA, thrombophlebitis. Mother: Died at 96, CHF, HTN. Siblings: Six sisters, one died of uterine cancer, one with HTN, two with severe thrombophlebitis. Husband: Died 9 years ago at 51 with MI. Children: Three girls, 1 with HTN, otherwise healthy.
Employment/insurance/income	Works part time as a cafeteria cook, has insurance through husband's employer. Gets husband's pension. Income adequate to meet needs.

2. *What are the key points on the review of systems?*

SYSTEM REVIEWED	DATA ANSWER
General	Feels healthy.
Skin	No other problems other than PI, except dry skin.
HEENT	Wears reading glasses, used to have migraines, but that is now gone.
Lungs	Has frequent cough. Has had this worked up, no lung cancer found. Comes and goes. Controls by cough drops/syrup.
Cardiac	No problems.

● PHYSICAL ASSESSMENT

What are the significant portions of the physical examination that should be completed for Nancy?

SYSTEM	RATIONALE	FINDINGS
Vital signs	Provides baseline data.	B/P: 138/88 HR: 72 R: 16 T: 98.2

(continued)

SYSTEM	RATIONALE	FINDINGS
		Ht: 5'5" Wt: 130 lbs
General appearance/skin	Provides overall view of Nancy.	White female, NAD. Pale, dry skin. Small red confluent papules with indistinct borders on the dorsal surface of the wrist, approx. 2 cm from radius toward the elbow. Lesion 1 to 1/2 cm in size. Scab visible. No drainage. Lesions localized to Lt. wrist. All skin surfaces examined, no other lesions found. No burrows seen. Rash present where watch is worn.
Lungs	Given history of smoking, wise to evaluate if you have not seen her before.	CTA.
Heart	Given history of HTN, wise to evaluate if you have not seen her before.	RRR, no MRG.

● DIFFERENTIAL DIAGNOSES

What are the significant positive and negative data that support or refute your diagnoses for Nancy?

DIAGNOSIS	POSITIVE DATA	NEGATIVE DATA
Lichen simplex chronicus	Localized lesions, erythematous papules/placques.	Denies itching or scratching, has only had for 3–4 weeks.
Contact dermatitis	Localized, acute lesions.	Denies itching, no known allergen, no vesicles.
Scabies	Papular lesions on wrist.	No burrows, no intense itching, no family members involved.
Tinea corporis	Lesion on wrist.	Not sharply marginated, no itching, not typical configuration.

(continued)

DIAGNOSIS	POSITIVE DATA	NEGATIVE DATA
Carcinoma, squamous cell	Lesion present 3–4 weeks, open area, sun exposed area, pale skin, history of lesions on face, age >50.	No indurated papule, with a firm elevated margin.
Atopic dermatitis	Poorly defined erythematous patch, dry skin.	No history of allergies, no affliction in childhood.

● DIAGNOSTIC TESTS

Based on the history and physical assessment, what, if any, diagnostic tests would you obtain?

DIAGNOSTIC TEST	RATIONALE	RESULTS
Patch test	Used to identify allergic reactions. A positive test shows erythema and papules confined to test site. Patch test should be delayed until dermatitis has subsided at least 2 weeks.	Not done at the present time due to dermatitis. May consider later if no improvement.
Skin scraping, KOH prep	Scraping of skin will reveal the presence of tinea.	Not done.

● DIAGNOSES

What diagnoses are appropriate for Nancy?

Contact dermatitis, irritant/toxic

Data Supporting the Diagnosis

Although Nancy can not identify an allergen, the symptoms are classic contact dermatitis. Since Nancy has a new watch, and the nickel sulfate in jewelry commonly causes contact dermatitis this is the likely cause. Because toxic irritant dermatitis is a toxic phenomenon, the rash was confined to the area of exposure, and did not spread. The rash was present where Nancy wears her watch (Fitzpatrick et al., 1997).

● THERAPEUTIC PLAN

1. What is acute management for contact dermatitis?

It is important to identify and remove the causative agent as the first line of treatment. A hydrative ointment such as a Eucerin or Aquaphor will help to rehydrate the skin (Uphold & Graham, 1994).

2. What medications are commonly prescribed for contact dermatitis?

A topical class 1 corticosteriod preparation is indicated. This includes such ointments as hydrocortisone $\frac{1}{2}$, 1, or 2.5%.

3. What follow up is needed for Nancy?

None is needed if the rash is cleared up by the hydrocortisone ointment and avoidance of the irritative item (i.e., watch).

REFERENCES

Fitzpatrick T, Johnson R, Wolff K, Polano M, Suurmond D. *Color Atlas and Synopsis of Clinical Dermatology*, 3rd ed. New York: McGraw-Hill; 1997.

Uphold C, Graham M. *Clinical Guidelines for Family Practice,* 2nd ed. Gainesville, FL: Barmarrae Books; 1994.

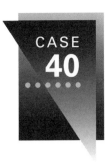

A 29-year-old woman with a bump on her vagina with itching and discharge

SCENARIO

Tonya is a 29-year-old Caucasian female. She presents with complaints of a "bump" on her vagina and itching with vaginal discharge. She is unemployed and has been divorced for 5 years with multiple sexual partners. She has sought medical care for vaginal infections and treated once for gonorrhea at local health clinic. She takes birth control bills for contraception, and does not usually use condoms.

TENTATIVE DIAGNOSES

Based on the information provided so far, what are potential diagnoses?

● HISTORY

1. *What are significant questions in Tanya's history?*
2. *What are the key points to cover on the review of systems?*

● PHYSICAL ASSESSMENT

What are the significant portions of the physical examination that should be completed for Tonya?

● DIFFERENTIAL DIAGNOSES

What are the significant positive and negative data that support or refute your diagnoses for Tonya?

● DIAGNOSTIC TESTS

Based on the history and physical assessment, what, if any, diagnostic tests would you obtain? Include your rationale for the tests.

● DIAGNOSIS

What diagnoses are appropriate for Tonya?

● THERAPEUTIC PLAN

1. *What is the treatment for external HPV?*
2. *What is the significance of HPV for females?*
3. *What is the treatment for internal HPV?*
4. *Should Tonya's partner be informed and treated?*
5. *How can the transmission of HPV be prevented? What self-care measures should be discussed with Tonya?*
6. *How should Tonya's yeast infection be treated?*
7. *When should follow up take place?*

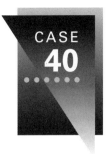

TUTORIAL

A 29-year-old woman with a bump on her vagina with itching and discharge

SCENARIO

Tonya is a 29-year-old Caucasian female. She presents with complaints of a "bump" on her vagina and itching with vaginal discharge. She is unemployed and has been divorced for 5 years with multiple sexual partners. She has sought medical care for vaginal infections and treated once for Gonorrhea at local health clinic. She takes birth control bills for contraception, and does not usually use condoms.

● TENTATIVE DIAGNOSES

Based on the information provided so far, what are the potential diagnoses?

DIAGNOSIS	RATIONALE
1. Condylomata acuminata	Single or multiple 2–3 mm. Fingerlike projections or flat-topped lesions with itching and vaginal discharge.
2. Syphilis: chancre/condylomata lata	Papule, rarely painful.
3. Chancroid	Papule or pustule, often painful.
4. Lymphogranuloma	Vesicle or papule, painless.
5. Herpes simplex	Vulvar vesicle, fever, malaise, lymphadenopathy, burning, painful.
6. Molluscum contagiosum	Wart-like papules 1–10 mm in size, asymptomatic.
7. Acrochordon (skin tag)	Soft sessile or pedunculated tags of skin, asymptomatic.
8. Folliculitis	Papule or pustule with central hair shaft, vulvar irritation or pain.

(continued)

DIAGNOSIS	*RATIONALE*
9. Bartholin cyst	Discrete swelling of the inferior aspect of the labium majus, vulvar irritation.
10. Epidermal cyst (sebaceous cyst)	Discrete swelling often 1 cm in diameter, vulvar irritation and pain if infected.

● HISTORY

1. What are significant questions in Tonya's history?

REQUESTED DATA	*DATA ANSWER*
Allergies	NKA.
Current medications	Oral contraceptives × 10 years.
Surgery	None.
Past medical history and hospitalizations/fractures/injuries/accidents	History of vaginal infections, hospitalized × 2 days for abdominal pain (patient unsure of diagnosis). Does not seek routine medical care. Cannot recall last care received or reason. Denies diabetes or immunosuppressed condition.
Adult illness	URI; one to two times per year.
OB/GYN history	GO, PO, LMP 3 weeks ago, last pap smear was >1 year ago, thinks it was normal, not sure.
Appetite	Poor; eats only one meal/day.
Sexuality	Multiple heterosexual partners; sexually active since 15 years old; denies sexual abuse.
Social history	Unemployed, 10th grade education, smoker of two packs/day; alcohol of 4–6 8 oz. beers/day plus occasional mixed drink or wine. Denies drug use.
Family history	Divorced; both parents alive; two younger brothers alive but all estranged; family history details unknown.
CAGE questionnaire	2/4 (concerned - 0; annoyed - 1; guilty - 0; eye opener - 1).

2. What are the key points on the review of systems?

SYSTEM REVIEWED	DATA ANSWER
General	Generally feels tired, restless sleep, denies fever.
Skin	No rash or other lesions.
HEENT	No lesions in or around mouth.
Abdominal	No complaint of pain.
Genitalia	"Bump" noticed over the last two weeks. Had unprotected intercourse with a new partner about three months ago who also had some bumps on genitalia. No history of HPV or herpes.

● PHYSICAL ASSESSMENT

What are the significant portions of the physical examination that should be completed for Tonya?

SYSTEM	RATIONALE	FINDINGS
Vital signs	Routine part of exam. Has not had medical care recently. Baseline data.	B/P; 120/82 P: 78 R:18 T:98.8
General appearance	Routine part of exam. Has not had medical care recently.	Alert, oriented, normally developed Caucasian female in NAD.
Skin/hair	To observe for other lesions or rashes, hair loss.	Warm and dry without other lesions or rashes, no alopecia.
Mouth	To observe for mouth lesions characteristic of syphilis.	No mouth lesions, poor dental condition.
Thyroid	No recent exam.	Nonpalpable.
Lungs	No recent exam.	CTA.
Heart	No recent exam.	RRR; no MRG.

(continued)

SYSTEM	RATIONALE	FINDINGS
Abdomen	To identify masses or tenderness.	Flat, soft, few bowel sounds; no organomegaly. No masses or tenderness.
Genitalia	Identify type of lump.	Small, soft, flesh-colored papule on right labia; nontender, negative lymphadenopathy.
Pelvic	To perform pap, cultures.	No other lesions, masses, or tenderness. Uterus anteverted, cervix WNL, no CMT.
Rectal	To check for additional lesions.	No lesions noted.

● DIFFERENTIAL DIAGNOSES

What are the significant positive and negative findings that support or refute your diagnoses for Tonya?

DIAGNOSIS	POSITIVE DATA	NEGATIVE DATA
Human papillomavirus	Single small lesion, itching and vaginal discharge; no complaint of pain, unprotected intercourse approximately 3 months ago with partner who may have had lesions. Incubation (3 weeks–8 months).	Solitary lesion, usually clusters.
Syphilis: chancre (primary) vs condylomata lata (secondary)	Chancre: indurated and painless vulvar ulcer; condylomata lata: pink-tan soft papule on the vulva. Potential exposure 3 months ago.	Chancre: lymphadenopathy and not 21 days after exposure, firm indurated; condylomata lata: lymphadenopathy, no alopecia, no splenomegaly, no mouth lesions.
Herpes simplex	Vulvar lesion.	Painful; + lymphadenopathy, fever, malaise, incubation in 2–12 days.
Molluscum contagiosum	Painless, wartlike papules.	Umbilical depression containing cheeselike core.

(continued)

DIAGNOSIS	POSITIVE DATA	NEGATIVE DATA
Acrochordon	Skin tag, soft skin colored papule.	Sessile or pedunculated polyps.
Folliculitis	Papule.	Central hair shaft, no pustule noted, no tenderness.
Bartholin cyst	Discrete swelling/papule on labia.	No painful lesion, lymphade-nopathy.
Epidermoid cyst (seba-ceous cyst)	Discrete swelling 1cm.	Cystic formation filled with ker-atin, nontender.

● DIAGNOSTIC TESTS

Based on the history and physical assessment, what, if any, diagnostic tests would you obtain?

DIAGNOSTIC TEST	RATIONALE	RESULTS
Wet smear	Identify vaginal drainage via microscope.	+ budding hyphae.
Gen probe	To rule out GC and chlamydia.	Negative for GC and chlamydia.
Pap smear	May note changes associated with HPV.	+ HPV, ASCUS.
Viral culture	Identify atypical lesion.	+ Human papilloma virus.
RPR	To rule out syphilis.	Negative.
Colposcopy	To identify lesions not visible with naked eye.	Not usually first line test, may be needed based on pap results.
Biopsy	To identify HPV or cervical changes.	+ HPV.
HIV	Presence of HPV is indicative of unsafe sexual practices: need to offer HIV testing.	Refused.

● DIAGNOSES

What diagnoses are appropriate after a review of the subjective and objective data?

Human papillomavirus
Vaginal candidiasis

Data Supporting the Diagnosis

1. Presents with history of new potentially infected partner.
2. Time frame of exposure consistent with incubation period.
3. Examination reveals soft flesh-colored lesion.
4. Pap smear reveals +HPV.
5. Vaginal discharge, itching, + budding hyphae on wet smear.

● THERAPEUTIC PLAN

1. What is the treatment for external HPV?

The goal of treatment is the removal of warts and amelioration of signs and symptoms, not eradication of HPV. Solitary lesions should be surgically excised and sent for pathologic examination. Treatment is more successful if warts are small and have been present for less than 1 year. Choice of available treatments is determined by cost and patient preference (Holmes et al., 1990).

- Podophyllin (Podofilox): 0.5% for self-treatment
  - apply to warts twice daily for 3 days, followed by 4 days of no therapy
  - cycle may be repeated for a total of four cycles
- total wart area treated should not exceed 10 cm^2 and a total volume of Podofilox should not exceed 0.5 mL per day
  - contraindicated in pregnancy
- Podophyllin: 10–25% in compound tincture of benzoin (Podofilox, Condylox)
  - apply petroleum to area surrounding lesion to protect skin from injury
  - apply Podophyllin solution carefully to wart
  - limit the total volume of Podophyllin solution to <0.5 mL or limit area treated to 10 cm^2 per session
  - instruct client to thoroughly wash off in 1–4 hours
  - repeat applications at weekly intervals for 3 weeks
  - contraindicated in pregnancy
- Trichloroacetic Acid (TCA): 80–90%
  - apply directly to lesions (5)
  - powder with talc or sodium bicarbonate (baking soda) to remove unreacted acid
  - does not require washing off later
  - repeat applications at weekly intervals

- if warts persist after six applications, consider other therapies
- consult physician regarding use in pregnancy
- Cryosurgery with liquid nitrogen
  - apply with cotton swab
  - repeat weekly or biweekly
  - relatively inexpensive, does not result in scarring (Fitzpatrick et al., 1997)

2. *What is the significance of HPV for females?*

At least 60 types of HPV have been identified; several of which have been found to cause cervical and vulvar cancer. Women who become infected before age 25, like Tonya, are 40 times more likely to develop cervical cancer than those who are not infected. In addition, for both men and women, lesions, if not treated, may become numerous and quite large, requiring more extensive treatment and frequent follow up (Barker et al., 1995).

3. *What is the treatment for internal HPV?*

Choices for removal of warts on the cervix consist of punch biopsy if small, electrodesiccation, cryotherapy, loop excision, or laser vaporization. Tanya should be referred to a provider who is experienced in treating cervical lesions. A colposcopy must be done to visualize the cervical area prior to treatment. Dysplasia associated with HPV should be treated according to the severity and extent of the dysplastic process (Decherney & Pernoll, 1994).

4. *Should Tonya's partner be informed and treated?*

Sexual partners need to be examined by a healthcare provider and treated if warts are noted. Role of reinfection, however, is probably minimal. Majority of partners are probably subclinically infected with HPV, even if no warts are visible.

5. *How can the transmission of HPV be prevented? What self-care measures should be discussed with Tonya?*

Abstinence or use of condoms should be practiced until both partners are cleared of the disease. Tanya should practice safe sex and use a condom with all partners. This practice will not only reduce her chance of contracting HPV but HIV, GC, chlamydia, and hepatitis (Uphold & Graham, 1994).

6. *How should Tonya's yeast infection be treated?*

Tonya should be given a prescription for Clotrimazole 1% cream. She should insert the cream once daily at HS for 7 days. Eating yogurt with live cultures might also assist in diminishing her symptoms.

7. *When should follow up take place?*

Follow up every 2–3 weeks after initial treatment, self-examination initiated, PAP smear in 3 months, and return to health care provider if warts reoccur. Women with history of genital warts and women partners of men with a history of genital warts should have PAP smears at least every 6 months.

REFERENCES

Barker LR, Burton JR, Zieve PD (eds). *Principles of Ambulatory Medicine,* 4th ed. Baltimore, MD: Williams & Wilkins; 1995.

Decherney AH, Pernoll ML (eds). *Current Obstetrics and Gynecologic Diagnosis and Treatment,* 8th ed. Norwalk, CT: Appleton & Lang; 1994.

Fitzpatrick TB, Johnson RA, Wolff K, Polano MK, Suurmond D. *Color atlas and Synopsis of Clinical Dermatology,* 3rd ed. New York: McGraw-Hill; 1997.

Holmes KK, Mardh P, Sparling PF, Weisner PJ, Cates W Jr, Lemon SM, et al. *Sexually Transmitted Diseases,* 2nd ed. New York: McGraw-Hill; 1990.

Uphold CR, Graham MV. *Clinical Guidelines in Family Practice,* 2nd ed. Gainesville, FL: Barnarrae; 1994.

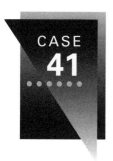

A 29-year-old woman with an abnormal menstrual cycle and diarrhea

SCENARIO

Sally is a 29-year-old obese African-American female presenting with complaints of abnormal menstrual cycle, abdominal bloating, diarrhea for 5 months with excessive flatulence and muscle tightness. Her previous menstrual cycle was 30 days previous to the office visit and only lasted 1 day. She had been having menstruation every other month for the past 6 months. Although she has had no menses she described mild ovarian cramping mainly in the left lower quadrant. She also complained of diarrhea consisting of alternating loose and watery stools intermittently combined with constipation. She also noted a swelling or out-pouching of the left upper abdominal quadrant, worse with constipation. Sally also indicated she had extreme fatigue in late afternoon, and muscle cramping in both legs.

TENTATIVE DIAGNOSES

Based on the information provided so far, what are potential diagnoses?

● HISTORY

1. *What are significant questions in the history for a woman with fatigue, menstrual abnormalities, and diarrhea?*
2. *What are the key points to cover on the review of systems?*

● PHYSICAL ASSESSMENT

What are the significant portions of the physical examination that should be completed for Sally?

● DIFFERENTIAL DIAGNOSES

What are the significant positive and negative data that support or refute your diagnoses for Sally?

● DIAGNOSTIC TESTS

Based on the history and physical assessment, what, if any, diagnostic tests would you obtain? Include your rationale for the tests.

● DIAGNOSIS

What diagnoses do you determine as being appropriate for Sally?

● THERAPEUTIC PLAN

1. *What pharmacological agents will be used to control Sally's hypothyroidism?*
2. *What are indications that Sally should be referred to a specialist?*
3. *What are signs and symptoms that Sally and the care provider should be alert to given her history?*
4. *When should Sally return for follow up?*
5. *How often should Sally have her TSH levels monitored?*
6. *How will you know if Sally is improving?*
7. *What patient education issues should be discussed with Sally?*

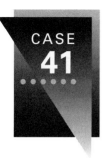

TUTORIAL

A 29-year-old woman with an abnormal menstrual cycle and diarrhea

SCENARIO:

Sally is a 29-year-old obese African-American female presenting with complaints of abnormal menstrual cycle, abdominal bloating, diarrhea for 5 months with excessive flatulence and muscle tightness. Her previous menstrual cycle was 30 days previous to the office visit and only lasted 1 day. She had been having menstruation every other month for the past 6 months. Although she has had no menses she described mild ovarian cramping mainly in the left lower quadrant. She also complained of diarrhea consisting of alternating loose and watery stools intermittently combined with constipation. She also noted a swelling or out-pouching of the left upper abdominal quadrant, worse with constipation. Sally also indicated she had extreme fatigue in late afternoon, and muscle cramping in both legs.

● TENTATIVE DIAGNOSES

Based on the information provided so far, what are the potential diagnoses?

DIAGNOSIS	RATIONALE
Pregnancy	One day of spotting without regular periods for 6 months. Pregnancy could be early, because last period was not normal or could be advanced and not noticed due to obesity. Pregnancy could contribute to abdominal pain and fatigue.
Secondary amenorrhea	Hormonal imbalance can contribute to menstrual irregularities. Uterine infection or endometriosis can contribute to pain and irregular menses. Young women on low-fat

(continued)

DIAGNOSIS	*RATIONALE*
	diets, less than approximately 30 grams of fat daily do not have the cholesterol to produce estrogen and progesterone.
IBS	Sally's complaints of alternating diarrhea/constipation, and outpouching of abdomen are symptoms of IBS.
Electrolyte imbalance	Electrolytes, specifically potassium, can be lost with diarrhea. Hypokalemia can contribute to fatigue. Young women who diet are prone to nutritional imbalance.
Anemia	Complaints of fatigue in women who menstruate should be evaluated for anemia.
Hypothyroidism	Impaired thyroid function contributes to fatigue, alopecia, and weight gain.

● HISTORY

1. *What are significant questions in the history for a woman with fatigue, menstrual abnormalities, and diarrhea?*

REQUESTED DATA	*DATA ANSWER*
Allergies	NKA.
Current medications	Demulin-135.
Surgery/transfusions	None/None.
Past medical history and hospitalizations/fractures/injuries/accidents	Childbirth 1990, 1991. No injuries. Had chicken pox as a child.
Adult illness	Gestational diabetes, 1990 and 1991. UTI, 1991. Gastroenteritis, 1993. Elevated serum triglycerides, 1993 (286). Sinusitis and bronchitis, 1993. Inhalant allergies, 1995. Hard palate abscess, 1995. Acute pharyngitis, 1995. Alopecia, 1996.
Last complete PE	Never.

(continued)

REQUESTED DATA	DATA ANSWER
OB/GYN history	LNMP: 5-15-96. Last pap: 7/95, dysplasia. SBE, monthly. G2P2A0.
Appetite	Various cravings, fad dieting, 20-lb weight gain over past 3 years with reduced caloric intake.
24-Hour diet recall	B: None. S: Rice cakes. L: Fries, roast beef sandwich, diet cola. S: Baked fish, broccoli, salad. S: Low-fat popcorn.
Sleeping	Sleeps 9–10 hours per night, awakens fatigued, falls asleep on couch in evening.
Social history	Tobacco: Denies. Alcohol: Twice per year. Caffeine: Three to four cups coffee, two glasses iced tea, Mt. Dew, 12 oz. Drug: Denies. Exercise: None regular.
Family history	Father: age 55, hypercholesterolemia. Mother: 54, good health. Sister: 31, good health. Two children: 7, 6, in good health.
Social organizations	Church group, otherwise too tired.
Finances/insurance	Private insurance—Sally and her husband are both employed.
Occupation	Secretary at local water company. No exposure to toxic chemicals or substances.

2. *What are the key points on the review of systems?*

SYSTEM REVIEWED	DATA ANSWER
General	C/o of being pale and fatigued.
HEENT	Noticed swelling through the eyes, and all over body, worse in morning, decreasing in afternoon.

(continued)

SYSTEM REVIEWED	DATA ANSWER
Neurologic	Denies numbness and tingling of extremities.
Mental	C/o being sad and depressed.

● PHYSICAL ASSESSMENT

What are the significant portions of the physical examination that should be completed for Sally?

SYSTEM	RATIONALE	FINDINGS
Vital signs	Provides baseline data. 59% of hypothyroid patients have weight gain. Tachycardia and atrial fibrillation may occur.	B/P: 102/80 P: 92 R: 18 T: 98.8 Ht: 64″ Wt: 164 lbs
General appearance/skin	97% of hypothyroid patients c/o coarse, dry skin, 67% c/o pallor, 76% have coarse hair, 57% have loss of hair, and 9% with fine hair (Brody & Reichard, 1995).	Loss of pigmentation on face, arms, legs. 1–2 cm patches of alopecia on scalp.
HEENT	Assess for edema of eyelids, edema of the face, pallor of the lips, decreased hearing, decreased vision, and thick or atrophic tongue, all symptoms of hypothyroidism.	WNL, PERRLA, thyroid not enlarged, periorbital edema.
Lungs	Baseline data. Many patients have dyspnea, need to evaluate.	CTA.
Heart	Evaluate heart sounds. Many hypothyroid patients have distant heart sounds and c/o palpitations.	Regular rhythm, S_1S_2 WNL, no MRG. Sally has a possible mitral valve click difficult to hear owing to distant heart sounds.
Breasts	Usually no breast involvement with thyroid problems.	Deferred.

(continued)

SYSTEM	*RATIONALE*	*FINDINGS*
Abdomen	Evaluate for masses or obesity. Hypothyroid patients c/o constipation and weight gain.	Moderate obesity, no masses or pulsations.
Rectum	Helpful to rule out obstructive cause of constipation.	Good anal sphincter tone. No masses or hemorrhoids. Stool tan.
Pelvic	Will need to evaluate for secondary amenorrhea.	Check for abnormal cervical cells. Uterus size WNL. No adnexal tenderness.
Neurologic	Thyroid problems have many neuro manifestations that need to be assessed.	DTRs 3+/4+ Alert and oriented, able to count backwards from 99 by 7's.
Extremities	Assess for peripheral edema.	1+ tibial edema.

● DIFFERENTIAL DIAGNOSES

What are the significant positive and negative data that support or refute your diagnoses for Sally?

DIAGNOSIS	*POSITIVE DATA*	*NEGATIVE DATA*
Pregnancy	None.	Uterus size WNL, no Chadwicks, Hegar signs.
Secondary amenorrhea	3 months without menses.	
IBS	Alternating diarrhea/constipation with excessive flatulence. Afebrile.	No melena or mucus in stool. No lower abdominal pain or tenderness. No history of prior attacks.
Electrolyte balance	Fatigue.	DTRs hyperreflexic.
Anemia	Fatigue.	HR WNL.
Hypothyroidism	Weight gain although dieting, fatigue, distant heart sounds, dry skin, patchy alopecia, periorbital edema, constipation, amenorrhea, lethargy, depression.	

● DIAGNOSTIC TESTS

Based on the history and physical examination, what, if any, diagnostic testing would you obtain?

DIAGNOSTIC TEST	RATIONALE	RESULTS
CBC	Rule out anemia.	H/H: 14.4/39.1% RBC: 4.2 WBC: 5.5 MCV: 103 MCH: 36.3 MCHC: 35.3 Platelets: 206 Two bands, 58 segs, 39 lymphs, 1 mono
Pregnancy test (urine)	Rule out pregnancy.	Negative
SMA-24	Provides baseline information about electrolytes, renal and liver function.	NA: 142 K: 3.6 CL: 101 CO_2: 25 Anion gap: 20 Glucose: 77 BUN: 11 Creatinine: 1.2 Ca: 9.8 Phosphorus: 4.1 Uric acid: 4.1 Total protein: 9/1, Albumin: 4.6 Globulin: 4.5, A/G ration: 1.0 Total bilirubin: 0.5, Cholesterol: 351, Triglyceride: 756, LDL: 298 AST: 93 ALT: 27 Alk phos: 62 G Gt: 16 Iron: 109

(continued)

DIAGNOSTIC TEST	*RATIONALE*	*RESULTS*
Thyroid profile	Provides baseline information of thyroid functioning. Because this is your most likely diagnosis, important to include in screening.	T_3 uptake 14.8 T_4 1.6 T_7 0.2 TSH 77.09
Radioactive iodine thyroid uptake scan	Provides more detailed information about thyroid gland. The high TSH indicates possibility of enlarged thyroid.	Order so test results are available if/when referred to specialist. Findings: Low 24-hour radioiodine uptake. Nonuniform radionuclide uptake raising the possibility of multinodular goiter. If clinically indicated, ultrasound may be useful for further evaluation (Brody & Reichard, 1995).

● DIAGNOSES

What diagnoses are appropriate after a review of the subjective and objective data?

Hypothyroidism

Data Supporting the Diagnosis

Sally has weight gain (although dieting), fatigue, distant heart sounds, dry skin, patchy alopecia, periorbital edema, constipation, amenorrhea, lethargy, depression. These symptoms were confirmed by the TSH and other thyroid tests.

In primary hypothyroidism the pituitary gland attempts to correct the failing thyroid through the biofeedback system by increasing the output of TSH, the thyroid fails to respond with an increase in the thyroid hormones. In secondary hypothyroidism, the cause is disease of the pituitary gland or hypothalamus, which causes a low level of TSH.

It is important to differentiate between primary and secondary hypothyroidism since the addition of thyroid hormone in secondary hypothyroidism may precipitate adrenal failure. In secondary cases, cortisol must be administered before thyroid hormone. Because Sally has an elevated TSH it was determined she has primary hypothyroidism (Pronovost & Parris, 1995).

● THERAPEUTIC PLAN

1. *What pharmacological agents will be used to control Sally's hypothyroidism?*

   Levothyroxine (Synthroid) 0.025–0.050 mg QD initially increasing every 2–4 weeks based on TSH levels in adults under 65 years of age. Sally needs to be warned not to increase the level independently and to observe for chest pain, tachycardia, cardiac arrhythmias, and palpitations. She should know it is important for her to report any of the above symptoms. The end maximal dose is 0.3 mg daily.

2. *What are indications that Sally should be referred to a specialist?*

   Indications for referral include chest pain or cardiac arrhythmias at the time of diagnosis or after initiation of therapy; TSH over 12. Lack of skin pigmentation and anemia in this patient warrant referral also.

3. *What are signs and symptoms that Sally and the care provider should be alert to given her history?*

   Myxedema is a severe form of hypothyroidism with deposits of mucopolysaccharides under the skin resulting in a pale, puffy appearance without pitting edema. Usually there bags unders the eyes and possibly a yellow-orange discoloration of the skin. Because Sally's TSH is over 50 U/mL she is considered to have severe hypothyroidism. Although many of the manifestations of hypothyroidism are "subclinical" each system in the body is affected, such as impaired cardiac output, increased SVR, bradyarrhythmias, and so on (Pronovost and Parris, 1995).

   Sally is at risk for myxedema due to her high TSH. She should be aware of the symptoms and should contact her provider if she is aware of any.

4. *When should Sally return for follow up?*

   Either with or without referral, Sally should be followed in 2-4 weeks after the initiation of pharmacological intervention.

5. *How often should Sally have her TSH levels monitored?*

   Sally should have her TSH level monitored every 2 months until stable and then every 3 months.

6. *How will you know if Sally is improving?*

   Sally will notice improvement in energy level and mild weight loss in the first month. Sally will not notice as quick of an improvement for the other symptoms. They will slowly resolve over time.

7. *What patient education issues should be discussed with Sally?*

   Compliance with medication and monitoring is particularly important. Thyroid hormones should be taken in the morning at the same time daily. Sally should be cautioned not to take more medication than indicated to get more energy or lose weight. If chest pain, palpitations, rapid heartbeat, sweating, nervousness, or dyspnea occur she should contact the office immediately.

Although there are some recent studies that indicate that a medication vacation or cycling is helpful, it is important for Sally to know that she will be taking this medication for the rest of her life. As she ages, it may be necessary for the dosage to be lowered.

Some other medications such as lipid-lowering agents, insulin, oral antidiabetic medications, phenytoin, and oral anticoagulants may interact with the levothyroxine and may require adjusting the doses of some of her medications (Uphold & Graham, 1994).

REFERENCES

Brody M, Reichard R. Thyroid screening. *Postgrad Med* 1995; 98(2): 54–68.

Pronovost P, Parris K. Perioperative management of thyroid disease. *Postgrad Med* 1995; 98(2): 83–98.

Uphold C, Graham M. *Clinical Guidelines in Family Practice,* 3rd ed. Gainesville, FL: Barmarrae Books; 1994.

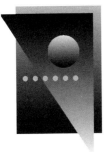

Index

A

Abdominal aortic aneurysm (AAA)
  vs. cholecystitis, 299–309
  vs. lumbosacral strain, 429–440
Abdominal bloating
  with diarrhea, 268–277
    diagnosis of, 275–276
    diagnostic tests for, 275
    differential diagnosis of, 274
    history of, 271–272
    physical assessment of, 273
    presenting symptoms of, 270
    tentative diagnoses for, 270
    therapeutic plan for, 276–277
  with hypothyroidism, 487–497
  in pregnancy, 46
Abdominal pain
  in cholecystitis, 299–309
    diagnosis of, 307
    diagnostic tests for, 306–307
    differential diagnosis of, 305
    history of, 302–303
    physical assessment of, 304
    presenting symptoms of, 301
    tentative diagnoses for, 301–302
    therapeutic plan for, 307–309
  left upper quadrant, 380–390
    diagnosis of, 388
    diagnostic tests for, 387–388
    differential diagnosis of, 386–387
    history of, 383–385
    physical assessment of, 385–386
    presenting symptoms of, 382
    tentative diagnoses for, 382–383
    therapeutic plan for, 388–390
  in pelvic inflammatory disease, 190–198
    diagnosis of, 196–197
    diagnostic tests for, 196
    differential diagnosis of, 195
    history of, 193–194
    physical assessment of, 194–195
    presenting symptoms of, 192
    tentative diagnoses for, 192
    therapeutic plan for, 197–198

Abortion, threatened, 36–47
  diagnosis of, 43–44
  diagnostic tests for, 42–43
  differential diagnosis of, 41–42
  history of, 39–40
  physical assessment of, 40–41
  presenting symptoms of, 38
  tentative diagnoses for, 38
  therapeutic plan for, 44–47
Abuse, physical, 308
Accidents, in children, 48–61
Accupril (quinapril), for congestive heart failure,
    147
Accuracy, 7
ACE (angiotensin-converting enzyme) inhibitor, for
    congestive heart failure, 146–147
Acetylsalicylic acid (ASA), for elderly, 125
ACL (anterior cruciate ligament) injury, *vs.* medial
    collateral ligament injury, 179–188
Acne, 167
Acoustic neuroma, *vs.* benign paroxysmal positional
    vertigo, 414–427
Acquired immunodeficiency syndrome (AIDS). *See*
    also Human immunodeficiency virus (HIV)
  indicator conditions for, 373–374
Acrochordon, *vs.* human papillomavirus, 477–486
Acyclovir (Zovirax), for herpes zoster, 176
Adderall, for ADHD, 59
ADHD. *See* Attention deficit hyperactivity disorder
    (ADHD)
Adolescent
  with abdominal pain, 190–198
  with knee pain, 179–189
  sports physical for, 157–158
    diagnostic tests for, 164–165
    history in, 159–161
    physical assessment in, 161–163
    therapeutic plan in, 165–168
AIDS (acquired immunodeficiency syndrome). *See*
    also Human immunodeficiency virus (HIV)
  indicator conditions for, 373–374
Alcohol dependence, 308
Alpha fetoprotein screen, 45
Alzheimer's disease, 199–214
  diagnosis of, 211–212

Alzheimer's disease, (*continued*)
diagnostic tests for, 209–211
differential diagnosis of, 208
history of, 204–205
physical assessment of, 206–207
presenting symptoms of, 201
resources for, 213
tentative diagnoses for, 202–204
therapeutic plan for, 212–214
Amenorrhea, secondary, *vs.* hypothyroidism, 487–497
Amniocentesis, 45
Amoxicillin
for peptic ulcer disease, 389
for streptococcal pharyngitis, 238
for urinary tract infection, 332
Analgesic rebound, *vs.* tension-type headache, 127–139
Anemia
vs. benign paroxysmal positional vertigo, 423
vs. congestive heart failure, 140–148
vs. COPD, 62–73
delirium with, 203
vs. depression, 74–90
vs. hepatitis, 402–413
vs. hypothyroidism, 487–497
vs. non-insulin dependent diabetes mellitus, 257–267
Aneurysm, abdominal aortic
vs. cholecystitis, 299–309
vs. lumbosacral strain, 429–440
Angina, *vs.* peptic ulcer disease, 380–390
Angiotensin-converting enzyme (ACE) inhibitor, for congestive heart failure, 146–147
Ankle laxity, 167
Antacids, for gastroesophageal reflux, 112
Anterior cruciate ligament (ACL) injury, *vs.* medial collateral ligament injury, 179–188
Antivert (meclizine), for benign paroxysmal positional vertigo, 426
Anxiety, *vs.* tension-type headache, 127–139
Anxiety disorder, *vs.* ADHD, 48–61
Aortic aneurysm, abdominal
vs. cholecystitis, 299–309
vs. lumbosacral strain, 429–440
Appendicitis, *vs.* pelvic inflammatory disease, 190–198
ASA (acetylsalicylic acid), for elderly, 125
Assumptions, in critical thinking, 2
Asthma, 10–26
vs. COPD, 62–73
diagnosis of, 20–21
diagnostic tests for, 18–20
differential diagnosis of, 17
history of, 13–15
physical assessment of, 15–16
presenting symptoms of, 12
resources for, 25–26
tentative diagnoses for, 12–13
therapeutic plan for, 21–26
Atopic dermatitis, *vs.* contact dermatitis, 469–476

Attention deficit hyperactivity disorder (ADHD), 48–61
diagnosis of, 57–58
diagnostic tests for, 56–57
differential diagnosis of, 55–56
history of, 51–53
physical assessment of, 54
presenting symptoms of, 50
resources for, 60–61
tentative diagnoses for, 50–51
therapeutic plan for, 58–61
Axid (nizatidine), for gastroesophageal reflux, 112
Azidothymidine (AZT), for human immunodeficiency virus, 376
Azithromycin (Zithromax), for gonorrhea and chlamydia, 100

B
Back pain
acute lower, 429–440
diagnosis of, 437
diagnostic tests for, 436–437
differential diagnosis of, 435–436
history of, 432–433
physical assessment of, 433–434
presenting symptoms of, 431
tentative diagnoses for, 431–432
therapeutic plan for, 437–440
chronic, 240–256
diagnosis of, 251–252
diagnostic tests for, 250–251
differential diagnosis of, 248–250
history of, 243–245
physical assessment of, 246–247
presenting symptoms of, 242
resources for, 255–256
tentative diagnoses for, 242
therapeutic plan for, 252–256
Bacteremia, neonatal, *vs.* failure to thrive, 215–229
Bacterial meningitis, *vs.* Kawasaki disease, 291–298
Bartholin cyst, *vs.* human papillomavirus, 477–486
Battering, 308
Behavior difficulty, in child, 48–61
Benign paroxysmal positional vertigo (BPPV), 414–427
diagnosis of, 425
diagnostic tests for, 423–425
differential diagnosis of, 422–423
history of, 418–419
physical assessment of, 420–421
presenting symptoms of, 416
resources for, 427
tentative diagnoses for, 416–417
therapeutic plan for, 425–427
Benign prostatic hyperplasia (BPH), 288
vs. non-insulin dependent diabetes mellitus, 262
vs. urinary tract infection, 441–454
Birth control, 310–323
diagnostic tests for, 318

history for, 313–315
with human immunodeficiency virus, 378–379
physical assessment for, 315–316
therapeutic plan for, 319–321
Bismuth subsalicylate, for peptic ulcer disease, 389
Bleeding, vaginal, during pregnancy, 36–47
Bloating
  with diarrhea, 268–277
    diagnosis of, 275–276
    diagnostic tests for, 275
    differential diagnosis of, 274
    history of, 271–272
    physical assessment of, 273
    presenting symptoms of, 270
    tentative diagnoses for, 270
    therapeutic plan for, 276–277
  with hypothyroidism, 487–497
  in pregnancy, 46
Blood sugar, decreased, *vs.* depression, 74–90
BPH. *See* Benign prostatic hyperplasia (BPH)
BPPV. *See* Benign paroxysmal positional vertigo
      (BPPV)
Brain tumor, *vs.* depression, 74–90
Breadth, 7
Breast cancer
  vs. fibrocystic breast disease, 149–156
  vs. human immunodeficiency virus, 362–379
Breast examination, clinical, 120
Breast lump, 149–156
  clinical presentation of, 151
  diagnosis of, 154
  diagnostic tests for, 154
  differential diagnosis of, 153–154
  history of, 151–152
  physical assessment of, 153
  tentative diagnoses for, 151
  therapeutic plan for, 154–156
Breast milk, poor fat content in, 218, 225–226
Breast nodule, 122
Breast self-examination (BSE), 155–156
Breath, shortness of
  with chronic cough, 10–26
  with cough and fever, 62–73
Bronchitis
  acute, *vs.* COPD, 62–73
  vs. asthma, 10–26
  chronic, 70
  vs. congestive heart failure, 140–148
BSE (breast self-examination), 155–156

C

Candida vaginitis, 485
  vs. gonorrhea and chlamydia, 91–103
Captopril (Capoten), for congestive heart failure,
      146
Carcinoma, squamous cell, *vs.* contact dermatitis,
      469–476
Cardiac disease
  vs. benign paroxysmal positional vertigo, 417, 423

congenital, *vs.* failure to thrive, 215–229
  vs. gastroesophageal reflux, 104–113
Cardiac event, delirium with, 203
Cardiovascular disease, diabetic, 266–267
Case studies, as teaching and learning tool, 8
Cataract, *vs.* non-insulin dependent diabetes
      mellitus, 257–267
Cauda equina syndrome, *vs.* lumbosacral strain,
      429–440
Cefadroxil (Duricef), for urinary tract infection,
      332
Ceftriaxone (Rocephin)
  for gonorrhea and chlamydia, 100
  for pelvic inflammatory disease, 197
Cerebellar disease, *vs.* benign paroxysmal positional
      vertigo, 423
Cerebral tumor, *vs.* tension-type headache, 127–139
Cerumen, impacted, 233, 236
Cervical erosion, *vs.* threatened abortion, 36–47
Cervical polyps, *vs.* threatened abortion, 36–47
Cervical spondylosis, *vs.* tension-type headache,
      127–139
Chancre, *vs.* human papillomavirus, 477–486
Chancroid, *vs.* human papillomavirus, 477–486
Checkup
  for adolescent sports, 157–158
    diagnostic tests for, 164–165
    history in, 159–161
    physical assessment in, 161–163
    therapeutic plan in, 165–168
  of elderly man, 279–289
    diagnostic tests in, 285–286
    history in, 281–283
    physical assessment in, 283–284
  of elderly woman, 114–126
    diagnostic tests in, 122–123
    history in, 116–118
    physical assessment in, 118–121
  of infant, 215–229
    history in, 218–220
    physical assessment in, 220–221
  for kindergarten, 335–344
    anticipatory guidance in, 343
    diagnostic tests in, 342
    history in, 337–339
    physical assessment in, 340–341
  of two-year-old, 455–468
    anticipatory guidance in, 466–468
    diagnostic tests in, 465
    history in, 458–461
    physical assessment in, 462–464
CHF. *See* Congestive heart failure (CHF)
Child(ren)
  behavior difficulty in, 48–61
  itchy red eye in, 27–35
  kindergarten physical for, 335–344
    anticipatory guidance in, 343
    diagnostic tests in, 342
    history in, 337–339
    physical assessment in, 340–341
  with knee pain, 179–188

Child(ren) (*continued*)
  with rash and fever, 291–298
  with sore throat and earache, 231–239
  sports examination for, 157–168
  well-child visit for two-year-old, 455–468
    anticipatory guidance in, 466–468
    diagnostic tests in, 465
    history in, 458–461
    physical assessment in, 462–464
Chlamydia, 91–103
  diagnosis for, 100
  diagnostic tests for, 98–99
  differential diagnosis of, 97–98
  history of, 94–96
  pelvic inflammatory disease due to, 190–198
  physical assessment of, 96–97
  presenting symptoms of, 93
  resources for, 101–102
  tentative diagnoses for, 93
  therapeutic plan for, 100–103
Cholecystitis, 299–309
  diagnosis of, 307
  diagnostic tests for, 306–307
  differential diagnosis of, 305
  history of, 302–303
  vs. peptic ulcer disease, 380–390
  physical assessment of, 304
  presenting symptoms of, 301
  tentative diagnoses for, 301–302
  therapeutic plan for, 307–309
Cholesterol level, 167, 288
Chorionic villus sampling (CVS), 45–46
Chronic fatigue syndrome
  vs. hepatitis, 402–413
  vs. human immunodeficiency virus, 362–379
Chronic obstructive pulmonary disease (COPD),
    62–73
  acute exacerbation of, 70
  diagnosis of, 70
  diagnostic tests for, 69–70
  differential diagnosis of, 67–68
  history of, 65–66
  with hypertension, 448, 450, 452
  physical assessment of, 66–67
  presenting symptoms of, 64
  tentative diagnoses for, 64–65
  therapeutic plan for, 71–72
Cigarette smoking, cessation of, 309
Cimetidine (Tagamet), for gastroesophageal reflux,
    112
Ciprofloxacin (Cipro), for urinary tract infection,
    332
Clarity, 6–7
Clinical decision making, 3–4
  critical thinking and, 4
  teaching of, 4–7
Clustering, of symptoms and data, 4
Colic, renal, *vs.* cholecystitis, 299–309
Colon cancer, *vs.* irritable bowel syndrome, 268–277
Condylomata acuminata, 477–486
  diagnosis of, 484

diagnostic tests for, 483
differential diagnosis of, 482–483
history of, 480–481
physical assessment of, 481–482
presenting symptoms of, 479
vs. scabies, 345–352
tentative diagnoses for, 479–480
therapeutic plan for, 484–486
Condylomata lata, *vs.* human papillomavirus,
    477–486
Confidentiality, with adolescent patient, 166
Confusion, in elderly, 199–214
  diagnosis of, 211–212
  diagnostic tests for, 209–211
  differential diagnosis of, 208
  history of, 204–205
  physical assessment of, 206–207
  presenting symptoms of, 201
  resources for, 213
  tentative diagnoses for, 202–204
  therapeutic plan for, 212–214
Congenital heart disease, *vs.* failure to thrive,
    215–229
Congestive heart failure (CHF), 140–148
  vs. asthma, 10–26
  clinical symptoms of, 142
  vs. COPD, 62–73
  diagnosis of, 145–146
  diagnostic tests for, 145
  differential diagnosis of, 144
  history of, 143
  physical assessment of, 144
  tentative diagnoses for, 142
  therapeutic plan for, 146–148
Conjunctivitis
  allergic, 32
  bacterial, 27–35
    diagnosis of, 34
    diagnostic tests for, 33
    differential diagnosis of, 32–33
    history of, 30
    physical assessment of, 31
    presenting symptoms of, 29
    tentative diagnoses of, 29
    therapeutic plan for, 34–35
  chemical, 32
  vs. corneal abrasion, 353–361
  vs. herpes zoster, 169–177
  viral, 32
Contact dermatitis, 469–476
  diagnosis of, 475
  diagnostic tests for, 475
  differential diagnosis of, 474–475
  vs. herpes zoster, 169–177
  history of, 472–473
  physical assessment of, 473–474
  presenting symptoms of, 471
  vs. scabies, 345–352
  tentative diagnoses for, 471
  therapeutic plan for, 476
Contact lenses, corneal abrasion due to, 356, 360

Contraception, 310–323
  diagnostic tests for, 318
  history for, 313–315
  with human immunodeficiency virus, 378–379
  physical assessment for, 315–316
  therapeutic plan for, 319–321
Corneal abrasion, 353–361
  vs. conjunctivitis, 29
  with contact lens wear, 356, 360
  diagnosis for, 359
  diagnostic tests for, 359
  differential diagnoses of, 358–359
  history of, 356–357
  physical assessment of, 357–358
  presenting symptoms of, 355
  tentative diagnoses for, 355–356
  therapeutic plan for, 360–361
Cough
  chronic, with shortness of breath, 10–26
  drug-induced, vs. asthma, 10–26
  and fatigue, 140–148
    clinical symptoms of, 142
    diagnosis of, 145–146
    diagnostic tests for, 145
    differential diagnosis of, 144
    history of, 143
    physical assessment of, 144
    tentative diagnoses for, 142
    therapeutic plan for, 146–148
  with fever and shortness of breath, 62–73
Critical thinking, 1–3
  and clinical decision making, 4
  teaching of, 4–7
CVS (chorionic villus sampling), 45–46
Cyst, epidermal or Bartholin, vs. human
          papillomavirus, 477–486
Cystitis, 329
Cytomegalovirus, vs. hepatitis, 408

D
ddC, for human immunodeficiency virus, 376
ddI, for human immunodeficiency virus, 376
Decision making, 3–4
  critical thinking and, 4
  teaching of, 4–7
Delirium, 199–214
  with anemia, 203
  with cardiac event, 203
  diagnosis of, 211–212
  diagnostic tests for, 209–211
  differential diagnosis of, 208
  with electrolyte imbalance, 203
  history of, 204–205
  with hyper/hypothyroidism, 203
  from medication side effects, 204
  with neurological event, 203
  with nutritional deficiencies, 203
  physical assessment of, 206–207
  presenting symptoms of, 201

  tentative diagnoses for, 202–204
  therapeutic plan for, 212–214
  with urinary tract infection, 203, 208, 211
Dementia, 199–214
  diagnosis of, 211–212
  diagnostic tests for, 209–211
  differential diagnosis of, 208
  history of, 204–205
  physical assessment of, 206–207
  presenting symptoms of, 201
  resources for, 213
  tentative diagnoses for, 202–204
  therapeutic plan for, 212–214
Dental abscess, vs. sinusitis, 391–401
Depo-Provera, 320–321
Depression, 74–90
  vs. dementia, 199–214
  diagnosis of, 85–86
  diagnostic tests for, 83–85
  differential diagnosis of, 82
  vs. hepatitis, 402–413
  history of, 77–79
  physical assessment of, 80–81
  presenting symptoms of, 76
  resources for, 89
  tentative diagnoses for, 76–77
  therapeutic plan for, 86–89
Depth, 7
Dermatitis
  atopic, 471, 475
  contact, 469–476
    diagnosis of, 475
    diagnostic tests for, 475
    differential diagnosis of, 474–475
    vs. herpes zoster, 169–177
    history of, 472–473
    physical assessment of, 473–474
    presenting symptoms of, 471
    vs. scabies, 345–352
    tentative diagnoses for, 471
    therapeutic plan for, 476
  nummular, 471
Dextroamphetamine (Dexedrine), for ADHD, 59
Diabetes insipidus, vs. non-insulin dependent
          diabetes mellitus, 257–267
Diabetes mellitus (DM)
  vs. depression, 74–90
  vs. gonorrhea and chlamydia, 91–103
  non-insulin dependent, 257–267
    cardiovascular disease with, 266–267
    diagnosis of, 263
    diagnostic tests for, 263
    differential diagnosis for, 262
    history of, 260–261
    with hypertension, 441–454
      diagnosis of, 449–450
      diagnostic tests for, 448–449
      differential diagnosis for, 447–448
      history of, 444–446
      physical assessment of, 446–447
      presenting symptoms of, 443

Diabetes mellitus (DM), non-insulin dependent,
  with hypertension (*continued*)
    tentative diagnoses with, 443–444
    therapeutic plan for, 450–454
  nephropathy with, 265–266
  neuropathy with, 266
  physical assessment of, 261–262
  presenting symptoms of, 259
  retinopathy with, 265
  risk factors for, 264
  tentative diagnoses for, 259
  therapeutic plan for, 264–267
Diarrhea
  with abnormal menstrual cycle, fatigue, and
    weight gain, 487–497
  with bloating, 268–277
    diagnosis of, 275–276
    diagnostic tests for, 275
    differential diagnosis of, 274
    history of, 271–272
    physical assessment of, 273
    presenting symptoms of, 270
    tentative diagnoses for, 270
    therapeutic plan for, 276–277
Diet. *See* Nutrition
Dimenhydrinate (Dramamine), for benign
  paroxysmal positional vertigo, 426
Diphenidol (Vontrol), for benign paroxysmal
  positional vertigo, 426
Diuretics, for congestive heart failure, 147
Diverticulosis, *vs.* irritable bowel syndrome,
  268–277
Dizziness, 414–427
  diagnosis of, 425
  diagnostic tests for, 423–425
  differential diagnosis of, 422–423
  history of, 418–419
  physical assessment of, 420–421
  presenting symptoms of, 416
  tentative diagnoses for, 416–417
  therapeutic plan for, 425–427
DM. *See* Diabetes mellitus (DM)
Domestic violence, 308
Doxycycline, for pelvic inflammatory disease,
  197
Dramamine (dimenhydrinate), for benign
  paroxysmal positional vertigo, 426
Drug-induced cough, *vs.* asthma, 10–26
d4T, for human immunodeficiency virus, 376
Duodenal ulcer, 380–390
  diagnosis of, 388
  diagnostic tests for, 387–388
  differential diagnosis of, 386–387
  vs. gastroesophageal reflux, 104–113
  history of, 383–385
  physical assessment of, 385–386
  presenting symptoms of, 382
  tentative diagnoses for, 382–383
  therapeutic plan for, 388–390
Duricef (cefadroxil), for urinary tract infection,
  332

E

Earache, 231–239
  diagnosis of, 237
  diagnostic tests for, 237
  differential diagnosis of, 236
  history of, 234–235
  physical assessment of, 235–236
  presenting symptoms of, 233
  tentative diagnoses for, 233
  therapeutic plan for, 238–239
Ectopic pregnancy
  vs. pelvic inflammatory disease, 190–198
  vs. threatened abortion, 36–47
EDC (estimated date of conception), 44
Elderly person
  confusion in, 199–214
    diagnosis of, 211–212
    diagnostic tests for, 209–211
    differential diagnosis of, 208
    history of, 204–205
    physical assessment of, 206–207
    presenting symptoms of, 201
    resources for, 213
    tentative diagnoses for, 202–204
    therapeutic plan for, 212–214
  dizziness in, 414–427
    diagnosis of, 425
    diagnostic tests for, 423–425
    differential diagnosis of, 422–423
    history of, 418–419
    physical assessment of, 420–421
    presenting symptoms of, 416
    tentative diagnoses for, 416–417
    therapeutic plan for, 425–427
  hypertension in, 441–454
    diagnosis of, 449–450
    diagnostic tests for, 448–449
    differential diagnosis of, 447–448
    history of, 444–446
    physical assessment of, 446–447
    presenting symptoms of, 443
    tentative diagnoses for, 443–444
    therapeutic plan for, 450–454
  perineal rash in, 345–352
  routine checkup of
    for man, 279–289
      diagnostic tests in, 285–286
      history in, 281–283
      physical assessment in, 283–284

Dyspnea, with cough and fatigue, 140–148
  clinical symptoms of, 142
  diagnosis of, 145–146
  diagnostic tests for, 145
  differential diagnosis of, 144
  history of, 143
  physical assessment of, 144
  tentative diagnoses for, 142
  therapeutic plan for, 146–148

for woman, 114–126
  diagnostic tests in, 122–123
  history in, 116–118
  physical assessment in, 118–121
Electrolyte imbalance
  delirium with, 203
  vs. hypothyroidism, 487–497
Elimite (permethrin cream), for scabies, 351
Emotions, in critical thinking, 2
Emphysema, 70
Enalapril (Vasotec), for congestive heart failure, 146
Endometriosis, *vs.* pelvic inflammatory disease, 190–198
Epidermal cyst, *vs.* human papillomavirus, 477–486
Epigastric pain, 299–309
  diagnosis of, 307
  diagnostic tests for, 306–307
  differential diagnosis of, 305
  history of, 302–303
  physical assessment of, 304
  presenting symptoms of, 301
  tentative diagnoses for, 301–302
  therapeutic plan for, 307–309
Epiglottitis, *vs.* streptococcal pharyngitis, 231–239
Epstein-Barr virus, *vs.* hepatitis, 408
Esidrix (hydrochlorothiazide), for congestive heart failure, 147
Estimated date of conception (EDC), 44
Eye
  itchy red, with drainage, 27–35
    diagnosis of, 34
    diagnostic tests for, 33
    differential diagnosis of, 32–33
    history of, 30
    physical assessment of, 31
    presenting symptoms of, 29
    tentatitive diagnoses of, 29
    therapeutic plan for, 34–35
  painful red, with facial rash, 169–177
    diagnosis of, 176
    diagnostic tests for, 175–176
    differential diagnosis of, 174–175
    history of, 172–173
    physical assessment of, 173–174
    presenting symptoms of, 171
    tentative diagnoses for, 171
    therapeutic plan for, 176–177
Eye injury
  vs. conjunctivitis, 29
  penetrating, *vs.* corneal abrasion, 353–361
Eye pain, 353–361
  diagnosis of, 359
  diagnostic tests for, 359
  differential diagnoses of, 358–359
  history of, 356–357
  physical assessment of, 357–358
  presenting symptoms of, 355
  tentative diagnoses for, 355–356
  therapeutic plan for, 360–361

F

Facial rash, with painful red eye, 169–177
  diagnosis of, 176
  diagnostic tests for, 175–176
  differential diagnosis of, 174–175
  history of, 172–173
  physical assessment of, 173–174
  presenting symptoms of, 171
  tentative diagnoses for, 171
  therapeutic plan for, 176–177
Failure to thrive (FTT), 215–229
  criteria for, 225
  diagnosis of, 225–226
  diagnostic tests for, 223–225
  differential diagnosis of, 222
  history of, 218–220
  physical assessment of, 220–221
  presenting symptoms of, 217
  resource for, 228
  tentative diagnoses for, 217–218
  therapeutic plan for, 226–229
Famciclovir (Famvir), for herpes zoster, 176
Family planning, 310–323
  diagnostic tests for, 318
  history of, 313–315
  with human immunodeficiency virus, 378–379
  physical assessment for, 315–316
  therapeutic plan for, 319–321
Famotidine (Pepcid), for gastroesophageal reflux, 112
Fat content, in breast milk, poor, 218, 225–226
Fatigue, 402–413
  with blurred vision and polyuria, 257–267
  with cough, 140–148
    fever, and shortness of breath, 62–73
  diagnosis of, 411
  diagnostic tests for, 409–410
  differential diagnosis of, 408–409
  with headaches, 74–90
  history of, 405–406
  physical assessment of, 407–408
  in pregnancy, 46
  presenting symptoms of, 404
  tentative diagnoses for, 404–405
  therapeutic plan for, 411–413
  with weight gain, diarrhea, and abnormal menstrual cycle, 487–497
Feeder, poor, *vs.* failure to thrive, 215–229
Fever
  with cough and shortness of breath, 62–73
  rash and, 291–298
Fibroadenoma, *vs.* fibrocystic breast disease, 149–156
Fibrocystic breast disease, 149–156
  clinical presentation of, 151
  diagnosis of, 154
  diagnostic tests for, 154
  differential diagnosis of, 153–154
  history of, 151–152

Fibrocystic breast disease (*continued*)
physical assessment of, 153
tentative diagnoses for, 151
Fibroma, ocular
vs. corneal abrasion, 353–361
vs. herpes zoster, 169–177
Flagyl (metronidazole)
for gonorrhea and chlamydia, 100
for peptic ulcer disease, 389
Folliculitis, *vs.* human papillomavirus, 477–486
FTT. *See* Failure to thrive (FTT)
Furosemide (Lasix), for congestive heart failure,
147, 148

G

Gastric cancer, *vs.* peptic ulcer disease, 380–390
Gastric pain. *See* Epigastric pain
Gastric ulcer, *vs.* gastroesophageal reflux, 104–113
Gastritis, *vs.* irritable bowel syndrome, 268–277
Gastroesophageal reflux disease (GERD), 104–113
vs. asthma, 10–26
vs. cholecystitis, 299–309
vs. congestive heart failure, 140–148
diagnosis of, 111
diagnostic tests for, 110–111
differential diagnosis of, 109
vs. failure to thrive, 215–229
history of, 107–108
vs. peptic ulcer disease, 380–390
physical assessment of, 108–109
presenting symptoms of, 106
tentative diagnoses for, 106
therapeutic plan for, 111–113
Generalized anxiety disorder, *vs.* ADHD, 48–61
Genital warts, 477–486
diagnosis of, 484
diagnostic tests for, 483
differential diagnosis of, 482–483
history of, 480–481
physical assessment of, 481–482
presenting symptoms of, 479
tentative diagnoses for, 479–480
therapeutic plan for, 484–486
GERD. *See* Gastroesophageal reflux disease (GERD)
Glaucoma, 121
vs. conjunctivitis, 29
vs. non-insulin dependent diabetes mellitus,
257–267
Glipizide (Glucotrol), for non-insulin dependent
diabetes mellitus, 264, 265
Gonorrhea, 91–103
diagnosis for, 100
diagnostic tests for, 98–99
differential diagnosis of, 97–98
history of, 94–96
pelvic inflammatory disease due to, 190–198
physical assessment of, 96–97
presenting symptoms of, 93
resources for, 101–102

tentative diagnoses for, 93
therapeutic plan for, 100–103
Gynecomastia, 168

H

Headache
fatigue and, 74–90
frontal, with rhinorrhea and maxillary tooth pain,
391–401
diagnostic tests for, 397–398
differential diagnosis of, 396–397
history of, 394–395
physical assessment of, 395–396
presenting symptoms of, 393
tentative diagnoses for, 393
therapeutic plan for, 398–401
migraine, without aura, 127–139
clinical presentation of, 129
diagnosis of, 135–136
diagnostic tests for, 135
differential diagnosis of, 134–135
history of, 130–132
physical assessment of, 132–134
tentative diagnoses for, 129–130
therapeutic plan for, 136–139
mixed, 127–139
clinical presentation of, 129
diagnosis of, 135–136
diagnostic tests for, 135
differential diagnosis of, 134–135
history of, 130–132
physical assessment of, 132–134
tentative diagnoses for, 129–130
therapeutic plan for, 136–139
steady, throbbing, 127–139
clinical presentation of, 129
diagnosis of, 135–136
diagnostic tests for, 135
differential diagnosis of, 134–135
history of, 130–132
physical assessment of, 132–134
tentative diagnoses for, 129–130
therapeutic plan for, 136–139
tension-type, 127–139
clinical presentation of, 129
diagnosis of, 135–136
diagnostic tests for, 135
differential diagnosis of, 134–135
history of, 130–132
physical assessment of, 132–134
tentative diagnoses for, 129–130
therapeutic plan for, 136–139
Heartburn, 104–113
diagnosis of, 111
diagnostic tests for, 110–111
differential diagnosis of, 109
history of, 107–108
physical assessment of, 108–109
presenting symptoms of, 106

tentative diagnoses for, 106
therapeutic plan for, 111–113
Heart disease. *See* Cardiac disease
Heart murmur, in infant, 226
Hepatitis, 402–413
  vs. cholecystitis, 305
  classification of, 411
  diagnosis of, 411
  diagnostic tests for, 409–410
  differential diagnosis of, 408–409
  history of, 405–406
  vs. human immunodeficiency virus, 362–379
  physical assessment of, 407–408
  presenting symptoms of, 404
  tentative diagnoses for, 404–405
  therapeutic plan for, 411–413
Herniated lumbar disc, *vs.* lumbosacral strain,
    429–440
Herpes simplex
  vs. herpes zoster, 169–177
  vs. human papillomavirus, 477–486
  vs. scabies, 345–352
  vs. urinary tract infection, 324–333
Herpes simplex blepharitis, *vs.* conjunctivitis, 29
Herpes zoster (HZ), 169–177
  diagnosis of, 176
  diagnostic tests for, 175–176
  differential diagnosis of, 174–175
  history of, 172–173
  physical assessment of, 173–174
  presenting symptoms of, 171
  tentative diagnoses for, 171
  therapeutic plan for, 176–177
HIV. *See* Human immunodeficiency virus (HIV)
Hormone replacement therapy (HRT), 125
HPV. *See* Human papillomavirus (HPV)
H$_2$-receptor antagonists, for gastroesophageal
    reflux, 112
HTN. *See* Hypertension (HTN)
Human immunodeficiency virus (HIV), 362–379
  birth control with, 378–379
  classification system for, 373
  diagnosis of, 372–374
  diagnostic tests for, 370–372
  differential diagnosis of, 369
  vs. hepatitis, 408
  history of, 365–367
  physical assessment of, 367–368
  presenting symptoms of, 364
  prognostic indicator for staging, 375
  resources for, 377
  tentative diagnoses for, 364–365
  therapeutic plan for, 374–379
  vaccination with, 377–378
Human papillomavirus (HPV), 477–486
  diagnosis of, 484
  diagnostic tests for, 483
  differential diagnosis of, 482–483
  history of, 480–481
  physical assessment of, 481–482
  presenting symptoms of, 479

tentative diagnoses for, 479–480
therapeutic plan for, 484–486
Hydrochlorothiazide (Esidrix, HydroDIURIL, for
    congestive heart failure, 147
Hypercholesterolemia, 167, 288
Hyperlipidemia, 288
Hypertension (HTN), 441–454
  diagnosis of, 449–450
  diagnostic tests for, 448–449
  differential diagnosis of, 447–448
  in elderly, 121, 123
  history of, 444–446
  physical assessment of, 446–447
  presenting symptoms of, 443
  vs. tension-type headache, 127–139
  tentative diagnoses for, 443–444
  therapeutic plan for, 450–454
Hyperthyroidism
  delirium with, 203
  vs. irritable bowel syndrome, 268–277
Hypoglycemia, *vs.* depression, 74–90
Hypotension, syncope due to, 417, 423
Hypothyroidism, 487–497
  vs. benign paroxysmal positional vertigo, 423
  with congestive heart failure, 140–148
  delirium with, 203
  vs. depression, 74–90
  diagnosis of, 495
  diagnostic tests for, 494–495
  differential diagnosis of, 493
  vs. gonorrhea and chlamydia, 91–103
  vs. hepatitis, 402–413
  history of, 490–492
  vs. non-insulin dependent diabetes mellitus,
    257–267
  physical assessment of, 492–493
  presenting symptoms of, 489
  tentative diagnoses for, 489–490
  therapeutic plan for, 495–497
HZ. *See* Herpes zoster (HZ)

I

IBD (inflammatory bowel disease)
  vs. cholecystitis, 299–309
  vs. irritable bowel syndrome, 268–277
IBS. *See* Irritable bowel syndrome (IBS)
Immunization, of elderly, 124
Impetigo, *vs.* herpes zoster, 169–177
Incontinence, with confusion, 199–214
Indinavir, for human immunodeficiency virus, 376
Infant
  with failure to thrive, 215–229
    diagnosis of, 225–226
    diagnostic tests for, 223–225
    differential diagnosis of, 222
    history of, 218–220
    physical assessment of, 220–221
    presenting symptoms of, 217
    resource for, 228

Infant, with failure to thrive (*continued*)
    tentative diagnoses for, 217–218
      therapeutic plan for, 226–229
    with heart murmur, 226
Infectious mononucleosis
    vs. hepatitis, 408
    vs. human immunodeficiency virus, 362–379
    vs. streptococcal pharyngitis, 231–239
Inflammatory bowel disease (IBD)
    vs. cholecystitis, 299–309
    vs. irritable bowel syndrome, 268–277
Influenza, chronic inflammatory viral, 397
Intellectual standards, 6–7
Intestinal infection, *vs.* irritable bowel syndrome,
    268–277
Iritis
    vs. conjunctivitis, 29
    vs. corneal abrasion, 353–361
Irritable bowel syndrome (IBS), 268–277
    diagnosis of, 275–276
    diagnostic tests for, 275
    differential diagnosis of, 274
    history of, 271–272
    vs. hypothyroidism, 487–497
    physical assessment of, 273
    presenting symptoms of, 270
    tentative diagnoses for, 270
    therapeutic plan for, 276–277

K

Kawasaki disease (KD), 291–298
KCl (potassium chloride), for congestive heart
    failure, 148
Keratitis, *vs.* corneal abrasion, 353–361
Kindergarten, physical examination for, 335–344
    anticipatory guidance in, 343
    diagnostic tests in, 342
    history in, 337–339
    physical assessment in, 340–341
Knee extensor mechanism, disruption of, *vs.* medial
    collateral ligament injury, 179–188
Knee pain, 179–188
    diagnosis of, 187
    diagnostic tests for, 186–187
    differential diagnosis of, 185–186
    history of, 182–183
    physical assessment of, 183–185
    presenting symptoms of, 181
    tentative diagnoses for, 181–182
    therapeutic plan for, 187–188

L

Lactose intolerance, 276
Lanoxin, for congestive heart failure, 147, 148
Laryngeal dysfunction, *vs.* asthma, 10–26
Lasix (furosemide), for congestive heart failure,
    147, 148

Lateral collateral ligament (LCL) injury, *vs.* medial
    collateral ligament injury, 179–188
Laxative abuse, *vs.* irritable bowel syndrome,
    268–277
Lead screening, 465
Learning disability, *vs.* ADHD, 48–61
Lentigo maligna melanoma, 285, 287, 289
Levothyroxine (Synthroid), for hypothyroidism,
    148, 495–496
Libido, decreased, with fatigue and headaches,
    74–90
Lichen simplex chronicus, *vs.* contact dermatitis,
    469–476
Lisinopril (Zestril), for congestive heart failure, 146,
    148
Logic, 7
Lumbar disc, herniated, *vs.* lumbosacral strain,
    429–440
Lumbosacral strain, 429–440
    diagnosis of, 437
    diagnostic tests for, 436–437
    differential diagnosis of, 435–436
    history of, 432–433
    physical assessment of, 433–434
    presenting symptoms of, 431
    tentative diagnoses for, 431–432
    therapeutic plan for, 437–440
Lump, under arm, 362–379
    diagnosis of, 372–374
    diagnostic tests for, 370–372
    differential diagnosis of, 369
    history of, 365–367
    physical assessment of, 367–368
    presenting symptoms of, 364
    tentative diagnoses for, 364–365
    therapeutic plan for, 374–379
Lung cancer, *vs.* COPD, 62–73
Lymphogranuloma, *vs.* human papillomavirus,
    477–486

M

Macrobid (nitrofurantoin macrocrystals), for
    urinary tract infection, 332
Macrodantin (nitrofurantoin macrocrystals), for
    urinary tract infection, 332
Malingering
    vs. lumbosacral strain, 429–440
    vs. opiate dependence, 240–256
Mammogram
    patient instructions for, 155
    recommendations for, 120
Mebendazole (Vermox), for pinworms, 343
Meclizine (Antivert), for benign paroxysmal
    positional vertigo, 426
Medial collateral ligament (MCL) injury, 179–188
    diagnosis of, 187
    diagnostic tests for, 186–187
    differential diagnosis of, 185–186
    history of, 182–183

physical assessment of, 183–185
presenting symptoms of, 181
tentative diagnoses for, 181–182
therapeutic plan for, 187–188
Medication side effects, delirium with, 204
Melanoma, lentigo maligna, 285, 287, 289
Meniere's disease, peripheral, *vs.* benign
paroxysmal positional vertigo, 414–427
Meningitis, bacterial, *vs.* Kawasaki disease, 291–298
Meniscal injury, *vs.* medial collateral ligament
injury, 179–188
Menopause, *vs.* depression, 74–90
Menses, irregular
with diarrhea, fatigue, and weight gain, 487–497
with fatigue and headaches, 74–90
Metabolism, inborn errors of, *vs.* failure to thrive,
215–229
Methylphenidate (Ritalin), for ADHD, 58
Metronidazole (Flagyl)
for gonorrhea and chlamydia, 100
for peptic ulcer disease, 389
MI (myocardial infarction), *vs.* cholecystitis,
299–309
Migraine headache, without aura, 127–139
clinical presentation of, 129
diagnosis of, 135–136
diagnostic tests for, 135
differential diagnosis of, 134–135
history of, 130–132
physical assessment of, 132–134
tentative diagnoses for, 129–130
therapeutic plan for, 136–139
Moexipril (Univasc), for congestive heart failure,
147
Molluscum contagiosum, *vs.* human papillomavirus,
477–486
Mononucleosis, infectious
vs. hepatitis, 408
vs. human immunodeficiency virus, 362–379
vs. streptococcal pharyngitis, 231–239
Mucocutaneous lymph node syndrome, 291–298
Murmur, in infant, 226
Myocardial infarction (MI), *vs.* cholecystitis,
299–309
Myxedema, 496

N

Nail biting, 48–61
Nares, mechanical obstruction of, *vs.* sinusitis,
391–401
Nausea
with peptic ulcer disease, 380–390
of pregnancy, 46
Nephropathy, diabetic, 265–266
Neurological disease
vs. ADHD, 48–61
vs. depression, 74–90
vs. failure to thrive, 215–229
Neurological event, delirium with, 203

Neuroma, acoustic, *vs.* benign paroxysmal
positional vertigo, 414–427
Neuropathy, diabetic, 266
Nitrofurantoin macrocrystals (Macrodantin,
Macrobid), for urinary tract infection, 332
Nizatidine (Axid), for gastroesophageal reflux, 112
Non-insulin dependent diabetes mellitus (NIDDM),
257–267
cardiovascular disease with, 266–267
diagnosis of, 263
diagnostic tests for, 263
differential diagnosis of, 262
vs. gonorrhea and chlamydia, 91–103
history of, 260–261
with hypertension, 441–454
diagnosis of, 449–450
diagnostic tests for, 448–449
differential diagnosis of, 447–448
history of, 444–446
physical assessment of, 446–447
presenting symptoms of, 443
tentative diagnoses for, 443–444
therapeutic plan for, 450–454
nephropathy with, 265–266
neuropathy with, 266
physical assessment of, 261–262
presenting symptoms of, 259
retinopathy with, 265
risk factors for, 264
tentative diagnoses for, 259
therapeutic plan for, 264–267
Nummular dermatitis, *vs.* contact dermatitis,
469–476
Nursing process, 3
Nutrition
for adolescent, 167
for elderly, 125
for failure-to-thrive infant, 226–227
for hypertension and diabetes mellitus, 451–452
for peptic ulcer disease, 389
during pregnancy, 44–45
Nutritional deficiencies, delirium with, 203

O

Obesity
with diabetes mellitus, 257–267
with hypertension, 441–454
with hypothyroidism, 487–497
Ocular fibroma
vs. corneal abrasion, 353–361
vs. herpes zoster, 169–177
ODD (oppositional defiant disorder), *vs.* ADHD,
48–61
Opiate abuse, 249
Opiate dependence, 240–256
diagnosis of, 251–252
diagnostic tests for, 250–251
differential diagnosis of, 248–250
history of, 243–245

Opiate dependence (*continued*)
   physical assessment of, 246–247
   presenting symptoms of, 242
   resources for, 255–256
   tentative diagnoses for, 242
   therapeutic plan for, 252–256
Opiate withdrawal, 249
Oppositional defiant disorder (ODD), *vs.* ADHD,
   48–61
Organic problems, *vs.* ADHD, 48–61
Osteochondral fracture, *vs.* medial collateral
   ligament injury, 179–188
Osteoporosis, 122, 124, 125
Otitis externa, *vs.* otitis media, 231–239
Otitis media, 231–239
   diagnosis of, 237
   diagnostic tests for, 237
   differential diagnosis of, 236
   history of, 234–235
   physical assessment of, 235–236
   presenting symptoms of, 233
   tentative diagnoses for, 233
   therapeutic plan for, 238–239
Ototoxic drugs, vertigo due to, 417, 422

P

Pain, assessment of, 245
Pain disorder, chronic, *vs.* opiate dependence,
   240–256
Pancreatitis
   vs. cholecystitis, 299–309
   vs. peptic ulcer disease, 380–390
Papillomavirus, human, 477–486
   diagnosis of, 484
   diagnostic tests for, 483
   differential diagnosis of, 482–483
   history of, 480–481
   physical assessment of, 481–482
   presenting symptoms of, 479
   tentative diagnoses for, 479–480
   therapeutic plan for, 484–486
PAP smears, for elderly, 120–121
PCL (posterior cruciate ligament) injury, *vs.* medial
   collateral ligament injury, 179–188
Pelvic examination, for birth control, 310–323
   diagnostic tests for, 318
   history for, 313–315
   physical assessment for, 315–316
   therapeutic plan for, 319–321
Pelvic inflammatory disease (PID), 190–198
   vs. cholecystitis, 299–309
   diagnosis of, 196–197
   diagnostic tests for, 196
   differential diagnosis of, 195
   vs. gonorrhea and chlamydia, 91–103
   history of, 193–194
   physical assessment of, 194–195
   presenting symptoms of, 192
   tentative diagnoses for, 192

   therapeutic plan for, 197–198
Penicillin, for streptococcal pharyngitis, 238
Pepcid (famotidine), for gastroesophageal reflux,
   112
Peptic ulcer disease (PUD), 380–390
   vs. cholecystitis, 299–309
   vs. congestive heart failure, 140–148
   diagnosis of, 388
   diagnostic tests for, 387–388
   differential diagnosis of, 386–387
   vs. gastroesophageal reflux, 104–113
   history of, 383–385
   physical assessment of, 385–386
   presenting symptoms of, 382
   tentative diagnoses for, 382–383
   therapeutic plan for, 388–390
Perineal rash, 345–352
Periodontal disease, *vs.* sinusitis, 397
Peripheral pulmonic stenosis (PPS), 226
Peripheral vestibulopathy, *vs.* benign paroxysmal
   positional vertigo, 414–427
Peritonitis, *vs.* cholecystitis, 299–309
Permethrin cream (Elimite), for scabies, 351
Pharyngitis
   streptococcal, 231–239
     diagnosis of, 237
     diagnostic tests for, 237
     differential diagnosis of, 236
     history of, 234–235
     vs. Kawasaki disease, 296
     physical assessment of, 235–236
     presenting symptoms of, 233
     tentative diagnoses for, 233
     therapeutic plan for, 238–239
   viral, 236
Phlegm, with chronic cough, 10–26
PHN (post-herpetic neuralgia), 177
Physical examination
   for adolescent sports, 157–158
     diagnostic tests for, 164–165
     history in, 159–161
     physical assessment in, 161–163
     therapeutic plan in, 165–168
   of elderly man, 279–289
     diagnostic tests in, 285–286
     history in, 281–283
     physical assessment in, 283–284
   of elderly woman, 114–126
     diagnostic tests in, 122–123
     history in, 116–118
     physical assessment in, 118–121
   of infant, 215–229
     anticipatory guidance in, 229
     history in, 218–220
     physical assessment in, 220–221
   for kindergarten, 335–344
     anticipatory guidance in, 343
     diagnostic tests in, 342
     history in, 337–339
     physical assessment in, 340–341
   of two-year-old, 455–468

anticipatory guidance in, 466–468
diagnostic tests in, 465
history in, 458–461
physical assessment in, 462–464
PID. *See* Pelvic inflammatory disease (PID)
Pinworms, 341, 343–344
Pneumonia
vs. asthma, 10–26
vs. COPD, 62–73
Podophyllin (Podofilox), for human
papillomavirus, 484
Polyuria, with blurred vision and fatigue, 257–267
Posterior cruciate ligament (PCL) injury, *vs.* medial
collateral ligament injury, 179–188
Post-herpetic neuralgia (PHN), 177
Potassium chloride (KCl), for congestive heart
failure, 148
PPS (peripheral pulmonic stenosis), 226
Precision, 7
Pregnancy
abdominal bloating in, 46
ectopic
vs. pelvic inflammatory disease, 190–198
vs. threatened abortion, 36–47
fatigue in, 46
vs. gonorrhea and chlamydia, 91–103
vs. hypothyroidism, 487–497
nausea and vomiting of, 46
nutrition during, 44–45
vaginal bleeding during, 36–47
warning signs in, 47
Presbyopia, *vs.* non-insulin dependent diabetes
mellitus, 257–267
Prokinetic drug therapy, for gastroesophageal
reflux, 112
Prostatic hyperplasia, benign, 288
vs. non-insulin dependent diabetes mellitus, 262
vs. urinary tract infection, 441–454
Proton pump inhibitors, for gastroesophageal
reflux, 112–113
Psoriasis, *vs.* scabies, 345–352
Psychiatric illness, *vs.* benign paroxysmal positional
vertigo, 417, 423
PUD. *See* Peptic ulcer disease (PUD)
Pulmonary disease, *vs.* failure to thrive, 215–229
Pulmonic stenosis, peripheral, 226
Pyelonephritis, 329

Q

Quinapril (Accupril), for congestive heart failure,
147

R

Ramsay Hunt syndrome, 177
Ranitidine (Zantac), for gastroesophageal reflux, 112
Rash
on arm, 469–476

child with fever and, 291–298
facial, with painful red eye, 169–177
perineal, 345–352
Reasoning, elements of, 5–6
Reflux, gastroesophageal, 104–113
vs. asthma, 10–26
vs. cholecystitis, 299–309
vs. congestive heart failure, 140–148
diagnosis of, 111
diagnostic tests for, 110–111
differential diagnosis of, 109
vs. failure to thrive, 215–229
history of, 107–108
vs. peptic ulcer disease, 380–390
physical assessment of, 108–109
presenting symptoms of, 106
tentative diagnoses for, 106
therapeutic plan for, 111–113
Relevance, 7
Renal colic, *vs.* cholecystitis, 299–309
Respiratory tract infection, upper, *vs.* sinusitis,
391–401
Retinopathy, diabetic, 265
Rhinitis
allergic, *vs.* sinusitis, 391–401
chronic inflammatory, *vs.* sinusitis, 397
vasomotor, with sinusitis, 391–401
Rhinitis medicamentosa, *vs.* sinusitis, 397
Rhinorrhea, with frontal headache and maxillary
tooth pain, 391–401
diagnostic tests for, 397–398
differential diagnosis of, 396–397
history of, 394–395
physical assessment of, 395–396
presenting symptoms of, 393
tentative diagnoses for, 393
therapeutic plan for, 398–401
Ritalin (methylphenidate), for ADHD, 58
Ritonavir, for human immunodeficiency virus, 376
Rocephin (ceftriaxone)
for gonorrhea and chlamydia, 100
for pelvic inflammatory disease, 197
Roseola, *vs.* Kawasaki disease, 291–298
Routine checkup
for adolescent sports, 157–158
diagnostic tests for, 164–165
history in, 159–161
physical assessment in, 161–163
therapeutic plan in, 165–168
of elderly man, 279–289
diagnostic tests in, 285–286
history in, 281–283
physical assessment in, 283–284
of elderly woman, 114–126
diagnostic tests in, 122–123
history in, 116–118
physical assessment in, 118–121
of infant, 215–229
anticipatory guidance in, 229
history in, 218–220
physical assessment in, 220–221

Routine checkup (*continued*)
  for kindergarten, 335–344
    anticipatory guidance in, 343
    diagnostic tests in, 342
    history in, 337–339
    physical assessment in, 340–341
  of two-year-old, 455–468
    anticipatory guidance in, 466–468
    diagnostic tests in, 465
    history in, 458–461
    physical assessment in, 462–464

S

Safety issues, with toddlers, 466
Saquinavir, for human immunodeficiency virus, 376
Scabies, 345–352
  vs. contact dermatitis, 469–476
  diagnosis of, 351
  diagnostic tests for, 351
  differential diagnosis of, 350
  history of, 348–349
  physical assessment of, 349–350
  presenting symptoms of, 347
  tentative diagnoses for, 347
  therapeutic plan for, 351–352
Scarlet fever, *vs.* Kawasaki disease, 291–298
School, difficulty in, 48–61
Sciatica, *vs.* lumbosacral strain, 429–440
Sebaceous cyst, *vs.* human papillomavirus, 477–486
Sepsis, neonatal, *vs.* failure to thrive, 215–229
Sequestered lobe, *vs.* failure to thrive, 215–229
Sexual intercourse, abdominal pain with, 190–198
Sexually transmitted disease (STD), 91–103
  diagnosis for, 100
  diagnostic tests for, 98–99
  differential diagnosis of, 97–98
  history of, 94–96
  physical assessment of, 96–97
  presenting symptoms of, 93
  resources for, 101–102
  tentative diagnoses for, 93
  therapeutic plan for, 100–103
Shaking, with fatigue and headaches, 74–90
Shingles, 169–177
  diagnosis of, 176
  diagnostic tests for, 175–176
  differential diagnosis of, 174–175
  history of, 172–173
  physical assessment of, 173–174
  presenting symptoms of, 171
  tentative diagnoses for, 171
  therapeutic plan for, 176–177
Shortness of breath (SOB)
  with chronic cough, 10–26
  with cough and fever, 62–73
Sinusitis, 391–401
  diagnostic tests for, 397–398
  differential diagnosis of, 396–397

history of, 394–395
  physical assessment of, 395–396
  presenting symptoms of, 393
  vs. streptococcal pharyngitis and otitis media, 231–239
  tentative diagnoses for, 393
  therapeutic plan for, 398–401
Skin cancer, *vs.* contact dermatitis, 469–476
Skin dryness, with fatigue and headaches, 74–90
Skin tag, *vs.* human papillomavirus, 477–486
Sleep disturbances, with fatigue and headaches, 74–90
Smoking cessation, 309
SOB (shortness of breath)
  with chronic cough, 10–26
  with cough and fever, 62–73
Sore throat, 231–239
  diagnosis of, 237
  diagnostic tests for, 237
  differential diagnosis of, 236
  history of, 234–235
  physical assessment of, 235–236
  presenting symptoms of, 233
  tentative diagnoses for, 233
  therapeutic plan for, 238–239
Sports injury, to knee, 179–188
Sports physical, 157–158
  diagnostic tests for, 164–165
  history in, 159–161
  physical assessment in, 161–163
  therapeutic plan in, 165–168
Spotting, during pregnancy, 36–47
Sprain, of medial collateral ligament, 179–188
  diagnosis of, 187
  diagnostic tests for, 186–187
  differential diagnosis of, 185–186
  history of, 182–183
  physical assessment of, 183–185
  presenting symptoms of, 181
  tentative diagnoses for, 181–182
  therapeutic plan for, 187–188
Sputum, with cough, fever, and shortness of breath, 62–73
Squamous cell carcinoma, *vs.* contact dermatitis, 469–476
STD. *See* Sexually transmitted disease (STD)
Stomach pain. *See* Epigastric pain
Strep throat, 231–239
  diagnosis of, 237
  diagnostic tests for, 237
  differential diagnosis of, 236
  history of, 234–235
  vs. Kawasaki disease, 296
  physical assessment of, 235–236
  presenting symptoms of, 233
  tentative diagnoses for, 233
  therapeutic plan for, 238–239
Substance abuse
  vs. depression, 74–90
  vs. lumbosacral strain, 429–440
Substance dependence, 240–256

Syncope, *vs.* benign paroxysmal positional vertigo, 414–427
Synthroid (levothyroxine), for hypothyroidism, 148, 495–496
Syphilis, *vs.* human papillomavirus, 477–486

T

Tagamet (cimetidine), for gastroesophageal reflux, 112
TB (tuberculosis), 122, 124
  vs. COPD, 62–73
  vs. human immunodeficiency virus, 362–379
3TC, for human immunodeficiency virus, 376
TCA (trichloroacetic acid), for human papillomavirus, 484–485
Tension-type headache, 127–139
  clinical presentation of, 129
  diagnosis of, 135–136
  diagnostic tests for, 135
  differential diagnosis of, 134–135
  history of, 130–132
  physical assessment of, 132–134
  tentative diagnoses for, 129–130
  therapeutic plan for, 136–139
Testicular self-examination, 165
Tetracycline, for peptic ulcer disease, 389
Throat, sore, 231–239
  diagnosis of, 237
  diagnostic tests for, 237
  differential diagnosis of, 236
  history of, 234–235
  physical assessment of, 235–236
  presenting symptoms of, 233
  tentative diagnoses for, 233
  therapeutic plan for, 238–239
Tinea corporis, *vs.* contact dermatitis, 469–476
TMP-SMZ (trimethoprim-sulfamethoxazole), for urinary tract infection, 332
Toddlers, anticipatory guidance for, 466–467
Toilet training, 467
Tooth pain, with rhinorrhea and headache, 391–401
  diagnostic tests for, 397–398
  differential diagnosis of, 396–397
  history of, 394–395
  physical assessment of, 395–396
  presenting symptoms of, 393
  tentative diagnoses for, 393
  therapeutic plan for, 398–401
Toxin exposure, *vs.* failure to thrive, 215–229
Tremor, with fatigue and headaches, 74–90
Trichloroacetic acid (TCA), for human papillomavirus, 484–485
Trimethoprim-sulfamethoxazole (TMP-SMZ), for urinary tract infection, 332
Tuberculosis (TB), 122, 124
  vs. COPD, 62–73
  vs. human immunodeficiency virus, 362–379

U

Ulcers, peptic, 380–390
  vs. cholecystitis, 299–309
  vs. congestive heart failure, 140–148
  diagnosis of, 388
  diagnostic tests for, 387–388
  differential diagnosis of, 386–387
  vs. gastroesophageal reflux, 104–113
  history of, 383–385
  physical assessment of, 385–386
  presenting symptoms of, 382
  tentative diagnoses for, 382–383
  therapeutic plan for, 388–390
Univasc (moexipril), for congestive heart failure, 147
Upper respiratory tract infection (URI)
  vs. gonorrhea and chlamydia, 91–103
  vs. sinusitis, 391–401
Urethritis, 329
Urinary frequency, 324–333
Urinary tract infections (UTIs), 324–333
  vs. benign prostatic hyperplasia, 441–454
  classification of, 330–331
  complicated *vs.* uncomplicated, 330–331
  with delirium, 203, 208, 211
  diagnosis of, 330
  diagnostic tests for, 329
  differential diagnosis of, 329
  vs. gonorrhea and chlamydia, 91–103
  history of, 327–328
  after intercourse, 333
  lower *vs.* upper, 329, 330
  in men, 331
  physical assessment of, 328
  presenting symptoms of, 326
  prevention of, 332–333
  tentative diagnosis of, 326
  therapeutic plan for, 330–333
Urinary urgency, 324–333
Urination, burning during, 324–333
Uveitis, *vs.* herpes zoster, 169–177

V

Vagina, "bump" on, 477–486
  diagnosis of, 484
  diagnostic tests for, 483
  differential diagnosis of, 482–483
  history of, 480–481
  physical assessment of, 481–482
  presenting symptoms of, 479
  tentative diagnoses for, 479–480
  therapeutic plan for, 484–486
Vaginal bleeding, during pregnancy, 36–47
  diagnosis of, 43–44
  diagnostic tests for, 42–43
  differential diagnosis of, 41–42
  history of, 39–40
  physical assessment of, 40–41
  presenting symptoms of, 38
  therapeutic plan for, 44–47

Vaginal discharge, 91–103
  diagnosis for, 100
  diagnostic tests for, 98–99
  differential diagnosis of, 97–98
  history of, 94–96
  physical assessment of, 96–97
  presenting symptoms of, 93
  tentative diagnoses for, 93
  therapeutic plan for, 100–103
Vaginitis, 485
Vaginosis, bacterial, 91–103
  vs. candidiasis, 93, 98
  diagnosis for, 100
  diagnostic tests for, 98–99
  differential diagnosis of, 97–98
  history of, 94–96
  physical assessment of, 96–97
  presenting symptoms of, 93
  tentative diagnoses for, 93
  therapeutic plan for, 100–103
Valacyclovir (Valtrex), for herpes zoster, 176
Vasotec (enalapril), for congestive heart failure, 146
Vermox (mebendazole), for pinworms, 343
Vertebral fracture, *vs.* lumbosacral strain, 429–440
Vertibrobasilar arterial disease, *vs.* benign paroxysmal positional vertigo, 414–427
Vertigo
  benign paroxysmal positional, 414–427
    diagnosis of, 425
    diagnostic tests for, 423–425
    differential diagnosis of, 422–423
    history of, 418–419
    physical assessment of, 420–421
    presenting symptoms of, 416
    resources for, 427
    tentative diagnoses for, 416–417
    therapeutic plan for, 425–427
  due to ototoxic drugs, 417, 422
  peripheral *vs.* central, 416–417
  post-traumatic, 417, 422
Vestibulopathy, peripheral, *vs.* benign paroxysmal positional vertigo, 414–427
Violence, domestic, 308
Viral infection
  vs. hepatitis, 402–413
  vs. Kawasaki disease, 291–298
Vision
  blurred, with polyuria and fatigue, 257–267
  in elderly, 123–124
Volume depletion, *vs.* benign paroxysmal positional vertigo, 423
Vomiting
  with peptic ulcer disease, 380–390
  in pregnancy, 46
Vontrol (diphenidol), for benign paroxysmal positional vertigo, 426
Vulvovaginitis, *vs.* urinary tract infection, 324–333

W

Warts, genital, 477–486
  diagnosis of, 484
  diagnostic tests for, 483
  differential diagnosis of, 482–483
  history of, 480–481
  physical assessment of, 481–482
  presenting symptoms of, 479
  tentative diagnoses for, 479–480
  therapeutic plan for, 484–486
Weight gain
  with abnormal menstrual cycle, fatigue, and diarrhea, 487–497
  with fatigue and headaches, 74–90
Well-child checkup
  with difficulty in school, 48–61
    diagnosis of, 57–58
    diagnostic tests for, 56–57
    differential diagnosis of, 55–56
    history in, 51–53
    physical assessment in, 54
    presenting symptoms of, 50
    therapeutic plan for, 58–61
  for infant, 215–229
    anticipatory guidance in, 229
    history in, 218–220
    physical assessment in, 220–221
  for kindergarten, 335–344
    anticipatory guidance in, 343
    diagnostic tests in, 342
    history in, 337–339
    physical assessment in, 340–341
  for sports participation, 157–168
    diagnostic tests in, 164–165
    history in, 159–161
    physical assessment in, 161–163
  for two-year-old, 455–468
    anticipatory guidance in, 466–468
    diagnostic tests in, 465
    history in, 458–461
    physical assessment in, 462–464
Wheezing, 10–26

Y

Yeast infection, 485

Z

Zantac (ranitidine), for gastroesophageal reflux, 112
Zestril (lisinopril), for congestive heart failure, 146, 148
Zithromax (azithromycin), for gonorrhea and chlamydia, 100
Zovirax (acyclovir), for herpes zoster, 176